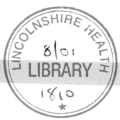

GU00992071

THE CAMBRIDGE

medical ethics w

This is a practical, versatile, case-based introduction to bioethics for anyone who is interested in the ethical issues raised by modern medicine. It is designed to be used both for individual reference and as a set text in group teaching or open learning environments.

The workbook is structured around a variety of guided activities designed to introduce and examine the major ethical questions. The activities are clustered around actual cases (provided by an international team of healthcare professionals), commentaries (from clinicians, ethicists and lawyers), and short papers. The range of problems covered includes ethical issues raised by new reproductive and genetic technologies, the rights of vulnerable groups, and allocation of scarce medical resources.

The workbook will be invaluable to practitioners, medical and nursing students, and anyone who needs to develop skills in ethical analysis for clinical practice or research.

Michael Parker is Clinical Ethicist at the John Radcliffe Hospital Trust, Oxford, and Lecturer in Medical Ethics, Ethox, University of Oxford
Donna Dickenson is the Leverhulme Reader in Medical Ethics and Law, and Head of the Medical Ethics Unit at Imperial College of Science, Technology and Medicine.

THE CAMBRIDGE

medical ethics workbook

Case studies

commentaries

and activities

Michael Parker

Donna Dickenson

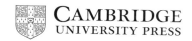

CAMBRIDGE
UNIVERSITY PRESS

PUBLISHED BY THE PRESS SYNDICATE OF THE UNIVERSITY OF CAMBRIDGE
The Pitt Building, Trumpington Street, Cambridge, United Kingdom

CAMBRIDGE UNIVERSITY PRESS
The Edinburgh Building, Cambridge CB2 2RU, UK
40 West 20th Street, New York, NY 10011-4211, USA
10 Stamford Road, Oakleigh, VIC 3166, Australia
Ruiz de Alarcón 13, 28014 Madrid, Spain
Dock House, The Waterfront, Cape Town 8001, South Africa

http://www.cambridge.org

First published 2001

Printed in the United Kingdom at the University Press, Cambridge

Typeface Utopia 9/12 pt   *System* QuarkXPress™   [SE]

A catalogue record for this book is available from the British Library

ISBN 0 521 78301 1 hardback
ISBN 0 521 78863 3 paperback

Every effort has been made in preparing this book to provide accurate and up-to-date information which is in accord with accepted standards and practice at the time of publication. Nevertheless, the authors, editors and publisher can make no warranties that the information contained herein is totally free from error, not least because clinical standards are constantly changing through research and regulation. The authors, editors and publisher therefore disclaim all liability for direct or consequential damages resulting from the use of material contained in this book. Readers are strongly advised to pay careful attention to information provided by the manufacturer of any drugs or equipment that they plan to use.

Although case histories are drawn from actual cases, every effort has been made to disguise the identities of the individuals involved.

Every effort has been made to reach copyright holders; the publishers would like to hear from anyone whose rights they have unknowingly infringed.

Contents

Cases

Papers

All papers are reproduced with permission.

Introduction

The *Cambridge Medical Ethics Workbook* is a practical, case-based introduction to medical ethics for anyone who is interested in finding out more about, and reflecting on, the ethical issues raised by modern medicine. It is designed to be flexible; suitable both to be read in its own right and also for use as a set text in group teaching or in open learning. It is aimed at the interested general reader, at practising healthcare professionals and at medical and nursing students studying ethics for the first time.

The workbook is able to be flexible in this way because it is based around the reading of and reflection upon real cases. It uses a variety of structured activities to introduce and to explore the major ethical issues facing medicine today. These activities are clustered around: (a) cases (which were provided by healthcare professionals from many countries); (b) commentaries on those cases by healthcare professionals, ethicists, lawyers and so on; and (c) short papers by experts in the area concerned. This is very much a workbook, designed to help readers think about, reflect upon and to work their own way through ethical problems, by deliberating on the issues raised by them either alone or together with others. In this way, the reader is guided through the core themes in medical ethics in a way which is appropriate for them and which is relevant to their own experience.

While a glance at the workbook's contents page shows that it covers most of the major themes in medical ethics, it does not aim to provide in itself a comprehensive survey of every issue. Our aim is rather, through the active and structured exploration of core themes and key cases, to develop skills of independent study and research in ethics. This is an increasingly important requirement of healthcare professionals. For a measure of good practice in medicine today is increasingly coming to be seen to be the extent to which such practice is 'evidence based'. An understanding of the ethical issues involved and of the way to balance and assess the validity of ethical arguments in relation to particular cases is a core skill in the development of an analytical approach to medicine. Good quality healthcare is ethical healthcare and a consideration of the ethical dimensions of decision making in healthcare practice must form a cornerstone of good evidence-based practice. This workbook helps practitioners and students to develop these skills and to have confidence in their use, not only in the context of research but also of teamwork within clinical practice.

Medical ethics is increasingly coming to be seen as an essential element of the education of any healthcare professional (GMC, 1993) and this is increasingly reflected in the medical and nursing schools themselves. Recently, teachers of medical ethics in UK medical schools published a joint statement on the core themes and topics which ought to form the basis of any ethics curriculum (Consensus statement by teachers of medical ethics and law in UK medical schools, 1998). Similar work is also currently being done by the Association of Teachers of Ethics in Australasian Medical Schools and developments are also proceeding apace in other countries. Whilst recognizing these developments and being to some extent a reflection of them, this workbook does not follow any of these curricula rigidly. (We do, however, provide a useful grid in Appendix 2, showing how the UK national core curriculum maps onto the chapters and subtopics of this workbook.) This workbook is intended to be a flexible educational resource which will enable those who teach medical ethics in any of these or any other educational setting to explore the core themes and issues in the ethics of medicine using cases and activities which will resonate with, and be engaging for, both medical and nursing students and those healthcare professionals who wish to develop their skills in this area. We would encourage teachers of medical ethics to pick and choose cases, activities and themes from the workbook in order to construct courses, workshops or training days appropriate to those they are teaching. The workbook is intended to be both a coherent approach to medical ethics and also a toolkit of resources for teachers and lecturers.

The workbook is divided into three parts. In Part I we explore some key ethical themes arising as a result of recent and ongoing technological developments in medicine. The first chapter is on ethical decisions at the end of life and explores ethical issues relating to the withholding and withdrawing of life-prolonging treatment and other ethical issues at the end of life. The chapter's focus is the extent to which the application of modern medicine at the end of life demands a reconsideration of the goals of medicine itself. When healing is no longer possible, what ought to be the goals of medicine and of the healthcare professional? The second chapter in Part I looks at the ethical issues raised by genetic testing and by the use of genetic information in clinical practice. The third chapter investigates the ethical implications of developments in reproductive technology. The fourth looks at the ethics of medical research itself and investigates the extent to which the research which is driving advances in medicine itself raises ethical issues – for those who organize and fund such research, for those clinicians who enrol their patients in research and for those of us who participate as research subjects.

In Part II of the workbook we look more specifically at four themes which permeate medical ethics: vulnerability, truth-telling, competence and confidentiality. We do so by looking at the ethical issues raised by medicine and healthcare with three particularly vulnerable groups of patients. In keeping with the UK national curriculum in medical ethics, we also consider the vulnerabilities of clinicians. In Chapter 5 we investigate the ethical issues that arise in long-term and daily care. In Chapter 6 we look at the ethics of mental health and of the treatment of psychiatric patients. And in Chapter 7 our attention turns to the ethics of work with children and young people. In each case the key issues are competence, vulnerability, truth-telling and confidentiality.

In Part III of the workbook we explore some of the generic ethical issues relating to healthcare. In Chapter 8, still by means of real cases, we investigate the ethical issues relating to the allocation of healthcare resources, questions of priority setting and just distribution. It hardly needs saying that these issues are increasingly important in all healthcare systems and across all clinical specialties. Finally, in Chapter 9 we reflect on a theme which emerges at several points throughout the workbook, the extent to which we ought to see autonomy and patient choice as the key measure of whether healthcare provision and treatment are ethical? What exactly are the limits of such patient-centredness? To what extent is an ethical approach based on the concerns of individual patients capable of addressing the role of relationships and the duty of care which appear to be central to ethical healthcare practice?

The existence of the workbook depends a great deal upon the willingness and enthusiasm of those who have provided us with cases, papers and commentaries and so on. We feel that this makes the workbook both up to date and vibrant as a way of learning about medical ethics. But times change and so do the ethical issues in medicine. It is our intention to update the workbook in the future and in order to do that we will need new cases and papers. If you have any comments on the workbook or any suggestions for how it might be improved, or if you have cases which would work well as educational tools, we would be very pleased to hear from you. You can contact us on michael.parker@ethox.ox.ac.uk.

We think the case-based approach, supported by activities and guided reading exercises has several advantages over other approaches to medical ethics. Firstly, such an approach cuts across disciplinary and cultural boundaries. Everyone can 'relate' in some sense to an actual case, even if they come from very distinct religious or cultural traditions, which dictate different principles of ethical conduct. The cases we have chosen are, wherever possible, 'everyday' cases. Similarly, different healthcare disciplines have increasingly evolved their own forms of healthcare ethics: nursing ethics, for example, sees its concerns and approach as quite distinct from those of medical ethics proper. But in a case-based approach, the different slants of different disciplines can be explicitly built in. Secondly, such an approach requires little previous knowledge of ethics and reassures students who think of philosophy as abstruse and difficult. It is, at the same time, an approach which is capable of facilitating the development of the skills necessary for a rigorous and consistent analytical approach to the ethics of healthcare practice. Thirdly, a guided, case-based approach encourages students to think of comparable cases of their own, and thus to generalize what they have learned from one case to another, comparing similarities and differences. Finally, given the approach adopted by this workbook, the case-based approach allows students to learn from practice in other countries.

We hope that you will agree and that these chapters will give you the necessary motivation and support for doing the important tasks of learning about medical ethics, for students/practitioners, and of teaching students and practitioners, for medical and nurse educators.

Acknowledgements

We owe thanks to a great many people for their help and advice with this workbook over the 3 years it has taken us to write it. The cases and papers used have been gathered from all over the European Union, the United States and Australia. Many of them were collected at a series of workshops held as part of the European Biomedical Ethics Practitioners Education project (EBEPE) which was funded by the European Commission's BIOMED II programme. We would like to acknowledge the European Commission's Directorate General 12 for their support during this period and Hugh Whittal in particular for his support and encouragement. We would also like to acknowledge the role of Imperial College London who supported us through the later stages of the EC project.

Michael Parker would like to thank Julian Savulescu, the University of Melbourne Visiting Scholars' Scheme and the Centre for Health and Society at the University of Melbourne for providing him with a Visiting Fellowship in summer 1999 which enabled him to work on this book and to write two additional chapters (and to see the Barrier Reef). Thanks too to Elena Iriarte-Jalle.

We would also like to acknowledge the contribution made by those who participated in the EBEPE workshops without whom this workbook would not have been possible. The success of the project was a result of the teamwork and support of our project partners. They are Ruud ter Meulen, Juhani Pietarinen, Raffaele Bracalenti, Carlo Calzone and Stella Reiter-Theil.

Many of the EBEPE participants and partners provided the commentaries, papers and cases which form the core of the workbook. Those who do not appear in print have influenced the workbook in other ways. Those who contributed papers or commentaries are acknowledged where their work appears in the workbook itself. Those who contributed cases are not acknowledged for reasons of confidentiality but we would like to take this opportunity to thank them for their contributions. A special thank you to Anne-Cathrine Mattiasson, however, for the cases she provided. The EBEPE participants were Ines Adriaenssen, Gwen Adshead, Steve Baldwin, Attilio Balestrieri, Loutfib Benhabib, Ron Berghmans, Dieter Birnbacher, Gunilla Bjorn, Stefano Boffelli, Paul van Bortel, Nico Bouwan, Raffaele Bracalenti,

Masja van den Burg, Arturo Casoni, Carlo Calzone, Abram Coen, Anne Crenier, Paula Daddino, P. Dalla-Vorgia, Joaquin Delgado, Paolo Deluca, Dolores Dooley, Ralf Dressel, Holger Eich, Dag Elgesem, Bart van den Eynden, Eduard Farthmann, Luis Simoes Ferreira, T. Garanis-Papadatos, Chris Gastmans, Wolfgang Gerok, Sandro Gindro, Diane De Graeve, Marco Griffini, Harald Gruber, Anja Hannuniemi, Jocelyn Hattab, Jean Marc Heller, Eckhard Herych, Christian Hick, Wolfgang Hiddemann, Rachel Hodgkin, Tony Hope, Franz Josef Illhardt, Giuseppe Inneo, Antti Jääskeläinen, Winfried Kahlke, Aristoteles Katsas, John Keown, Valeria Kocsis, Kristiina Kurittu, Raimo Lahti, Veikko Launis, Kristiina Lempinen, Jerome Liss, Salla Lötjönen, Giuseppe Magno, Caroline Malone, Elina Männistö, Glauco Mastrangelo, Simonetta Matone, Anne-Cathrine Mattiasson, Susan Mendus, Roland Mertelsmann, Ruud ter Meulen, Michael Mohr, Emilio Mordini, Maurizio Mori, Dimitrios Niakas, Marti Parker, Valdar Parve, Stephen Pattison, John Pearce, Filimon Peonidis, Juhani Pietarinen, Gideon Ratzoni, Marjo Rauhala-Hayes, Dolf de Ridder, Stella Reiter-Theil, Klaus Schaefer, Renate Schepke, Alrun Sensmeyer, Jaana Simula, Sandro Spinsanti, Karl-Gustav Södergård, Randi Talseth, Maxwell Taylor, Mats Thorslund, Ulrich Tröhler, Mauro Valeri, Maritta Välimäki, Kristiane Weber, Sander Welie, Vera Wetzler-Wolff, Hugh Whittal, Guy Widdershoven, Rainer Wolf.

First drafts of all the chapters were sent to critical readers in several countries for comment. Their comments and criticisms have been central to the success of the workbook. The critical readers were Ann Sommerville, Tony Hope, Richard Ashcroft, Carmen Kaminsky, Mark R. Wicclair, Chris Milet, Mairi Levitt, Ruth Chadwick, Chris Barnes, Martin Richards, Julian Savulescu, Ainsley Newson, Udo Schüklenk, Peter Rudd, Judy McKimm, Dieter Birnbacher, Alastair Campbell, Rowan Frew, Don Chalmers, Ajit Shah, Corrado Viafora, Peter Kemp, Robin Downie, Dolores Dooley, Win Tadd, Margareta Broberg, Alan Cribb, John Keown and Richard Lancaster, along with many of the EBEPE participants listed above.

Our thanks also to Richard Barling and Joe Mottershead of Cambridge University Press, who helped us to develop what may have appeared to them a rather unwieldy collection of materials into this present work. And, finally, the authors would like to acknowledge the administrative and other support of Yvonne Brennan and Helen Watson of Imperial College London and Caroline Malone of the Open University – for always being calm and positive in a crisis.

Michael Parker and Donna Dickenson

Part I

Ethical issues raised by developments in modern medicine

End of life decision-making

Introduction

A medical man does not have to use all the techniques of survival offered him by a constantly creative science. In many cases would it not be useless torture to impose vegetative resuscitation in the final stages of an incurable sickness? The doctor's duty here is rather to ease the suffering instead of prolonging as long as possible, by any means whatsoever, a life no longer human (Cardinal Jean Villot, Vatican Secretary of State, 1970, quoted in Maguire 1975, p. 75).

Death is an intrinsic part of life. Increasingly, however, the techniques of modern medicine are making it possible for us to delay death and in many cases to enable those who would have previously died prematurely to recover and to live full and healthy lives. However, such techniques also allow us to exert a greater degree of control over the processes of dying even when full recovery is not possible. This means that, in addition to those who recover, there are people who would previously have died of their injuries, or condition, who can now be kept alive by medical interventions but who will never recover sufficiently to live an independent, or in some cases even a conscious, life as a result. The use of these techniques raises important ethical questions about the withholding and withdrawing of such life-prolonging treatment at the end of life. Indeed, the application of modern medicine at the end of life raises a wide range of ethical questions, many of which require a reconsideration of the purpose of medicine itself. When healing is no longer possible, what ought to be the goal of medicine and of the healthcare professional? In this chapter we investigate some of these questions by means of a series of real cases. We look particularly at the ethics of palliative medicine and attempt to answer the question: to what extent are the ethical implications at the end of life different from, or the same as, the ethics of medicine more generally?

Section 1: Withdrawing treatment

We begin this chapter on 'Decisions at the end of life' with a case from Greece. We decided to use this case as the starting point both because it raises important ethical questions in itself and also because it brings to the fore questions about how we ought to define the goals of medicine at the end of life. Are there important morally significant differences between palliative medicine and medicine at other periods of life? If so, what are their implications for the practice, and indeed the goals, of medicine?

THE CASE OF MARIA

Maria was an 82-year-old woman who lived in Athens. She had been seriously incapacitated by arthritis for over 2 years, and was also virtually blind following recent unsuccessful cataract and glaucoma treatment. As is very common in Greece, Maria was being cared for by her family in the family home. Although Maria's family found this quite difficult, they were coping reasonably well.

However, Maria's condition deteriorated drastically when she suffered a severe cerebral vascular accident (or stroke) and was admitted into hospital. The result of the stroke was that Maria was left in what her physicians called a 'semi-coma'. The doctors at the hospital immediately began to provide Maria with artificial nutrition and hydration by means of a naso-gastric tube, but they told the family that they felt that no other treatment was appropriate as Maria was very unlikely to recover.

Maria's family visited her regularly at the hospital, but they found these visits very upsetting. Maria found it extremely difficult to speak and was clearly very distressed. Whilst recognizing the severity of Maria's condition, her relatives, who cared for her a great deal, and the staff at the hospital were careful not to discuss this in her presence. Despite this, it was clear from the start that Maria herself found her situation intolerable and, during the first 6 weeks of her hospitalization, repeatedly expressed her wish to be allowed to die. She did this through the use of signs and hard-fought words, even though this was itself extremely difficult and distressing for her. As she became increasingly frustrated, Maria also made several repeated attempts to remove her feeding tube.

Clearly, this was also very upsetting for Maria's children, who were spending quite a lot of time with her at this stage. They knew that their mother had a lifelong aversion to hospitals and medicine, and they felt also a duty to respect her clearly expressed wish to die. After having discussed this among themselves, Maria's children together decided to approach her physician about the possibility of withdrawing treatment and allowing her to die, as she wished.

At their meeting with the physician, however, he made it very clear to the family in no uncertain terms that he would not consider acceding to such a request. He said that he felt that this would go against his responsibilities as a doctor to his patient. He also argued that Maria's requests to be allowed to die should not be taken at face value as Maria had a recent history of mild depression. Maria's family were unhappy with this decision and with the doctor's reasoning, but felt that they had no choice other than to accept it.

After a further week, however, Maria's condition had deteriorated to such an extent that she was now in a full and irreversible coma and, after further discussion with the family, the physician agreed to withdraw nutrition but continued to refuse absolutely to withdraw the supply of hydration.

Maria survived for another 2 weeks without respiratory or other complications, but then died rather suddenly when she suffered a second stroke.

After the death of his mother, Maria's son complained bitterly to the physician about the way his mother had been dealt with. He argued that, had the physician agreed with the family's request for the withdrawal of all kinds of treatment when this was originally requested, his mother would have died sooner and would have suffered a great deal less than she did. He argued that, when it is clear that a patient is going to die, the doctor's duty is to alleviate their suffering, and that this means that it can sometimes be wrong to keep a patient alive for as long as possible and at all costs.

ACTIVITY: Maria's son felt that the doctor in this case was being paternalistic and ignoring the wishes of both Maria and her family. This raises the question of who should decide in this kind of case. Stop here for a moment and write down all the reasons you can think of both for and against withdrawing treatment when it was first requested by the family.

If one comes to the conclusion that the patient has the moral right to be allowed to die, it is tempting to jump from here to the claim that it is the doctor's duty to allow the patient to die, but clearly this need not be the case (we will be returning to this point in Sections 2 and 4 of the chapter). The doctor in the case of Maria continued to argue that, in his opinion, hydration was not simply another 'form of treatment' and was in fact the most fundamental form of care that he as a physician felt it his duty to provide to *any* patient. He argued that, whilst he was not in favour of prolonging unnecessarily a dying patient's life, he felt that allowing a patient to die from lack of hydration was not what he considered to be a dignified and peaceful death and would, in fact, contravene his duty of care as a doctor. Moreover, he argued, to do so would have been against any medical and religious tradition of his country, Greece, and against his personal beliefs.

ACTIVITY: To what extent do you agree with the doctor? What counts as treatment? Does hydration? Is the withdrawal of hydration a violation of the doctor's fundamental duty of care for the patient?

The dispute between the doctor and Maria's family appears to come down to one about what the goals of medicine ought to be in cases like that of Maria. The family argued that, in situations where healing is no longer possible the central goal of medicine ought to be the alleviation of suffering. They ask, what was the aim of preserving Maria's life, when in the event she had another stroke and died? Did she suffer more than she would have done were she simply allowed to die after the first stroke? The doctor's view, on the other hand, appears to be that both the with-

drawal of hydration and allowing a patient to die constitute violations of the deepest kind of the goals of medicine and of his duty of care to his patient.

ACTIVITY: Stop here for a moment and consider what you think of as the goals of medicine. Make a list of activities and attitudes which you consider to be part of the goals of medicine in general as you see them (i.e. not simply at the end of life) and another of those which you would consider to constitute an absolute violation of these goals. Then spend some time reflecting on your list and ask yourself which of these is no longer appropriate at the end of life, in palliative medicine, if any. In this context which of the list would you remove and what new activities and attitudes would you add?

After you have done this, we would like you to go on to read the following extract from a paper called 'Physician-assisted death, the moral integrity of medicine, and the slippery slope', by Dr Ron Berghmans from the Netherlands. The reason we introduce the paper at this point is because it raises and attempts to address this question of whether the goals of medicine in the broadest sense are in tension with, and perhaps even conflict with, what we would consider ethical treatment or care at the end of life. Are the ethical and moral dimensions different when questions of life and death are at issue in this setting? Whilst you are reading Berghmans's paper we would like you to bear these questions in mind as they will form an important thread throughout the chapter.

Physician-assisted death, violation of the moral integrity of medicine, and the slippery slope

Dr Ron Berghmans

Those who take the view that physician-assisted death involves a violation of the moral integrity of medicine argue that doctors must never be a party to intentional killing, because that would go against the very essence of the medical profession (Singer & Siegler, 1990; Pellegrino, 1992; Momeyer, 1995). The essence of medicine from this perspective is considered to be healing and the protection of life. This view is opposed to the possibility of physician-assisted death in all circumstances. Those who defend this view refer to categorical claims such as the inalienability of the right to life, the sanctity of life, the absolute prohibition against killing other human beings, and to healing as the single and ultimate goal of medicine. I want to focus on this last claim.

On this view, the essence of medicine is to be found in the *telos* of benefiting the sick by the action of healing. It is worth asking, however, just what is the status of this claim. It should be recognised that the practice of medicine and the ends it serves are of human invention, and not 'naturally given' activities deriving from the structure of natural order. The practice of medicine is shaped by human beings in order to serve human purposes. It involves human choice with regard to value systems, and choosing such a value system requires moral argument and justification, not an appeal to the 'nature of things'. Whatever the goals of medicine are, or should be, is thus a matter which is open to rational debate, and cannot be decided without reference to value considerations.

But even if, for the sake of argument, we agree that the *telos* of medicine is healing – and not, for instance, the relief of human suffering or the promotion of the benefit of patients – then we still are left with the question of exactly what moral force such an end or goal of medicine has. If we look at the actual practice of medicine, it is clear that healing is more an ideal than an unconditional goal of medical endeavour. Take for instance the case of refusal of treatment by the patient. A well-considered refusal of treatment ought to be respected, even if the physician takes the view that treatment would be beneficial to the patient. The reasons for respecting competent refusals of treatment are twofold. The first reason is that non-consensual intervention where a person has decision-making capacity invades the

integrity of the person involved. The second is that competent persons ought to be considered the best judges of their own interests. Only the competent person himself can assess the benefits, burdens and harms of treatment in view of his or her wishes, goals, and values. So, if a person refuses treatment because he or she does not value treatment in his or her personal life, then such a refusal ought to be respected, even if this might result in an earlier death. Thus, as this example shows, healing as an ideal in medical practice implies that other goals and values can and do operate as constraints upon medical actions serving this ideal.

More directly related to the issue of physician-assisted death is the consideration that the ideal of healing can become illusory, for instance in cases of severe and unbearable suffering in which no prospect of alleviation exists. The goal of relieving the suffering of the patient then becomes the primary goal of the physician, rather than healing.

Part of the moral integrity argument is the claim that, if physicians assist in suicide or euthanasia, then the public will begin to distrust the medical profession, and as a result the profession itself will suffer irreparable harm (Pellegrino, 1992; Thomasma, 1996). Against this objection it can be argued that, if physician-assisted death is categorically rejected, the result may also be a loss of trust in the medical profession. The public may experience this as a lack of compassion and personal engagement on the part of physicians in those cases where no adequate means of relieving the suffering of the patient are available and the patient wants some control over how to die, but is left alone by the doctor.

My conclusion is that, in principle as well as in practice, euthanasia and physician-assisted suicide do not necessarily go against the goal or goals of medicine, or the moral integrity of the medical profession. The Hippocratic vow of 'helping the sick' and of exercising medical skills for the benefit of patients does not prohibit the co-operation of physicians with requests for euthanasia and assisted suicide, so long as they are convinced that this is what is in a patient's best interests and to the degree that the physician is committed to respecting a patient's own values.

The involvement of doctors in the dying of patients is inescapable. In many cases, a decision of a doctor leads to a hastening of death, although that decision may not always be considered the direct cause of the death of the patient (i.e. the decision to respect the treatment refusal of a patient). In euthanasia and assisted suicide, the causal role of the actions of the doctor is more clear-cut, and the practice of physician-assisted death raises a number of issues regarding the proper role of the physician and the self-understanding of the medical profession. Although the primary task of the physician is to preserve the life of the patient, preservation of life is not an absolute goal. This would demand an unconditional obligation to preserve life by all possible means and under all circumstances. If the relief of suffering is also a proper goal of medicine, then in particular circumstances a weighing or balancing of the goal to preserve life and the goal of relieving suffering becomes inescapable.

Euthanasia and assisted suicide do not necessarily violate the moral integrity of medicine.

> ACTIVITY: Ron Berghmans's argument for the claim that the withdrawal of treatment in palliative care does not violate the *telos* or goal of medicine is a powerful one. But can you think of any counter-arguments to this?

Two of those which Berghmans mentions are, firstly, the claim that if the public sees the medical profession engaged in 'letting die' it may undermine the way in which the medical profession is perceived, and, secondly, that allowing the withdrawal of treatment under certain circumstances will lead to a slippery slope in which it is allowed in more and more cases which were not envisaged as being appropriate at the beginning. In his article Ron Berghmans rejects each of these criticisms, but we will be coming back to explore them in more detail later on in the chapter.

In this first section of the chapter we have raised the question of the goals or 'telos' of medi-

cine at the end of life. Both Berghmans and Maria's son have proposed the hypothesis that the goals of palliative care ought to be the alleviation of suffering, even if this sometimes goes against our sense that, in general, medicine ought to concern itself with healing. In the rest of this chapter we shall be going on to explore the ethical implications of this claim in a variety of different ways. In Section 2 we shall be going on to consider the ethical implications of a decision not to resuscitate a patient.

> ACTIVITY: Stop for a moment and make a list of the key points raised by this section.

Section 2: Deciding not to resuscitate

In the Greek case study examined in Section 1, the patient was semi-comatose, although she appeared to express her wish to have the feeding tubes withdrawn by trying to pull them out, making signs, and uttering a few hard-fought words. In this section we will begin with another case in which the patient lacks capacity to consent to treatment. Here the issue is not whether to continue intravenous feeding and hydration, but whether to resuscitate a severely disabled patient if he suffers a cardiac arrest. Although the clinical picture is very different in this case, however, the same theme arises. Because this patient, known as 'Mr R', appeared to be in considerable suffering, this case gives rise to the same question as did the Greek case: is it part of the *telos* of medicine to avoid the imposition of unnecessary suffering by treating at all costs? Is it actually in the best interests of a suffering patient to impose treatment? Even in terms of the doctor's values and the *telos* of medicine, rather than the rights of the patient, we will need to draw boundaries that avoid a form of *iatrogenic* harm:

imposing burdens without corresponding benefits of treatment. In the case of patients who are not competent to accept or refuse treatment, doctors' main concern will be to avoid the imposition of unnecessary suffering.

THE CASE OF MR R

(Re R [1996] 2 FLR 99)
R was born with a serious malformation of the brain and cerebral palsy. At 8 months of age he developed severe epilepsy. At the age of 23 he was spastic, incontinent, and apparently deaf and blind (with possible vestigial response to a buzzer and to light). He was unable to walk, to sit upright, or to chew; food had to be syringed to the back of his mouth. His bowels had to be evacuated manually because his limited diet resulted in serious constipation. He suffered from thrush and had ulcers 'all the way through his guts', according to testimony. When cuddled he did indicate pleasure, and he also appeared to respond to pain by grimacing. Although he was not comatose, nor in a persistent vegetative state, his awareness on a scale of 1 to 10 was rated somewhere between 1 and 2 in an assessment by Dr Keith Andrews of the Royal Hospital for Neurodisability at Putney, London, who said:

It is my opinion that he has very little, if any, real cognitive awareness at a level where he can interpret what is going on in his environment. He reacts at the most basic level by responding to comfort, warmth and a safe environment by being relaxed and producing the occasional smile. He responds to discomfort, pain and threatening situations by becoming distressed and crying. These are very basic level responses and do not imply any thought processes.

Until he was 17 R lived at home, where he was totally dependent on his devoted parents. He then moved to a residential home, but continued to return home at weekends. Now his condition was beginning to deteriorate: his weight had dropped to just over 30 kg, and he was extremely frail, suffering from recurrent chest infections, bleeding from ulceration of the oesophagus, and continued epileptic fits. In 1995 he was admitted to hospital

on five occasions, each time for a life-threatening crisis. After the last crisis Dr S, the consultant psychiatrist for learning difficulties who was responsible for his care, wrote:

To hospitalize R if he had another life-threatening crisis would, in my clinical judgement, be nothing more than striving officiously to keep him alive for no gain to him. In my opinion, this is tantamount to a failing against a basic duty of humanity. Indeed, at the last few admissions to hospital, I have had real concern as to whether it was ethical to treat him actively. That said, I would never withhold treatment against the wishes of his parents. In summary, taking R's best interests into account and whilst taking into account the basic premise of the sanctity of human life, it is in my judgement unquestionably in R's best interests to allow nature to take its course next time he has a life-threatening crisis and to allow him to die with some comfort and dignity. That would relieve him of physical, mental and emotional suffering.

ACTIVITY: Go through the consultant's opinion again and write down the ethically charged terms or concepts that are being used to construct an argument. After each term, write down the consultant's apparent interpretation of it. Do you agree with this interpretation? If not, write down your own. For example, 'withhold treatment' is crucial to the argument, and the consultant seems to be saying that withholding treatment is ethically acceptable provided that R's parents agree. Nothing is said about actively ending R's life; rather the emphasis is on 'passively' withholding treatment which could be undertaken, but which it would actually be ethically wrong to administer. We shall return later in this section to arguments about the ethical validity of the distinction between withholding care and actively initiating death. The British Medical Association published guidance on withholding and withdrawing life-prolonging treatment in 1999 in which they asserted that:

Although emotionally it may be easier to withhold treatment than to withdraw that which has been started, there are no legal, or necessary morally relevant, differences between the two actions (BMA, 1999).

What do you think about this claim? Can you think of
any arguments in favour or against it?
See also the Government's White Paper 'Making
Decisions', 1999.

How did you get on with the list of ethically
charged terms? In addition to withholding treatment, we identified these key underlying con-
cepts/arguments:

(a) Best interests of the patient
(b) Sanctity of life
(c) Relief of suffering
(d) 'Basic duty of humanity'
(e) 'Gain' or benefit to the patient
(f) Treating actively (as against the implied alter-
    native of allowing nature to take its course)
(g) Wishes of the parents
(h) Death with dignity
(i) Medical futility: the question of how to judge
    when treatment is no longer effective

Quite a full list for one paragraph. This exercise
illustrates how tightly packed with ethical concepts an apparently clinical judgement can be.

Now please continue reading the case of Mr R.

THE CASE OF MR R (*cont.*)

The immediate question now was whether to
resuscitate R in the event of another acute admission resulting in cardiac arrest. He was so frail that
it was feared CPR (cardio-pulmonary resuscitation) might crush his ribcage. In addition, there
was a risk of further brain damage from resuscitation. A subsidiary question was whether to
administer antibiotics if he developed pneumonia. After R's fifth hospital admission, in
September 1995, the consultant. Dr S, discussed
the position with R's parents. They agreed that R
would not be subjected to CPR if he suffered a
cardiac arrest in future. Accordingly, Dr S signed a
DNR (do not resuscitate) direction, signed by R's
mother under the heading 'next of kin'.

This decision was opposed by staff at the day
care centre which R had been attending; they felt
that he did, in fact, have some 'quality of life'. In

addition they interpreted Dr S's decision as a 'no
treatment' policy, which Dr S denied: the only
treatment which she was withdrawing, she
argued, was cardio-pulmonary resuscitation.
Agreement could not be reached, and a member
of the day care centre staff applied for review of
the decision by a court, on the basis of information provided by social workers involved in R's day
care. The basis of the application was that the
DNR (do not resuscitate) decision was irrational
and unlawful in permitting medical treatment to
be withheld on the basis of an assessment of the
patient's quality of life. The hospital sought a
court judgement that despite R's inability to give a
valid refusal of treatment, it would be lawful and
in his best interests to withhold cardio-pulmonary
resuscitation and the administration of antibiotics. A proposed gastrostomy would be performed, however, underlining that there was no
question of comprehensive refusal to treat R.
Likewise, the hospital decided that it would venti-
late R and provide artificial nutrition and hydration if applicable, although initially it had
indicated it would not. The application made it
clear that the hospital intended 'to furnish such
treatment and nursing care as may from time to
time be appropriate to ensure that [R] suffers the
least distress and retains the greatest dignity until
such time as his life comes to an end'.

At the High Court hearing, where R was represented by the Official Solicitor (who acts on behalf
of incompetent patients), discussion centred on
guidelines for resuscitation issued by the British
Medical Association in 1993 (Revised, 1999) in a
joint statement with the Royal College of Nursing.
Resuscitation, originally devised to be used in a
small minority of cases, is now overused, it has
been argued (Hilberman et al., 1997). Although
the technique can be very successful in the right
context, at least in some US states it has become
the default response to cardiac arrest, required
unless it is explicitly refused or clearly 'futile'. Yet
cardiac arrest is part of death. But was R dying?

The 1993 BMA/RCN guidelines, as used in the R

decision, did not actually say that resuscitation must always be attempted unless the patient is clearly in a terminal condition. Instead, they suggest three types of case in which it is appropriate to consider a DNR decision:

(a) where the patient's condition indicates that effective cardio-pulmonary resuscitation (CPR) is unlikely to be successful
(b) where CPR is not in accord with the recorded sustained wishes of the patient who is mentally competent
(c) where successful CPR is likely to be followed by a length and quality of life which would not be acceptable to the patient.

> **ACTIVITY: Which, if any, of these conditions might apply to R? Note down the reasons for your answer.**

Condition (a) is the most obviously clinical of the three. It focuses solely on the medical facts of the matter. Certainly R is gravely ill, but he has come through five acute admissions in the past year, so that it is difficult to say that he is definitely unlikely to survive CPR. Condition (b) cannot be met, because R is not mentally competent to record a wish. Although the consultant says that she would never terminate his care against his parents' wishes, in English law the parents of an adult have no power to accept or refuse treatment on his behalf (although at the time of writing, this was open to change after consultation on proposals for appointment of proxy decision-makers as put forward by the Law Commission (Law Commission, 1995: Lord Chancellor's Department, 1997)). (In most other European jurisdictions – for example, Greece – and in many American states, proxy decision-making on behalf of an incompetent adult is in fact possible.) The BMA guidelines merely noted that the opinions of relatives 'may be valuable' – not determining. Finally, we have condition (c), focusing on unacceptable quality of life – but again, acceptable or unacceptable to the patient. It is very hard to know whether R gets any enjoyment out of life: he seems to respond to being cuddled, and to react to pain, but that is really all we can say. Again, the

BMA guidelines did note that: 'If the patient cannot express a view, the opinion of others close to the patient may be sought regarding the patient's best interests.' But the guidelines do not say that opinion has anything more than advisory value as to what the patient would regard as reasonable quality of life. They also appear to envision a different kind of situation – where a previously competent patient, who (unlike R) had expressed definite views about good and bad quality of life, is no longer able to enunciate his or her wishes, but where the family will remember his or her preferences. (We will return to the important issue of quality of life in Section 6.)

So, strictly speaking, it is possible to make a case for arguing that none of these conditions applies to R. But that was not the opinion of the Court. Prompted by guidance from Keith Andrews as an expert witness, the Court agreed that conditions (b) and (c) were not applicable – ruling out the quality of life arguments both for and against. Only condition (a) was to be considered, that is, the likelihood rather than the desirability of successful CPR. Even in hospital settings only about 13 per cent of patients receiving CPR survive to discharge, Dr Andrews testified; in a residential home such as the one R lived in, the chances would be virtually nil. Accordingly, the case turned on the futility of treatment, rather than on quality of life. On the basis of medical futility, the Court accepted the DNR order, but not a global policy against other interventions by the consultant when, and if, a potentially life-threatening infection arose.

> **ACTIVITY: Stop here for a moment and try to devise a possible counter-argument to this view. What might be the pitfalls of using medical futility to decide whether or not to resuscitate?**

There is quite widespread distrust of the concept of medical futility (e.g. Gillon, 1997) as excessively paternalistic. Because it purports to be a purely 'scientific' criterion, it allows the doctor to decide, rather than in consultation with the patient. It is never possible to say that, in this particular case, a treatment will or will not be completely futile; rather, it is a question of what levels of probability are acceptable. That decision should rest with the patient, it can be argued, and not with the doctor alone. Of course, in the case of R, no consultation with the patient was possible, and Dr S's decision was accepted by the parents. But we have already seen that the parents' opinion is only advisory in English law. And it might be argued that precisely because Dr S couldn't know whether R would have thought resuscitation futile, she should have erred in favour of administration of CPR, rather than a DNR order.

One argument in favour of using medical futility as a criterion is that it is simply unavoidable. Unless we want to say that treatment should always be provided to a competent patient who requests it, or to an incompetent patient whatever the circumstances, then someone has to draw the line somewhere. That person is most likely to be the doctor (Brody, 1997).

Whichever you believe, the R case centres on what duties doctors have to avoid imposing suffering, unless suffering has a point. It is when suffering is pointless, in the face of unacceptable burdens for little benefit, that the decision not to resuscitate appears valid. The issue is who decides what is unacceptable, and on what basis.

Acts, omissions and the doctrine of double effect

The R judgement emphasized that 'there is no question of the Court being asked to approve a course aimed at terminating life or accelerating death. The Court is concerned with circumstances in which steps should not be taken to prolong life.' The distinction here is between acts and omissions, a distinction originating in Catholic moral theology and also found in other contexts. The wording in the Anglican creed, for example, asks God to pardon believers for two separate matters: that 'we have done those things we ought not to have done' (wrongful acts) and that we have 'left undone those things we ought to have done' (wrongful omissions). In the medical context, this Catholic tradition would hold that a decision to withhold treatment 'is not the equivalent of suicide; on the contrary, it should be considered as an acceptance of the human condition, or a wish to avoid the application of a medical procedure disproportionate to the results that can be expected' (in the words of the Vatican's 1980 Declaration on Euthanasia).

It is often difficult to distinguish between acts and omissions in practice. For example, is turning off a ventilator a positive act, or merely omitting to perform the treatment any longer? More radically, however, some philosophers, those who concentrate on the consequences of actions, do not accept the acts/omissions distinction, not even in principle. This is true of utilitarians such as James Rachels (Rachels, 1986), who argues that there is no significant moral difference between killing and letting die, and Jonathan Glover, who uses this example:

A man who will inherit a fortune when his father dies, and, with this is mind, omits to give him medicine necessary for keeping him alive, is very culpable. His culpability is such that many people would want to say that this is not a mere omission, but a positive act of withholding the medicine. Supporters of the acts and omissions doctrine who also take this view are faced with the problem of explaining where they draw the line between acts and omissions. Is consciously failing to send money to [charity] also a positive act of withholding? (Glover 1977, p. 96).

Supporters of the distinction might answer Glover's challenge by saying that the point at which to draw the line is the doctor's duty to care. It is because the son has a duty to care for the father that failing to give the medicine is wrong. (It might also be wrong to fail to give it to anyone who needed it, if we think we have a generalized 'Good Samaritan' duty to others.) In the context of a doctor's duty to care, both acts and omissions may indeed be wrongful: treating without consent would be a wrongful act, whilst failing to treat someone who had consented and who needed treatment might be a wrongful omission.

This may explain why doctors are often reluctant to rely on the distinction between acts and omissions, why they feel a duty to treat at all costs – sometimes against relatives' wishes. This sort of scenario is illustrated by a 1995 Irish case, known for reasons of confidentiality only as 'in the matter of a ward of court'.

THE CASE OF A WARD OF COURT

The case concerned a young woman who, at the age of 22, underwent a minor gynaecological diagnostic procedure under general anaesthetic. During the procedure she suffered three cardiac arrests, resulting in serious anoxic brain damage. Doctors continued to maintain her in what they termed 'a near-persistent vegetative state' for over 20 years, feeding her first by nasogastric tube and then by gastrostomy. (She continued to breathe normally; ventilation was not required, except briefly after her cardiac arrests.) For many years she was in a rehabilitation centre, and was then transferred to a hospice, whose philosophy would not allow withdrawal of feeding tubes.

After almost 23 years her family sought an order that all artificial hydration and nutrition should cease, and that the Court should give such directions as to her care. Against public expectations, they succeeded in obtaining a Supreme Court judgement allowing treatment to be withdrawn. Non-treatment of any possible infections was also granted. With the Court's authorization, the Ward was brought home from the hospice, where volunteer nurses and doctors assisted in withdrawing the feeding tubes and caring for her until she died a week later. (They did so in contravention of guidelines from the Irish Medical Council and Irish Nursing Board, which refused, even after the Supreme Court judgement, to retreat from their insistence that 'feeding is a universal requirement in the care of human beings, and whether or not this feeding is done through tube mechanisms does not alter this moral position.') (Irish Medical Council Guidelines of 4 August 1995)

The prayer card for the Ward's memorial mass gave two dates of death: the first in 1972, the time of the accident, and the second in 1995, when she was finally allowed to die.

Although the Supreme Court judgement eventually upheld the notion that the Ward's best interests did not require active treatment which had little chance of success, the family were angered by doctors' refusal to listen to this argument earlier – as Dolores Dooley of University College Cork makes plain.

Following a minor diagnostic procedure under anaesthetic, Ms X was left severely brain-damaged. She would, in all probability, never recover cognitive functioning, never be able to move voluntarily, and never be able to communicate by choice. The family wanted life-support therapies to be ended when the prognosis became clear.

But they were baffled and angered by the marginalization they experienced as many decisions were taken unilaterally and without consultation. They tried to ask: why resuscitate her on numerous occasions when all bodily evidence indicated she was trying to die? Why reinsert an abdominal feeding tube under anaesthetic only 6 months before her death, when their daughter had been in a 'near-persistent vegetative state' for 22 years? Why not provide the best of pain relief care (if she knew pain) and allow her dying to proceed naturally? What were the healthcare goals for this patient, and why were they not discussed with the family? What was the objective of such aggressive life-support measures? What moral imperatives were guiding these decisions?

> **ACTIVITY: Which of the procedures in the previous paragraph is an act, and which is an omission?**

We would say that resuscitation is clearly an act, and a medical procedure. Insertion of an abdominal feeding tube is likewise active medical treatment, according at least to the decision in *Airedale NHS Trust v. Bland* (1993). (In this, one of the first such cases in Europe, withdrawal of feeding tubes was authorized for a young man left in a persistent vegetative state, although basic nursing care continued to be required.) Providing pain relief is a more difficult issue, even though it is an act rather than an omission.

Suppose that the issue in R had not been resuscitation, but the administration of pain relief in such quantities as were likely to accelerate death – again, with the intention of avoiding unnecessary suffering. The final words in the R judgement stress this: 'His parents, his doctors and the devoted and selfless care workers will continue to spare no effort to make his life as bearable and as comfortable as possible until a crisis occurs which will result in Nature taking its course and R being relieved of intolerable suffering.' Could this care rightfully include pain relief? Clearly it could; the hospital stressed that it had never sought a 'no-treatment' order, and that it intended to make R's death as comfortable and dignified as possible. But could it include pain relief at levels which might actually hasten R's death? (Of course, it is a misconception to believe that pain relief always necessarily shortens life.) That seems a different matter from letting nature take its course: it is an active step. So far, we have distinguished between not doing everything that could be done – passively accepting the inevitability of death – and actively trying to bring it about. But this example lies uncomfortably between the two. It begins to sound more like active euthanasia and less like 'letting die'.

ACTIVITY: Another concept from Catholic moral theology, the doctrine of double effect, describes this situation. In the paragraphs which follow, John Keown, a medical lawyer at Cambridge University, outlines the doctrine. Read the account through, writing down the various claims underlining the principle (Keown, 1997).

According to the principle of 'double effect' it is sometimes perfectly proper if one's conduct unintentionally has the effect of shortening, or of not lengthening, life. For example, the doctor who, with the intention of easing pain, administers morphine to a terminally ill cancer patient may foresee that this will shorten the patient's life. But the shortening of life is merely an unintended side-effect of the doctor's intention to alleviate pain, and there is a very good reason (namely the alleviation of pain) for allowing that bad side-effect to happen. He is not attacking the patient's life but the patient's pain.

Similarly, a doctor may sometimes properly withhold or withdraw treatment even though the doctor foresees that the patient's life will be shorter than it would be with the treatment. [In this view] a doctor is under no

duty to administer (and patients are fully entitled to refuse) disproportionate treatments, that is, treatments which would either offer no reasonable hope of benefit or would involve excessive burdens on the patient. Even if the doctor foresees that the patient's life will not be as long without the treatment as it would have been with it, the patient's earlier death is merely an unintended side-effect of the doctor's intention to withhold or withdraw a disproportionate treatment.

ACTIVITY: What is the weakest spot in this argument?

Perhaps one candidate is the concept of an 'unintended side-effect'. Must we take a doctor's word that the side-effect was merely foreseen and not intended? Surely there is a risk of hypocrisy here? Against that charge, it can be argued – convincingly, in our view – that if the doctor is not disappointed when the unintended side-effect fails to occur, it really is unintended. That is, if the patient's pain is relieved, and the patient does *not* die, the doctor genuinely abiding by the doctrine of double effect should be pleased rather than disappointed. He or she has truly intended the good effect and merely tolerated the possibility of the bad one.

Put in Keown's terms, the unifying factor between the withdrawal of treatment and the administration of possibly fatal pain relief is intention, rather than the action itself. In both cases the intended effect (the relief of suffering) is good. However, one might argue that is also the intention in active euthanasia. We will return to that problem in Section 4, where we discuss a case of actively assisting suicide. For now, we would like you to undertake one final activity before finishing this section.

ACTIVITY: Thinking back to the case of Mr R. in the light of the arguments you have explored thus far, do you think it would have been justifiable for Dr S to administer pain relief to R in the knowledge that his death might be accelerated? Jot down any conditions that you would want to impose on her power to do so.

In Catholic doctrine there are four conditions which must be fulfilled if a good action with a bad side-effect is to be allowed:

(a) The action, considered by itself and independently of its effects, must not be morally wrong.

(b) The bad effect must not be the means of producing the good effect.

(c) The bad effect must be sincerely unintended, and merely tolerated.

(d) There must be a proportionate reason for performing the action in spite of its bad potential consequences (Veatch, 1989).

In the case of R it seems to us that all these conditions can be met. There is nothing morally wrong with administering pain relief, in itself; indeed, it is morally good to relieve others' suffering. Death, if defined as the bad effect, is not the means of producing the good effect of pain relief, as would be the case if, say, Dr S administered a lethal dose of potassium chloride – whose only function would be to bring about R's death. We have already considered the third condition: if Dr S is not disappointed in the event that R does not die, then she genuinely does not intend his death. Finally, there is clearly a proportionate reason for performing the action, that is, the relief of suffering. All this is premised on Dr S's own feelings about the ethical acceptability of such a course.

> ACTIVITY: Is it always up to the doctor's individual moral beliefs? Should doctors have the right to refuse to carry out treatments that contradict their own moral beliefs?

Although the answer to this question might obviously seem 'yes', you might also like to consider the opposite point of view: that patients can be harmed if doctors exercise their rights of conscience. In an American case, Beverley Requena, a competent woman of 55 who was on a ventilator in a church-affiliated hospital, decided to refuse tube feeding (Miles et al., 1989). This contradicted the hospital's ethical code, but hospital management offered to transfer her to another institution which would honour her refusal. Ms Requena refused the transfer; in all other respects she was happy with the care she was receiving in the church-affiliated hospital, and it was there that she wanted to die. The hospital brought a suit to force Ms Requena to transfer, but failed in court. There the judge directed the hospital to reconsider its beliefs in a more flexible manner. The case of Beverley Requena makes a good link to the next section of this chapter, in that it concerns a legally competent patient.

In this section, as in Section 1, we have looked at ethical issues in the care of patients who cannot express a preference in their own end-of-life decisions. In the next section we move on to the competent patient. How comprehensive is the duty to relieve suffering there?

> ACTIVITY: Make a list of the key points raised by this section.

Section 3: Refusal of treatment and advance directives

In the previous two sections we looked at the goals of medicine in the care of dying patients who are not competent to choose or refuse treatment. There, the clinician's main concern was to avoid imposing unnecessary suffering, in the best interests of the patient. But what happens when doctors also have to take into account the views of patients? Here and in Section 4 we move on to cases of competent patients – although in both these cases the patient's competence was borderline, for reasons of mental illness. In Section 3 we consider the UK case of Mr C, a long-term mental patient who was allowed to refuse amputation of a gangrenous leg; in Section 4, we look at the Dutch case of Dr Chabot, who assisted the suicide of a clinically depressed but otherwise healthy woman.

Even if healing and/or the relief of suffering are taken to be the unquestionable goals of medicine, that does not justify the doctor's imposing his or her goals and values on those of the competent patient. Treating patients without their informed consent, even in the name of their best interests, is an unacceptable invasion of personal integrity, in this argument about what is ethically right and wrong – and that is also the legal position in most European jurisdictions. Even at the end of life, or at the risk of death, a competent adult patient has an absolute right to refuse treatment, as Ron Berghmans explains.

A well-considered refusal of treatment ought to be respected, even if the physician takes the view that treatment is beneficial to the patient. The reasons for respecting competent refusals of treatment are twofold. The first reason is that non-consensual intervention where a person has decision-making capacity invades the integrity of the person involved. The second is that competent persons ought to be considered the best judges of their own interests. Only the competent person himself can assess the benefits, burdens and harms of treatment, in view of his or her wishes, goals and values. So, if a person refuses treatment because he or she does not value treatment in his or her personal life, then such a refusal ought to be respected, even if this might result in an earlier death. Although healing is an ideal in medical practice, other goals and values can and do operate as constraints on medical actions serving this ideal (Berghmans, 1997a).

But what does Berghmans mean by 'a well-considered refusal of treatment'? Might one argue that refusing treatment which is medically advisable is automatically ill-considered? That this kind of reasoning does occur in practice has been extensively documented (e.g. Roth et al., 1977; Faulder, 1985; Culver and Gert, 1982) and, in the case of young people under 18, it has actually been upheld in law (*Re R* [1991]). The argument here is that refusal should carry a heavier 'tariff' than consent to treatment, because it goes against medical opinion. But that is different from saying that a refusal can never be 'well considered', even

if it flies in the face of medical opinion. As another court ruled in an earlier decision, 'the patient is entitled to reject [medical] advice for reasons which are rational, or irrational, or for no reason' (*Sidaway v. Bethlem RHG*, 1985).

We will now look briefly at a case which illustrates the criteria for competence. (This case is considered at greater length in the mental health chapter.)

THE CASE OF MR C

Mr C, aged 68, had been detained in a secure mental hospital for 30 years as a paranoid schizophrenic. His delusions included the belief that his doctors were torturers, whilst he himself was a world-famous specialist in the treatment of diseased limbs. When his own foot became infected, he therefore hid his condition from medical personnel until it had actually become gangrenous. His doctors believed that unless his foot was amputated, he stood an 80 to 85 per cent chance of dying.

Mr C, however, refused to consent to the amputation, saying that he would rather die intact than survive with only one foot. He sought reassurances from the hospital that his foot would not be amputated without his consent if he slipped into a coma. The health authority in charge of the hospital refused to give an undertaking not to amputate his foot without his consent. Mr C then sought a High Court order to prevent amputation if he became unconscious.

ACTIVITY: Do you think Mr C was competent to refuse consent to treatment? Jot down the principal reasons why, or why not.

As Mr C's solicitor, Lucy Scott-Montcrieff, explained:

The issue at the heart of all of this was whether or not Mr C had the capacity to refuse the treatment that was being offered to him. Mental illness doesn't of itself mean that a person doesn't have capacity; you could have capacity for some things and not other things. We had to establish whether Mr C could understand and retain the information about the advantages and disadvantages of amputation and the advantages and disadvantages of not having amputation. The surgeon who'd been treating Mr C gave evidence; what he said was that he believed that Mr C did have capacity, because Mr C's views about capacity fitted in a very normal sort of way with the views of other elderly people with vascular disease who got gangrene more or less at the end of their lives. They didn't want to spend their last few years either coping with an amputation or possibly coping with repeated amputation as the vascular system fails all round the body. So the order was made that the hospital trust shouldn't amputate his foot without his permission (BBC, 1995).

In the event, Mr C survived, and his case made legal history in the UK for two reasons which are very important to the wider concerns of this chapter. Firstly, it established a clear set of criteria for competence.

(a) Capacity to comprehend and retain information about the proposed treatment. Mr C was found to have this capacity, in part because it was shown that, in other aspects of everyday prudence, such as budgeting, he was able to take 'sensible' decisions. Further, it was held that what mattered was the narrowly construed ability to comprehend and retain information about this particular decision, on a functional basis, not capacity in some general sense. Given the general presumption of competence in adults, the doctors had to establish that Mr C did not possess this capacity; the court held that this had not been proved.

(b) Belief in the validity of the information (see also Re MB, 1997). It might be thought questionable whether Mr C really believed what the doctors told him; after all, he thought they were torturers. Perhaps he also believed, in his delusions about his own medical 'stardom', that he knew better than the hospital physicians. Nevertheless, the court held that Mr C also met this criterion.

(c) Ability to weigh up the information so as to arrive at a choice. Mr C had balanced the risks and benefits differently from the doctors, but that did not invalidate his decision, particu-

larly because an expert witness had testified that many other elderly people came to the same conclusion.

Secondly, the C case concerned the validity of advance directives, sometimes called living wills: statements made while a patient is competent, concerning what forms of treatment he or she would wish to refuse in the event of becoming incompetent, e.g. through coma or persistent vegetative state (Law Commission, 1995; Lord Chancellor's Department, 1997). (Because the general purpose of advance directives is to specify treatment which would not be considered acceptable, they are also sometimes known as 'advance refusals'.) They can be either written or oral, Mr C's was a witnessed verbal refusal. Advance directives illustrate in practical form the distinction introduced in the previous section between acts and omissions. They rest on the legal and ethical distinction between acting to do everything which could be done to relieve suffering – regardless of what the patient wants – and respecting the patient's right to request that certain forms of treatment should be omitted.

In the UK, at the time of writing (early 2000), it has been emphasized that *'certain forms of advance statement already have full effect at common law'* (Lord Chancellor's Department, 1997, p. 23). The conditions are that an advance refusal must be 'clearly established' and 'applicable in the circumstances'. In that case the refusal is as binding as that of a competent, conscious adult. 'An advance refusal made with capacity simply survives any supervening incapacity.' (Law Commission, 1995). However, because there was no statutory provision at the time of writing – although a consultation document was laying the grounds for such legislation – it was still necessary to go to court in order to establish the validity of an advance directive, as Mr C had to do. None the less, advance directives are generally recognized as an important part of patient choice and autonomy. Although they no longer apply only to terminal conditions, as they did when first introduced in the United States during the late 1970s, they may be particularly important in planning a treatment programme for dying people. In the US there are both 'information directives' which specify what treatments are not acceptable to the patient and 'proxy directives' which authorize another individual to make the decision.

Advance directives also illustrate the difference between acts and omissions in another sense. They cannot direct the clinician to undertake acts against his or her clinical judgement: only to refrain from treatment which the patient finds unacceptable. Resource limitations will also determine what an advance directive can specify. Someone dying of kidney failure cannot obtain dialysis or a kidney transplant merely by taking out an advance directive demanding it. English case law has held that there is no specific liability on the Secretary of State to provide any particular level of health care (*ex parte Hincks*, 1980). Furthermore, an advance directive cannot direct what is unlawful. Thus in the UK at present, no one can take out an advance directive requesting euthanasia or assisted suicide. The position in the Netherlands is different in relation to euthanasia, as we shall see in the next section.

ACTIVITY: Take a few moments to write down the key points raised by this section.

Section 4. Euthanasia and physician-assisted suicide

Can euthanasia and physician-assisted suicide ever be a rightful part of the goals of medicine? Can it ever be ethical to inflict death in the name of avoiding suffering? Or is this a violation of the moral integrity of medicine (Singer and Siegler, 1990; Pellegrino, 1992; Momeyer, 1995)? Can 'the best interests of the patient' extend to ceasing to exist, or is that logically impossible? Is trust in the medical profession so radically undermined if

doctors are allowed to kill that we ought to rule out euthanasia and physician-assisted suicide altogether? Or does the possibility of euthanasia and of assisted suicide where suffering is intractable actually meet what patients want?

This section will explore these questions in the context of practice in the Netherlands, where euthanasia and assisted suicide are prohibited by the Penal Code but may lawfully be performed if the doctor follows certain guidelines laid down by the courts and the medical profession. Those guidelines, and Dutch public opinion about euthanasia and physician-assisted suicide, were severely tested in a case involving a doctor who assisted the suicide of an otherwise healthy woman who was deeply depressed over the deaths of her two sons: the case of Dr Boudewyn Chabot (Berghmans, 1997a). Dr Chabot felt that he would be letting his patient down, and increasing her suffering, if he failed to grant her request for assisted suicide. His deep commitment to his patient – which no one questioned – led him to feel that assisting her suicide was indeed part of his medical duty, and of the goals of medicine as he construed them.

Chabot's critics, however, denied that he would be failing in his duty to the patient if he refused her request. It was also argued that the Chabot case dramatically illustrated the 'slippery slope' argument against euthanasia and physician-assisted suicide: that once introduced, it allows physicians to 'kill off' patients who are not terminally ill, and indeed not even ill at all. At most, Dr Chabot's patient was mentally ill, clinically depressed; but should such a request from a mentally ill patient be respected? This relates back to the C case, which you examined in the previous section, and to the criteria for competence.

In this section we concentrate on a further extract from Ron Berghmans's article on 'Physician-assisted suicide in the case of mental suffering', which you began reading in Section 1. This part of the paper concerns the Chabot case explicitly, but it also sets that case in the wider context of euthanasia and physician-assisted suicide in Dutch practice. Before you begin, you should note the difference between the two:

- In physician-assisted suicide, the doctor provides the means and guidance, e.g. a prescription for a lethal dose of medicine, and counselling on doses and methods. Although the physician may be present at the end, he or she does not perform the final act: the patient does.
- In voluntary euthanasia, a physician administers a drug injection or other agent at the patient's request, thereby performing the final act that results in the patient's death (Berghmans, 1997a). Euthanasia is more common than physician-assisted suicide: about 2.4 per cent of deaths in a recent Dutch research project resulted from euthanasia, against 0.3 per cent from physician-assisted suicide. In 0.7 per cent of cases, life was ended without the explicit, concurrent request of the patient, even though in the Netherlands euthanasia is defined as voluntary euthanasia (Van der Maas et al., 1996). In many of these cases the patient was comatose or otherwise incapable of making a request. The Dutch Remmelink Commission of 1992 estimated that up to 1000 instances of euthanasia every year were unasked for, and that some of these included competent patients. This is a frightening statistic, and, if accurate, a powerful argument against euthanasia; but it is not our principal concern here. Rather, we proceed from the assumption, *in arguendo,* that euthanasia is valid when requested by a competent patient; but we test that argument to the utmost by looking at a particularly troubling case.

Now continue with your reading of Berghman's paper.

Physician-assisted suicide in the case of mental suffering

Ron Berghmans

The debate concerning physician-assisted suicide and euthanasia is broadening: along with patients suffering from terminal illness, other groups of patients are also being considered as potential candidates for assistance in dying. One of these groups is the mentally ill. I will concentrate on the case of physician-assisted suicide for the mentally ill, offering some background to the debate concerning the practice of assisted suicide and euthanasia in the Netherlands, and presenting opinion as it is developing in the Dutch context.

Although the point is sometimes misunderstood by foreign commentators, physician-assisted suicide and euthanasia remain criminal offences in the Netherlands. Assisting in the suicide of a person, which includes providing the means for someone to take his life, is a crime under Article 294 of the Penal Code. This article also applies to physicians acting on the request of a patient (Gevers, 1995).

The legal acceptability of euthanasia and assisted suicide is based on recognition on a case-to-case basis of the physician's defence of necessity (*force majeure*). To have this defence accepted, the doctor performing euthanasia or assisting with suicide must act according to the five following criteria, as set down by the Royal Dutch Medical Association:

(a) There must be a voluntary, competent and enduring request on the part of the patient.
(b) The patient's request must be based on full information.
(c) The patient must be in a situation of intolerable and hopeless suffering.
(d) All acceptable treatment alternatives must have been attempted.
(e) The physician must consult an independent colleague before performing euthanasia or assisting with suicide.

ACTIVITY: Which of these criteria would be the easiest to fulfil, in your opinion, and which would be the most problematic?

We rated criterion (e) as the least problematic, and the easiest to prove or disprove in practice. (After you have read the case of Dr Chabot below, you might want to return to this list: you will see that his case hinged on this factor.) The other four criteria all seemed problematic to us for different reasons.

(a) How do we judge whether the doctor's influence lessens the voluntariness of the action? What about patients who are unable to give a voluntary consent, because they are in a coma? We have already seen that there are instances of euthanasia being performed on such patients in the Netherlands.

(b) Full information is almost never available: no one can say for certain how long the patient will have to suffer. It is largely in B-grade films that doctors give a definite estimate such as 'You only have six months to live'.

(c) The same caveat applies to 'hopeless'. The palliative care movement would deny that any suffering is 'hopeless'; palliation can almost always be achieved. Does 'hopeless' refer to the possibility of cure or of good palliative care?

(d) 'No acceptable treatment alternatives' begs the question, insofar as the existence of euthanasia itself contaminates this decision. If it weren't available, the patient couldn't rule out all other alternatives.

These requirements were developed in the context of persons suffering from a terminal, or at least fatal or incurable, disease, such as patients with advanced cancer (Gevers, 1995). In the 1980s and 1990s, through a series of court decisions, reports and opinions from bodies such as the Dutch Society of Psychiatrists, the Royal Dutch Society of Medicine, the Inspectorate for Mental Health, and the Dutch Association for Voluntary Euthanasia, attention was extended to the issue of physician-assisted suicide for psychiatric patients. Lower courts took the view that, in exceptional circumstances, assisting a mentally ill person to commit suicide might be acceptable practice.

A landmark in this respect has been the so-called Chabot case (Griffiths, 1995). The defendant was a psychiatrist named Boudewyn Chabot, who in September 1991 supplied to Mrs Boomsma, at her request, lethal drugs which she consumed in the presence of the defendant, her GP, and a friend. She died half an hour later.

Mrs Boomsma was 50 years old; she had married at 22, but from the beginning the marriage was unhappy. In 1986 her eldest son committed suicide. From that time on her marital problems grew worse and her husband more violent; her wish to die began to take shape, but she said that she remained alive only to care for her younger son. In 1988 she left her husband, taking her younger son with her. In 1990 her son was admitted to hospital in connection with a traffic accident, and was found to be suffering from cancer, from which he died in May 1991. That same evening Mrs Boomsma attempted suicide with drugs she had put by, but did not die. She then approached the Dutch Association for Voluntary Euthanasia, which put her in touch with Dr Chabot.

Mrs Boomsma was diagnosed as suffering from an adjustment disorder, consisting of a depressed mood, without psychotic signs, in the context of a complicated bereavement process. Although her condition was in principle treatable, treatment would probably have been protracted and the chance of success small. But she rejected therapy, despite Dr Chabot's best efforts to persuade her. He became convinced that she was experiencing intense, long-term psychic suffering which was unbearable for her, and which held out no prospect of improvement. Her request for assistance with suicide in his opinion was well considered. In letters and discussion with him, she presented the reasons for her decision clearly and consistently, showing that she understood her situation and the consequences of her decision. In his judgement, her rejection of therapy was also well considered. Chabot consulted seven experts. None of them believed that there was any realistic chance of success, given Mrs Boomsma's clear refusal of treatment.

In its ruling of 21 June 1994, the Dutch Supreme Court used the Chabot case to clarify a number of important issues in the euthanasia debate. First, it held that assistance with suicide was justified in the case of a patient whose suffering is not somatic, and who is not in the terminal phase of an illness – but only if the physician has acted 'with the utmost carefulness'. The court took the view that what matters is the seriousness of the patient's suffering, not its source.

Secondly, the court stated that it was incorrect, as a general legal proposition, to claim that a psychiatric patient's request for assistance with suicide cannot be voluntary. A person's wish to die can be based on an autonomous judgement, even in the presence of mental illness.

> ACTIVITY: How does this judgement compare with the C case we considered earlier?

The basic proposition appears similar on the surface: both courts agree that mental illness does not in itself bar a patient from making a valid medical decision. If you believe that killing is different from letting die, however, the Chabot case is more serious: Dr Chabot was being asked not to refrain from doing everything which could be done, but to actively assist Mrs B in her suicide – an act rather than an omission. There is also considerable doubt about whether Mrs B actually was mentally ill, or simply grief-stricken – whereas there is no doubt that C was the victim of gross psychotic delusions. Finally, in English mental health law a patient is allowed to refuse treatment for a physical disorder, but not treatment for mental disorder. The C case is consistent with that principle. Mrs Boomsma, however, had rejected treatment designed to mitigate her depression, that is, treatment concerning her mental health. It is certainly arguable that, if she was adjudged mentally ill, she should have been forcibly treated by anti-depressant medication. If she was not mentally ill, but rather deeply bereaved and yet sane, there were no medical grounds for assisting her suicide.

The Supreme Court also took the view that a patient's condition cannot be considered hopeless if he or she freely rejects a meaningful treatment option. In such a case, assisted suicide is not justified. The difficult question is what counts as a meaningful option. The court followed the viewpoint of a committee of the Dutch Royal College of Medicine, which laid down the following three conditions:
- the patient's condition can be alleviated if proper treatment is given, on current medical opinion
- alleviation is possible within a reasonable time period
- the relationship of benefits to burdens of treatment should be proportionate.

Finally, the Supreme Court took the view that an independent expert must be consulted on all relevant aspects of the case, and must himself examine the patient before assistance with suicide can be given. This was the respect in which Chabot was adjudged to have failed. The seven experts whom he consulted had not themselves examined the patient. Therefore Chabot was convicted by the Court, although he was given a suspended sentence. After the Supreme Court decision, Chabot was also cautioned by the Dutch Medical Council, which took the view that he should have considered treating his patient with anti-depressants, even if she refused consent.

> ACTIVITY: The implication of the Dutch Medical Council ruling is that most psychiatrists would have treated Mrs Boomsma with anti-depressants, and that Dr Chabot's decision was aberrant practice. But how often do such cases arise? If they are rare, how can we know what is typical practice? – and how useful is the Chabot case for 'ordinary practice'? How common do you think such cases are?

Two large-scale research projects into the practice of medical decision-making at the end of life have provided reliable data on the types of decisions being made, the motives of physicians, and other characteristics of Dutch practice on euthanasia and assisted suicide (Van der Maas et al., 1991, 1996). Another project, conducted in 1996, after the Supreme Court ruling in the Chabot case, also gives insight into the incidence of physician-assisted death in psychiatric practice (Groenewoud et al., 1997). Explicit requests for physician-assisted suicide are not uncommon in psychiatric practice, but these requests are rarely granted. On the basis of Groenewoud's data, we can estimate that physician-assisted suicide in psychiatric practice occurs two to five times per year in the Netherlands. The total incidence of explicit requests for physician-assisted suicide by psychiatric patients was estimated to be about 320 annually. Most of the psychiatric patients who received suicide assistance suffered from both a mental disorder and a serious physical illness (unlike Mrs Boomsma, who was physically well). The most frequently mentioned reasons for assisting in suicide were that the patient's suffering was unbearable or hopeless, and that all previous treatment had failed. Two-thirds of Dutch psychiatrists surveyed consider assisted suicide in mental illness to be acceptable, and 46 per cent could envisage a case in which they themselves would be prepared to assist the patient in suicide.

After the Supreme Court's ruling in the Chabot case, the Dutch Society of Psychiatrists established a committee to advise on guidelines for dealing with requests for assisted suicide by patients who suffer from mental illness. The committee began from the following premises:

- A request for assistance in suicide in someone with mental illness ought to be assumed to be a request for help. The presumption should be that suicidal wishes are a sign of psychopathology, in the first instance, requiring suicide prevention, not suicide assistance.

ACTIVITY: Compare this premise with the argument made below by two medically trained practising psychoanalysts from Italy, Raffaele Bracalenti and Emilio Mordini:

A request for suicide assistance from a terminally ill patient should always be considered a reflection of bad practice. There is something wrong with the diagnostic or therapeutic process which has led to such a strong refusal to carry on with life (Bracalenti and Mordini, 1997).

Bracalenti and Mordini do not confine their statement to patients with mental illness: that is a key

difference from the Dutch guidelines. However, in both cases clinicians are advised to make a *prima facie* assumption against honouring a request for suicide. But the Dutch psychiatrists' association goes on to state that:

- Suicidality should not *a priori* be considered as a psychopathological phenomenon. Although many death wishes in mentally ill people have a temporary, transitory character, in exceptional cases a request for suicide assistance may be the result of a careful weighing process, and may be enduring.
- In exceptional cases, physician-assisted suicide may be responsible practice, but it can *never be* a general duty. Individual psychiatrists have no moral or legal obligation to practise assisted suicide, although they do have a duty to deal responsibly and carefully with every request for suicide assistance.

ACTIVITY: What does this imply about goals of medicine? Think back to the original premise with which this chapter began, that the principal goal of medical care at the end of life is the relief of suffering. Throughout this section we have been testing that premise to the utmost, by asking whether it is a duty in cases of hopeless and unbearable suffering to relieve that suffering by assisting the patient to die. On this alternative view, relieving suffering by assisting suicide is not part of the *telos* of medicine; rather, the proper goal is to deal carefully and responsibly with any request for suicide, and thereby to take the patient and her suffering seriously.

There is no duty to kill implied in the relief of suffering, nor in the patient's right to die. As the American bioethicist Daniel Callahan succinctly puts it, 'Your right to die doesn't imply my duty to kill'.

The Chabot case illustrates the 'slippery slope' problem about euthanasia and physician-assisted suicide, in that it seems unlikely that this was the sort of case envisioned when the current guidelines were first established (Keown, 1995a, 1997). Have the Dutch gone too far? Within the Netherlands, the Chabot case occasioned widespread doubts to that effect. Outside the country, some commentators even surmised the Chabot cases demonstrated that euthanasia and physician-assisted suicide risk becoming a kind of social control and medical abuse (Bracalenti and Mordini, 1997). If there was no medical problem in Mrs Boomsma's case, this argument runs, it becomes clear that Chabot's action instantiates social rather than medical judgements. If we look at a hypothetical case of a healthy 50-year-old Indian woman who 'requests' *suttee* on her bereavement, surely we would think this an instance of dreadful social pressure, not a free choice.

Terminal illness, however, had never been a requirement in the Dutch system, and it can certainly be argued that mental suffering is no less unendurable than physical pain. Although mental illness may undermine autonomy and competence – thereby casting the request for euthanasia from a mentally ill person into doubts about validity – it does not automatically make the decision to refuse treatment invalid, as we saw in the C case.

On the other hand, by focusing on the doctor's duties rather than the patient's competence, it becomes irrelevant as to whether Mrs B's illness was mental or physical. As one of his critics pointed out at the Dutch Medical Association hearing, if Mrs B was mentally well enough to make a valid request for physician-assisted suicide, Dr Chabot, as a psychiatrist, should not have been acting in the first place. (Although he also viewed himself as her friend, he would have had no access to the lethal drugs if he were acting merely in his private capacity.) If Mrs B was mentally ill, Dr Chabot's duty was to cure her mental illness rather than assist her suicide. In fact Dr Chabot recognized that Mrs B was not mentally ill; the 'illness' from which she suffered was intractable grief. But that takes us back to the question of whether euthanasia was intended as a 'remedy' for human tragedy. Surely not – and if not, then this case shows that the Dutch have indeed slid too far down the slope.

A different sort of argument against euthanasia and physician-assisted suicide draws attention to the regrettable practical consequences of focusing on its legalisation, rather than pressing for improvements in palliative care. This view, typical of the hospice movement, asserts that proponents of euthanasia and assisted suicide encourage the widespread public misapprehension that nothing can be done about suffering at the end of life except to end it by death. This is pernicious, they argue, and indeed ethically wrong. In the next section we will look at an example of good palliative care and dialogue with the patient. The purpose of this example is twofold: to provide an ordinary case from everyday hospice practice, in contrast to the highly dramatic and unusual case of Dr Chabot, and to show how doctors may respond to what their patients want without feeling, as Dr Chabot did, that he would be letting his patient down if he did not assist her suicide.

> ACTIVITY: Take a few moments to list the key points from this section.

Section 5: Ethics at the end of life: a case

We began this chapter on ethical issues at the end of life with a consideration of the *telos* of medicine and of the role of the physician in situations where it seemed clear that 'healing' was no longer possible. In the introductory section we made the tentative hypothesis that the *telos* of medicine under these circumstances might perhaps best be characterized as something like the 'alleviation of suffering'. As you have worked your way through the various sections of the chapter since then, we have asked you to consider whether this is in fact an adequate expression of the ethical dimensions of decision-making in palliative care. Together, we have explored what the ethical and practical implications of this conceptualization might be through the consideration of a range of 'hard cases'.

One thing that has already become clear, it seems to us, is that the interpretation of the *telos* of medicine at the end of life as the 'alleviation of suffering' is not a panacea enabling physicians to avoid the ethical problems related to the practice of medicine at the end of life. If anything, such a conceptualization brings with it a further unique range of ethical dilemmas relating, at least in part, to the tensions which are created between the more usual conception of the *telos* of medicine in terms of healing and the expression of the particular goals of medicine at the end of life in terms of the relief of suffering. In Section 1, for example, we considered the question of whether it is ever ethical to relieve suffering by the withdrawal of treatment. In Section 2 we went on to consider whether it might be ethical to relieve suffering by deciding not to resuscitate a patient. In Section 3 we looked at whether it might be ethical to alleviate suffering by respecting a patient's wish to refuse treatment, either in contemporaneous expression or as expressed in the form of an advance directive. Lastly, in Section 4 we considered the same question in relation to euthanasia and physician-assisted suicide.

Each of these investigations into ethical issues at the end of life has focused on one of the very many demanding and critical decisions which pose difficult ethical questions for physicians working in this area, that is, on hard cases. The dramatic nature of these dilemmas and cases gives them a distinctive power which forces us to reconsider the ethical and moral assumptions with which we began the chapter and which underpin our conception of the *telos* of medicine. The ethical discussion of medicine at this period of life and in particular of decisions relating to death and dying is very usefully expressed in this way, via the use of hard cases. It is a good way of bringing out the importance of the issues at hand. But how do such cases and how does such discussion relate to the more everyday, even if no less dramatic, cases with which practitioners are faced on a more frequent basis?

In this section we would now like you to go on to look at a very ordinary case which contrasts usefully with the ones we have heard about thus far. This is the case of Helena and it comes from Belgium.

> ACTIVITY: Before you do so, however, we would like you to reconsider this question of the goals of medicine at the end of life. Go back to the definition you came up with in Section 1. In the light of the four sections you have completed thus far, we would like you to reflect upon whether the relief of suffering is an adequate definition of the *telos* of medicine at the end of life. Make a list of other features of medicine which you consider to be important elements of good medicine in this area.

When we thought about this, we wondered whether it might be possible to identify some features of the end of life which are both morally significant and also different from other stages of life. One thought we had was that if Dan Callahan is right in his claim in *Setting Limits* (1995a) that the period at the end of life in a 'good life' will be one of reflection upon one's life as a whole, of coming to terms with one's mortality and of saying goodbye to the people around us, this might have ethical implications for those who care for the elderly and the dying. It might, for example, conceivably mean that it is important for practitioners to respect the unique features of this period of life by attempting, whenever they have the opportunity to do so, to allow this process of 'coming to terms' to take place. Often, as in many of the cases described thus far, this may not in fact be easy or indeed possible. However, in more ordinary and everyday cases, this might be an important joint goal for both the patient and those caring for her.

We would now like you to go on to read the following case and whilst you do so to bear these questions in mind, noting down in particular any elements of the case which suggest that the *telos* of medicine at the end of life is broader than the relief of suffering.

THE CASE OF HELENA

Helena was a robust 63-year-old woman. She had formerly been a gymnastics teacher and continued to be both physically fit and actively involved in a leading gymnastics organization for children and young people even after her retirement. Helena had never been married and lived alone in a first-floor apartment in central Antwerp. She was an independent woman of strong character who was considered to be very kind by those who knew her well.

In 1994 Helena began to suffer from a pain in her lower back which persisted for several weeks. She informed a relative, her nephew, about this at a family reunion. The nephew, who was a neurologist, advised Helena to rest and to seek some physiotherapy. This did not seem to help and in fact the pain appeared to get worse over subsequent weeks. When Helena informed her nephew of this, he arranged for some X-rays to be taken. The X-rays appeared normal and the nephew advised his aunt to go to her usual GP about her back pain.

The pain in Helena's back, which she described as having a constant burning character and which now radiated to her leg, continued and seemed in fact to be getting worse day by day. The pain was such that it made it increasingly difficult for Helena to walk. Helena's GP arranged for her to have a CAT scan and whereas the X-rays had revealed very little the CAT scan showed that Helena had cancer of the ovaries with metastasis spreading to the lumbar spine. Helena was immediately referred to an oncologist at the local hospital where she was given a 'debulking' operation followed by chemotherapy and radiotherapy.

From the start, Helena followed her course of treatment courageously and without complaint. This changed, however, when Helena began to develop a polyneuropathy (a disorder of the peripheral nerves) of her arms and legs which made it extremely difficult for her to move about. Soon Helena could hardly walk at all and it took her a great and increasing amount of effort and time to climb the steps to her apartment. She was also as a result of the pain in her fingers no longer able to do the needlework which had until now been the way she had tended to fill the long evenings. Helena found these symptoms and the side-effects of the chemotherapy very upsetting and was very unhappy. Helena informed her oncologist that the pain in her hands and fingers was getting progressively worse. The therapeutic relationship between Helena and those caring for her deteriorated rapidly.

> ACTIVITY: Stop for a moment and make a list of what you consider to be the ethical questions which have emerged in the first few paragraphs of the case study. We shall be returning to this in a moment. Add to this list as you continue to read about the case.

At this point Helena was clearly very unhappy with the way she had been treated. Over and above the distress which she felt as a consequence of her illness Helena, as an active and independent woman, was finding it very difficult to come to terms with her increased and progressive disablement. What seems to have angered her most is the fact that she believed this to be caused not by her condition directly but as a side-effect of the treatment she was receiving. As we read this, we wondered if she had been adequately informed about the likely side-effects of her chemotherapy. She seems to have been surprised by them. It is difficult to tell from this account of the case whether or not this was in fact the case but it shows how important it is, ethically, for the physician to ensure, as far as is possible, that the patient shares an ongoing understanding of, and an agreement about, the treatment programme. Iatrogenic harm – harm done unintentionally by doctors – is always a possibility in any intervention, and when getting consent doctors should make patients aware of its possibility while also remaining alert to the implications for the course of the treatment. This does not excuse them, of course, from trying to minimize this harm both in the first place and by rethinking their treatment plan accordingly during the course of treatment and we will see that, as the case progresses, this is what happens in the case of Helena. This serves to remind us that the ethical dimensions of healthcare are broader than those which arise in crisis situations and decision-making. The relationships between carers, patients, families and so on have an ongoing, relationship-centred ethical dimension which is perhaps not well expressed in terms of autonomy, choice and so on but may perhaps be best captured by the concepts of 'responsibility', 'duty of care', 'authenticity' and so on. Interestingly, this made us think about how closely tied up our sense of autonomy is with the sense we have of being related to others in particular kinds of ways.

We would now like you to continue reading the case.

Notwithstanding her unhappiness with the treatment she had received, Helena's condition gradually stabilized and remained stable for several months and this seems to have helped the relationship between Helena and those who cared for her. However, the pain and symptoms of the neuropathy did not decrease and after a few months they began to get worse once again, causing Helena more and more pain and progressively disabling her further.

At this point there was some difference of opinion between the two oncologists responsible for Helena's treatment. One of them considered the increasing pain being experienced by Helena to be due principally to the progression of the disease. The other disagreed and felt that it was being caused by the treatment itself. He felt that, by changing the form of Helena's treatment, some of her discomfort might be relieved. After some discussion it was proposed that Helena should be put on a new chemotherapy cocktail, which, it was felt, would present less risk of the side-effects of which Helena had complained. By this point, however, Helena had decided that she no longer wanted to be treated and refused these new drugs too.

ACTIVITY: Imagine that you had an opportunity to interview the oncologist, Helena and her nephew at this point. What questions would you ask them and how would their answers affect the way you feel about the case and about what ought to happen next?

Then continue reading the case.

For a while Helena received no treatment but after a few months she returned to her GP complaining of abdominal pain, vomiting and problems with defaecation: an obstruction appeared to have complicated her condition. In addition to this, Helena's neuropathy was getting worse and she was no longer able to leave her apartment alone.

Helena was immediately admitted into hospital and following the administration of fluids and medication she began to show signs of improvement. A meeting was arranged between Helena, her oncologist, a social worker and her GP at which Helena was offered several possible alternative ways forward:

(a) The first option was a surgical intervention to bypass the obstruction

(b) The second was continued chemotherapy, and

(c) The third was to receive no further treatment other than the management of the symptoms such as the pain.

At the end of the meeting Helena asked for 2 or 3 days to consider these options. She decided that she would prefer to forego any further treatment other than pain and symptom management and was transferred into a palliative care unit because the lack of space at her own apartment meant that good care would be difficult.

After 3 weeks Helena's condition suddenly deteriorated. She became anorexic and was vomiting several times a day. It was clear to her physician that she had entered the terminal stages of her illness. At this point, however, Helena requested another meeting with her doctors and expressed a desire to be given some more time in order to be able to say 'goodbye'.

ACTIVITY: Stop here for a moment. What do you think the doctors ought to have done at this stage? Earlier, Helena had refused treatment and had opted for the management of her pain only. Now she has changed her mind. What do you consider the goals of medicine ought to be under these circumstances? It seems that the suffering which is most acute for Helena is related not to the pain of her condition in itself but to the sense she has that her process of 'making sense' and of coming to terms with her death is incomplete. But what is the responsibility of medical practitioners here? If the doctors operate on Helena, this will not save her life but it may prolong it for a short time, time in which, perhaps, Helena would be able to 'say goodbye'. Is this what medicine ought to be doing? How does this situation differ from those in the other sections of this chapter? Take a moment to look back at the definition of the *telos* of medicine which you came up with in Section 1 and reworked at the beginning of this section; how does it apply to this case?

Later Helena met with her doctors and following this discussion it was agreed that a surgical intervention (Option (a)) would be carried out.

The operation was successful and after recovering from it Helena got a further 3 months of what her GP called 'good comfort and good quality of life'. Helena felt that this was important because it gave her the time to make some arrangements which were important to her and to say goodbye to the people she loved. Helena died peacefully 3 months later.

When he was reflecting on the case, after Helena's death, her GP said that he felt that there were three important principles which had informed his decision-making during this case.

Firstly, he argued that,

In palliative care the autonomy of the patient, his or her choices, options and ideas are extremely important and ought to be respected as much as possible.

Secondly, he claimed that,

It must be recognized that palliative care is not static but is a dynamic process. At each stage the caregiver must listen to the patient's requests and be willing to consider new options.

Thirdly, he suggested that,

Good and ethical palliative care depends upon an interdisciplinary approach in which a range of possibilities can be considered. However, the teamwork

required can present a challenge to caregivers and demands unique skills and attitudes.

ACTIVITY: Taking each of these in turn we would like you to read through the case again and consider the extent to which the practitioners in this case adhered to these principles. How do you feel about the way Helena's illness and ultimately her death were dealt with? Below is the definition of palliative care drawn up by the European Association for Palliative Care in Milan in 1988 and adopted by the World Health Organization in 1989. How do you feel Helena's treatment compared to this standard?

Palliative care is the active total care of patients whose disease is not responsive to curative treatment. Control of pain, of other symptoms, and of psychological, social and spiritual problems is paramount. The goal of palliative care is achievement of the best possible quality of life for patients and their families (WHO, 1989).

In the next section of the chapter, we will be going on to attempt to pull together all the various strands of our wide-ranging consideration of the goals of medicine at the end of life.

ACTIVITY: Take a few moments to list the key points raised by this section.

Section 6: The goals of medicine in palliative care (revisited)

The incompetent patient – sanctity of life, quality of life and vitalism

This section takes the form of a reading exercise based on a paper written by John Keown, who is a medical lawyer at Cambridge University. In it he addresses, through the use of a fictional case, the ethical issues raised by the case of a terminally ill patient who is incompetent and has no family. He explores these issues through the voices of three doctors, each of whom offers a different opinion on what ought to happen in the case.

The case concerns Mary, who is a frail woman, aged 75, who has advanced senile dementia. She has just been admitted to hospital after her third major heart attack and is examined by three consultant physicians, Keown calls them Dr V, Dr Q and Dr S, who respectively represent 'Vitalist', 'Quality of Life' and 'Sanctity of Life' views. All three agree about the diagnosis: Mary is suffering from severe coronary disease and advanced Alzheimer's disease. They also agree about the prognosis: Mary's condition is terminal. The coronary disease is progressive and irreversible and she is likely to suffer further heart attacks and to die within weeks if not days. The only way of attempting to extend her life when she suffers her next heart attack would be by cardio-pulmonary resuscitation (CPR).

The doctors discuss among themselves (since Mary is incompetent and has no relatives) the right ethical course to take when she suffers her next heart attack. Each doctor explains his ethical approach to the other two. As will appear in Keown's description, the doctors' disagreement about ethics is as pronounced as is their agreement about the medical facts.

ACTIVITY: Whilst you read through John Keown's account of the three perspectives expressed by Drs V, Q and S we would like you to attempt to pick out and list under three headings the various ethical and moral terms which relate to each of the views. Keown begins with the Vitalist perspective, as expressed by Dr V.

The incompetent patient – sanctity of life, quality of life and vitalism

John Keown

Dr V(italism) explains to Dr Q and Dr S that he thinks that human life is an absolute good and that it should be preserved at all costs, regardless of the expense of medical treatment or any pain and discomfort imposed by the treatment. It matters not, he says, whether the patient is young or old, able-bodied or disabled, curable or incurable: the life of every patient has to be preserved as long as possible. In short, Dr V is of the view that it is always unethical to shorten human life or to fail to lengthen it. He describes his ethical approach as 'Vitalism'. His motto is, he proclaims, 'Long live Vitalism! Keep everyone alive!'

Applying this vitalistic approach to Mary's case, he recommends that when she suffers her next heart attack, CPR should be administered. Indeed, he adds, any treatment necessary to preserve her life must be administered to her, regardless of its expense and regardless of any suffering the treatment may cause her.

ACTIVITY: Stop for a moment and make a note of any effective counter-arguments you can think of to the Vitalist perspective as exemplified by Dr V. As you read the rest of Keown's paper, add a list of arguments for and against each perspective under the headings you have already started.

While we were reading this section, we came to the conclusion that the vitalist perspective, whilst it might seem attractive on first sight, is counter-intuitive when taken seriously. Whilst it is undoubtedly true that we value human life as a good, when we do so we tend to be thinking about life which is more than simply organic. Would we really want to claim that such life is an absolute good? If we were asked to make a resource allocation decision between the preservation of the life of a patient whose life was 'merely' of this form and other forms of treatment, how would we decide?

In reply, Dr Q(uality of Life) explains that his views are at the opposite ethical extreme to those of Dr V. Dr Q states that, for him, human life is not an absolute good but only an instrumental good. It is not absolutely good in itself but is only good in an instrumental way, as a means to an end. That end is leading a 'worthwhile' life, a life of a minimum 'Quality'. 'For of what value is life', asks Dr Q, 'unless as a vehicle for a life which is worth living?'

Serious disability can, he adds, preclude a worthwhile life, particularly if it is a mental disability. For an essential requirement of a 'worthwhile' life is the ability to reason. And if the mental disability is sufficiently serious to deprive the individual of the ability to think rationally, what is to distinguish the life of that human being from that of a brute animal?

Indeed, he adds, a human being who lacks the ability to reason does not even qualify as a 'person' and is of no more intrinsic worth than a cat. Consequently, young children who have not yet developed the ability to reason (such as babies) and adults who have never had it (such as those with severe congenital mental handicap) or adults who have lost it (such as those with advanced senile dementia), do not count as 'persons' and killing them is not, in itself, any worse than killing a cat. His motto is 'It is wrong to kill persons with worthwhile lives, but not non-persons or persons with worthless lives'.

Applying this ethical approach to Mary's case, Dr Q recommends that, given Mary's serious mental disability which renders her unable to think rationally, Mary does not now, nor will she ever again, qualify as a 'person' and that her life is not worth living or preserving. Another reason for allowing Mary to die is, he continues, that her continuous care is a waste of healthcare resource.

Consequently, Dr Q advises that Mary should not be resuscitated when she suffers her next heart attack and should instead be 'allowed to die'. Dr Q adds that the ideal option would be intentionally to hasten her death immediately by lethal injection, but that, as this is illegal, the most appropriate course is simply to withhold resuscitation when it becomes necessary.

> **ACTIVITY:** The argument from Quality of Life considerations, as exemplified by Dr Q, suggests that the Vitalist is wrong to argue that life is always and under all circumstances worth preserving at any cost. In order to do so, however, it needs to depend upon a claim that there are certain key features which mark the difference between a life worth living and one which is not and Dr Q suggests that these include, for example, the ability to reason. Do you think that it is possible to establish such a distinction? If you think it is, make a list of five or ten qualities the absence of which would make a life not worth living. If you don't think that such a distinction is possible, what would you do in the case of Mary?

Dr S(anctity of Life) disagrees with both Dr V and Dr Q, and claims that his approach offers an ethical middle way between their two unethical extremes.

Dr S explains that human life is neither an absolute good nor merely an instrumental good but is, rather, a basic good. It is a necessary condition of leading a fulfilled life, and is undoubtedly good in itself. But there is more to a flourishing life than life itself. Life is not the only basic good. There are others, such as friendship, knowledge and the enjoyment of art and beauty. Someone leading a fully flourishing life is not simply alive: he or she also has friends, understands things and appreciates art and beauty, etc. Dr S calls these ingredients of a fulfilled life basic to emphasize that they are all equally important aspects of a fulfilled life: none is more important than another.

That is why Dr S rejects Dr V's elevation of the good of life to the status of an absolute good, which takes priority over the other basic goods. Were life such an absolute good, it would require us to devote all our time, energies and resources to the mere preservation of life instead of cultivating friendships, learning, and an appreciation of art and beauty. That would be a stunted rather than a fulfilled life. It would be no different from singling out one of the other basic goods, such as knowledge, for special attention and devoting all one's time, energies and resources to buying and reading books at the expense of one's other obligations such as looking after the health and welfare of oneself, one's family and one's community.

There is more to life than merely trying to extend one's lifespan just as there is much more to life than trying to learn everything one could. Placing an absolute value on human life would require individuals (including doctors) and societies to do nothing else but produce and preserve life. Unless they could make an adequate contribution to the preservation of life, schools, libraries and art galleries would be torn down to provide for more hospitals, and in those hospitals, patients would be given life-prolonging treatments, regardless of pain, regardless of cost, and regardless of their wishes.

It is not the role of the doctor, says Dr S, to squeeze every possible second of life out of patients, but to seek to restore patients to a state of health and, if that is not possible, to alleviate any suffering. There is, moreover, no duty to treat if the treatment is 'disproportionate', that is, if its burdens significantly outweigh its benefits. A treatment may be disproportionate either because it is futile (that is, offers no reasonable hope of benefit) or because it would involve excessive burdens to the patient (such as excessive pain or too much expense).

Interestingly, Dr S's conception of the *telos* of medicine where the restoration of health is no longer possible is not very different from the hypothesis with which we began this chapter, i.e. 'the alleviation of suffering'. One thing we liked about the account of Dr S was the way he made a distinction between life as a good in itself, which ought to be respected and life as an absolute good, which ought to take priority over every other consideration. But this brings us back, does it not, to the question we asked earlier of how one ought to decide when it is right for other priorities to take precedence over the preservation of life. Surely, this must come back once again to the question of the 'quality of life'. And this is, in fact, what Keown goes on to argue also.

In short, in Dr S's view, the doctor's duty to treat is much more limited than Dr V thinks. There is only a duty to treat if treatment is likely to improve the patient's condition or, in other words, 'quality of life'. In deciding whether a proposed treatment would improve the patient's condition or 'quality of life', Dr S asks:

'Given the patient's present condition, would this treatment improve it?'

If it would not, or if it would but it would impose excessive burdens on the patient, then the patient is under no duty to request it or the doctor to provide it.

Dr S goes on to explain that, just as he avoids Dr V's absolute notion of human life at one extreme, he also avoids Dr Q's instrumental notion of human life at the other extreme. He repeats that human life is a basic good, a basic aspect of a flourishing life. It is not, like money, of merely instrumental value. Human life is good in itself, must be respected as such, and must never be intentionally taken. And although both he and Dr Q use the words 'quality of life', Dr S stresses that he uses it to mean something entirely different from what Dr Q uses it to mean.

Dr Q uses 'Quality of Life' to distinguish between 'worthwhile' and 'worthless' patients. That is, Dr Q asks:

'Given this patient's "Quality of Life", that is, his or her disabilities, is the patient's life worth living or would the patient be better off dead?'

But Dr S, who believes that all patients are worthwhile, uses it to distinguish between worthwhile and worthless treatments:

'Given the patient's present "quality of life", that is, the patient's condition, would this treatment be worthwhile?'

In other words, says Dr S, the phrase 'quality of life' needs to be used very carefully as it can be used to mean two radically different things (which is why in this article Dr Q's use of the phrase is distinguished from Dr S's by the use of capital letters). Dr S stresses that whenever the words 'quality of life' are used, it is important to ask whether they are being used (as by Dr S) to discriminate between worthwhile and worthless treatments or (as by Dr Q) between worthwhile and 'worthless' patients.

ACTIVITY: How possible do you think it is to separate the two meanings of 'quality of life' described above? What might the difficulties with such a separation be? In reading this we wondered whether it is really possible to make a clear distinction between the worthwhileness of a treatment (when conceptualized in relation to a patient's quality of life) and the patient's quality of life. Were you convinced by this point? If not, why not? But let's go on now with Keown's paper.

As international declarations of human rights (and traditional codes of medical ethics) recognise, adds Dr S, every human being enjoys, simply because of his or her membership of the human family, an inalienable right to life, that is, a right not to be intentionally killed. Human life is a basic value, not a disposable commodity; it is an end in itself, not a mere means to an end. Intentionally to kill another, whether for some financial or political end, or because that other has some characteristic, whether racial, sexual, religious, physical or mental, is to deny that human life is an end in itself. Unfortunately, he points out, history is not short of examples of the intentional killing of people because they were thought to be leading 'inferior' lives, whether because of their race, sex, religion or physical or mental disability.

In short, says Dr S: 'Because human life is a basic good, it is always wrong intentionally to kill (innocent) human beings.' (Dr S adds the qualification 'innocent' to leave aside killing in war and self-defence, cases which can, in any event, have no relevance to the doctor–patient relationship.)

This is so whether it is an armed robber killing his victim in order to get his money, or a doctor killing his patient in order to relieve his suffering. As a good motive cannot justify a bad action, the doctor's good motive of relieving suffering no more justifies his treating his patient's life as a means to an end than would the robber's motive of donating his loot to charity.

And as all intentional killing of patients is wrong,

it can make no moral difference, if the doctor intends to shorten life, whether the doctor does so by an act, such as choking the patient, or by an omission, such as omitting to stop the patient from choking.

In short, Dr S says that human life is not a mere means and it must never be intentionally taken. But neither is it an absolute good to be preserved at all costs. Dr S's motto is 'Life must never be intentionally taken, but it need not be preserved at all costs.'

It is sometimes, he explains (citing the principle of 'double effect') perfectly proper if one's conduct sometimes unintentionally has the effect of shortening, or of not lengthening, life. For example, the doctor who, with the intention of easing pain, administers morphine to a terminally ill cancer patient may foresee that this will shorten the patient's life. But the shortening of life is merely an unintended side-effect of the doctor's intention to alleviate pain, and there is a very good reason (namely, the alleviation of pain) for allowing that bad side effect to happen. He is not attacking the patient's life but the patient's pain.

Similarly, a doctor may sometimes properly withhold or withdraw a treatment even though the doctor foresees that the patient's life will be shorter than it would be with the treatment. For, Dr S repeats, a doctor is under no duty to administer (and patients are fully entitled to refuse) disproportionate treatments, that is, treatments which would either offer no reasonable hope of benefit or would involve excessive burdens to the patient. Even if the doctor foresees that the patient's life will not be as long without the treatment as it would have been with it, the patient's earlier death is merely an unintended side-effect of the doctor's intention to withhold or withdraw a disproportionate treatment.

ACTIVITY: Stop for a moment and look back at the part of Section 4 when you were asked to identify the weak spots in the arguments about double effect. What are the implications of your consideration of the double-effect argument earlier for Dr S' argument? Let's go on now to see what Dr S recommends for Mary, in the light of his reflections.

Applying this reasoning to Mary, Dr S advises that, contrary to Dr Q's opinion, it would be wrong intentionally to shorten her life, whether by an act or by withholding CPR. There is no moral difference, says Dr S, between withholding a treatment with intent to kill Mary and administering a lethal injection to her. Either course of conduct denies her basic human right not to be intentionally killed and treats her life in a merely instrumental way, as a mere means to the end of living a life of a certain 'Quality'. Dr S criticizes all such judgements as flagrant discrimination on the ground of disability. And arbitrary, too, for who is to decide what disability, and what degree of disability, supposedly makes life worthless?

But just because it is wrong to kill Mary does not mean one must preserve her life at all costs, which is why he disagrees with Dr V's simplistic and absolutist approach. Dr S advises that the doctor's duty is not to preserve life at all costs but to restore the patient to health if that can be done by treatment which is not disproportionate. Would the treatment be disproportionate? Would it, in other words, offer any reasonable hope of benefit or impose excessive burdens on Mary?

Given that Mary is dying, CPR would offer no prospect of restoring her to health; it would, in fact, serve only to prolong her dying. It would, therefore, be quite futile. Moreover, the treatment could well impose grave burdens on her. Not only could it prove very distressing to her, but it could easily, in view of her age and frail condition, result in fractures. Dr S therefore agrees with Dr Q that CPR should be withheld, though for reasons quite inconsistent with those advanced by Dr Q.

ACTIVITY: You should now have three lists of ethical and moral terms associated with the perspectives of vitalism, quality of life and sanctity of life, along with points for and against each of them. Stop for a moment before finishing Keown's article and consider what you would do in the case of Mary. Do you accept any of the perspectives as expressed by Keown or do you find none of them entirely satisfying? If none of these perspectives by themselves is capable of enabling us to decide what to do in cases such as that of Mary, what can the law tell us? In order to look at this Keown introduces another character, Mrs Counsel.

Having discussed their different ethical approaches, the doctors decide to discover whether the implementation of their respective recommendations might, in English law, result in criminal liability.

Mrs Counsel informs the doctors that, in English law, a doctor must obtain consent from competent adult patients before treating them. If an adult patient is incompetent to consent (that is, is unable, like Mary, to understand the nature of the proposed treatment), no one, whether relative, partner, or even court, can consent on the patient's behalf. However, treatment may lawfully be given, provided it is in the best interests of the patient. But what ethical approach does the law adopt in determining what is in the patient's best interests?

Mrs Counsel informs the doctors that the law has never adopted the approach advocated by Dr V: doctors are not under a legal duty to preserve life at all costs.

Nor has the law historically accepted the approach advocated by Dr Q, that only those with 'worthwhile' lives have a right not to be killed.

The law has, however, traditionally incorporated the third approach, advocated by Dr S. Accordingly, the law has long prohibited the intentional killing of patients by doctors, by act or omission, regardless of the patient's condition or wishes. It is as much the crime of murder intentionally to kill a patient dying from incurable cancer who pleads to be killed as it is intentionally to kill a disabled baby, or a person in the prime of life who wishes to live.

Reflecting the principle of 'double effect', the law has also historically distinguished between intentionally and foreseeably shortening patients' lives. While it has long been unlawful intentionally to shorten a patient's life, it has long been lawful to administer palliative drugs or to withdraw disproportionate treatments, even if, as an unintended side-effect, the patient's life is thereby shortened.

Although it remains the crime of murder intentionally to kill a patient by an act, adds Mrs Counsel, the courts have, in a number of decisions from the early 1980s concerning both disabled babies and adult patients who are in a 'persistent vegetative state' (PVS), moved from the 'middle way' advocated by Dr S toward the position advocated by Dr Q. The courts have decided that it is now lawful for doctors to withhold life-prolonging treatment, not only on the ground that the treatment would be disproportionate (in the sense explained by Dr S), but even on the ground advocated by Dr Q, namely, that because of physical and/or mental disability the patient's life is not worth preserving.

In other words, the law has shifted from an ethical approach which asks whether the treatment is worthwhile, to one which asks whether the patient's life is worthwhile. And in one important case concerning an adult patient in PVS, the court evidently decided that, even though it remains murder intentionally to kill such a patient by an act, it is lawful intentionally to kill him by an omission. English law seems, therefore (like the law in many other countries), to be in a radically unprincipled, inconsistent and unstable condition, prohibiting doctors from intentional killing by an act but, at least sometimes, permitting them to kill by omission.

Mrs Counsel advises that whereas until the early 1980s, it seemed reasonably clear that the views of Dr S represented the law, it now seems that, in the light of the decisions of the courts since that time, it is lawful to withhold or withdraw treatment from a patient on the basis of a judgement, not that the treatment is worthless but that the patient is worthless, and to do so even with intent to kill the patient. In short, it would be lawful to withhold the CPR from Mary, not only for the reasons given by Dr S but even for those given by Dr Q.

ACTIVITY: Stop for a moment. Before you go on to the next section, find an example of a real case which is like the fictional one in which Mary finds herself and which has been the subject of legal controversy, either from your own practice or from the media. Find out what the judgement was and the reasoning given. Compare and contrast this with Keown's account of the law in England and also with each of the three ethical perspectives Keown describes.

Stop here and make a list of the key points raised in this section.

Section 7: Decisions at the end of life involving children

Most of the cases we have presented in this chapter have been related to ethical questions at the end of life in the elderly and, whilst many of the ethical questions posed by decisions at the end of life at other ages are very similar, there are also important differences. This is particularly the case in relation to young children, and in this final section of the chapter we shall be going on to explore the ethical questions which arise in relation to decisions at the end of life involving children. Firstly, we will ask you to critically appraise a set of guidelines concerning when it is acceptable to withdraw or withhold treatment from children and then, secondly, we shall go on to look at a case in which the practitioner's perception of the child's best interest is in conflict with that of the family.

ACTIVITY: In September 1997, the Royal College of Paediatrics and Child Health issued a 'Framework for practice in relation to the withholding or withdrawing of life-saving treatment in children' (RCPCH, 1997). Below is the summary page of the document. As you read it through, make a note of the appearance of any of the three approaches described by John Keown, i.e. Vitalism, Quality of Life and Sanctity of Life.

There are five situations where the withholding or withdrawal of curative medical treatment might be considered:

(a) The brain-dead child. In the older child where criteria of brain-stem death are agreed by two practitioners in the usual way, it may still be technically feasible to provide basic cardio-respiratory support by means of ventilation and intensive care. It is agreed within the medical profession that treatment in such circumstances is futile and the withdrawal of current medical treatment is appropriate.

(b) The permanent vegetative state. The child who develops a permanent vegetative state following insults, such as trauma or hypoxia, is reliant on others for all care and does not react or relate with the outside world. It may be appropriate both to withdraw current therapy and to withhold further curative treatment.

(c) The 'no chance' situation. The child has such severe disease that life-sustaining treatment simply delays death without significant alleviation of suffering. Medical treatment in this situation may thus be deemed inappropriate.

(d) The 'no purpose' situation. Although the patient may be able to survive with treatment, the degree of physical or mental impairment will be so great that it is unreasonable to expect them to bear it. The child in this situation will never be capable of taking part in decisions regarding treatment or its withdrawal.

(e) The 'unbearable' situation. The child and/or family feel that, in the face of progressive and irreversible illness, further treatment is more than can be borne. They wish to have a particular treatment withdrawn or to refuse further treatment, irrespective of the medical opinion on its potential benefit. Oncology patients who are offered further aggressive treatment might be included in this category.

In situations that do not fit with these five categories, or where there is dissent or uncertainty about the degree of future impairment, the child's life should always be safeguarded by all in the healthcare team in the best way possible.

> **ACTIVITY: How many did you find? The Royal College document received a lot of media coverage when it was first published in the UK and a certain amount of criticism. Can you identify counter-arguments to any of the points? One thing we noticed about this as a framework was that it seemed to be very doctor orientated with little role for the child's parents or family (except under point (e)).**

A further question which these guidelines raise is this: in what ways are decisions at the end of life different in the cases of children and the elderly and to what extent does this depend upon the age and understanding of the child? This will depend to a great extent upon the features of the particular case, but one way in which a contrast is sometimes drawn between children and adults in ethical decision-making is between the competence of adults and the incompetence of children. Clearly, this is a distinction which is open to question and has been challenged by many theorists of childhood (it is explored more fully in the chapter on Children and Young People). Nevertheless, the physician's concern about the competence of the patient and about the possibility that relatives' decisions might not be in the patient's best interest is particularly sharply defined in relation to children. For this reason we shall end this chapter, as we started it, with a case. This is a case involving these kinds of questions in relation to childhood but, as you read it, we would also like you to consider the extent to which such conflicts and dilemmas might arise in the elderly too.

Throughout this chapter we have been exploring the ethical issues which arise in decisions at the end of life and have examined the degree to which the *telos* of medicine in palliative care is different to those in other areas of medicine, whether it raises any particular and unique ethical questions.

We began by taking as our working hypothesis that the *telos* of medicine in palliative care might usefully be captured by the relief or alleviation of suffering. Since then we have put this hypothesis to the test by applying it in a variety of settings. In Section 1 we considered the ethical questions raised by the withdrawing of treatment. In Section 2 we considered the ethical implications of making a decision not to resuscitate a patient and in Section 3 we investigated whether or not it is ethical under certain circumstances to relieve suffering by respecting a patient's refusal of treatment. In Section 4 we took this further into the questions of euthanasia and physician-assisted suicide. Finally, in Section 6 of this section we have considered the situation in which the patient is incapable of expressing their wishes and has not made an advance directive. One of the central aims of this chapter has been to provide a wide-ranging investigation into the *telos* of medicine at the end of life and the ethical implications of such decisions and situations.

ACTIVITY: In this final section we offer you an account of a case. In the light of all that you have already considered in this chapter we would like you to read this case and attempt to analyse it ethically. As you read it through, make a note of what you consider to be the main ethical questions which it poses, drawing as much as possible on the concepts we have addressed in the earlier parts of this chapter.

THE CASE OF JW

JW was a 12-year-old boy who had cystic fibrosis. Since his condition was diagnosed, JW had been visiting the same hospital and physicians regularly for many years. Both he and his family were well known to the staff there and enjoyed a good relationship with them. In recent months, however, the boy's condition had become very serious. He had developed extensive varices of the oesophagus which brought with them an accompanying risk of serious bleeding which would put the boy's life in danger.

When the doctor informed the family that the seriousness of the boy's condition might require a blood transfusion in order to save his life, both the boy and his family refused to consider such an option because of their faith. The whole family were devout and active Jehovah's Witnesses.

The paediatricians involved in the case disagreed about how they ought to proceed and asked a child psychiatrist to assess the child's competence to make the decision to refuse treatment. One possible option which was considered was to make an application for a court order to take custody of the boy away from his parents in order to allow the transfusion to take place.

The psychiatrist reported that the boy was intelligent and sensitive, that he was in no sense emotionally or socially disturbed and that he had a good relationship with his parents. He also had a clear understanding of his illness and of the treatment and was conscious of the consequences of his decisions to refuse a blood transfusion. He stuck to his decision and said that his parents had exerted no pressure on him. He simply wanted to live according to the principles of his faith.

After interviewing the parents also, it seemed clear that they cared very much for their son and indeed for all of their children. On the whole they were rational about the decision to refuse the transfusion and appeared, as the boy himself had said, not to have put any explicit pressure on the boy to refuse the treatment.

It seemed clear that this was a caring family who, in the light of their religious beliefs, had come to a reasoned decision to refuse this particular form of treatment.

ACTIVITY: In the light of your analysis of this case, using the various arguments and perspectives you have covered as you have worked your way through the chapter, what do you think ought to be done in this case and why? Do you know what would be the legal situation in a case such as this? This case is discussed in more detail in the chapter on Children and Young People.

As we read the case we wondered about what the likely increasing influence and sophistication of technological developments might be in this kind of case. The use of so-called 'cell-savers' has been given the approval of the Jehovah's Witness community in New York, for example. Furthermore, there are in many cases multiple alternatives to blood transfusions. Might such developments mean that we will be increasingly able to avoid this particular kind of ethical conflicts in the future? Do you know of any such developments? If you are interested in following this further, you might like to take a look at the Jehovah's Witness volume on 'Family Care and Medical Management for Jehovah's Witnesses' (Watchtower Bible and Tract Society of New York, 1992) which is in the bibliography.

Nevertheless, setting this question aside for a moment, as we considered the ethical issues raised by the actual case in front of us, we wondered what the psychological (and perhaps the physical) consequences would be for the family and the child if custody were to be taken from the parents.

What, too, of the psychological consequences for the hospital and other staff who are confronted with, and must deal with, such dilemmas on a regular basis?

Thinking of the experience of moral dilemmas as bereavement seems justified. . . . When [healthcare professionals] experience moral dilemmas, they lose the self that they thought of as caring, the self that does the right thing for patients, the self who will not do wrong to others, their whole self. They lose their integrity. With each moral dilemma that is thrust upon [healthcare professionals], a bit of them dies: to themselves, to the world and to their patients (Fairbairn and Mead, 1990, p. 23).

Clearly, as Fairbairn and Mead suggest, the experience of confronting the ethical dilemmas which arise at the end of life can sometimes be very difficult for healthcare professionals both emotionally and in relation to the problematic nature of the decisions to be taken, and it may well be that among these decisions those involving young children are the most difficult. Nevertheless, it seems to us that, by the use of the kinds of analytic and ethical tools which we have been developing in this chapter, and the others in this series, it is possible for healthcare professionals to work towards the practical resolution of some of the most difficult of these dilemmas in ways which are challenging without being threatening.

ACTIVITY: Now make a list of key points raised by this chapter.

Suggestions for further reading

British Medical Association (1999). *Withholding and Withdrawing Life-prolonging Medical Treatment*. London: British Medical Journal Publishing Group.

Glover, J. (1977) *Causing Death and Saving Lives*. Harmondsworth: Penguin.

Keown, J. (1995). *Euthanasia Examined*. Cambridge: Cambridge University Press.

Kuhse, H. (1991). Euthanasia. In *Companion to Ethics*, ed. P. A. Singer. Oxford: Blackwell.

Rachels, J. (1980). Active and passive euthanasia. In *Killing and Letting Die*, ed. B. Steinbock. Englewood Cliffs, NJ: Prentice-Hall.

2

Genetic testing

Section1: Living with risk   **Section 2:** Living with certainty   **Section 3:** Genetics and reproductive choice
Section 4: The use of genetic information

Introduction

The continuing development of genetics has profound implications for the future of medicine. In
the medium to longer term the impact is perhaps
most likely to be felt in the development of more
effective treatments for the major diseases:
cancer, heart disease and so on. These treatments
will raise ethical dilemmas of their own, but such
developments are still some way off. What are the
practical ethical questions raised by genetics
today? In this chapter we focus on the ethical
issues surrounding the availability and use of
genetic testing. The chapter begins with a short
case about genetic testing for the BRCA1, breast
cancer, gene. This is followed by a personal
account of what it is like to live with the risk of
inherited breast cancer. It is becoming increasingly clear that, like breast cancer, most genetically related conditions will turn out to be the
result of a variety of factors, both genetic and
environmental. This means that genetic tests for
these conditions, when used presymptomatically
will give imperfect information about the likelihood of the condition occurring. This raises
important ethical questions about the availability
of such tests and the ways in which the results
ought to be interpreted. As you read through this
first section, consider what these ethical questions might be. Following this first section, we go
on to look at the ethical questions raised by those
tests which provide information which is more

certain by means of some cases relating to
Huntington's disease. Finally, we investigate the
use of genetic information more broadly, both in
reproductive choice and in the creation of large
commercial computerized databases.

Section 1: Living with risk

A CASE OF BREAST CANCER GENETICS

Barbara is from a family with an inherited risk of
ovarian and breast cancer. She does not know if
she herself has the BRCA1 gene, however. She
says,

*I don't think about cancer when I get up in the morning.
I'll probably be knocked down by a bus first.*

Barbara knows, however, that in the future her
daughter, her sons and her five female grandchildren will all face difficult dilemmas over whether
to be tested and what to do with the information.
In addition to the health risks themselves, those
who have a test result which shows them to be at
risk of developing the disease could face
difficulties getting life insurance or a mortgage.
    If Barbara was to take the test and it turned out
to be negative, this would reduce the worry for
both her and her descendents. On the other hand,
if the test turned out to be positive, Barbara, who

has no symptoms at present, would face the difficulty of knowing that she has a high risk of developing the cancer and would have to decide what to do about this.

A geneticist who is studying inherited breast cancer comments,

If a woman really wants the test, it would be unethical to withhold it. The first principle is that every woman has the right to know about her genotype.

This case was adapted from one in the *New Scientist* 18.9.93.

> ACTIVITY: What would you do if you were Barbara or one of her children? One of the most difficult features of genetic testing for most conditions is that the information gained is imperfect. For example, breast cancer is a multifactorial disease and only about 10 per cent of cases are thought to be due to an inherited risk. Also, a positive test for the BRCA1 gene indicates an 80 per cent chance of developing breast cancer by the age of 65. Another factor which has important ethical implications is the fact that it is possible for the results of tests for BRCA1 to be either falsely negative or falsely positive.
>
> In the light of these facts, should a genetic test like this be marketed as soon as possible or only when there is a proven treatment?
>
> A testing kit for the BRCA1 gene is currently available on the internet. Do you agree with the geneticist in the case that the BRCA1 test should be openly available for those who want to use it? If not, why not?

We would now like you to read the following account by June Zatz of what it is like to live with the risk of developing breast cancer after having come across the information by chance. Although her initial contact with information about her risk did not come about through a genetics test, her case has interesting parallels with the case of genetic testing. As you read it, continue to ask yourself whether or not there are particular ethical questions related to the availability of this kind of genetic information and whether any limitations ought to be put on its availability. What are the possible benefits and harms of such availability?

I am definitely having it done

June Zatz

I remember in 1973, when I was 23 years old, sitting in the hairdresser's, reading some obscure American magazine. I came across an article about a 19-year-old girl from New York where every female on her mother's side had contracted breast cancer, going back two or three generations. A decision was taken that she have both breasts removed as this was the only way to ensure that she would not contract the disease herself. I was absolutely aghast when I read this article. This was the first time I learnt that breast cancer was hereditary. My mother, her two sisters and her first cousin had had breast cancer but I never really thought of it as being a threat to me. And the thought of a 19-year-old having such a drastic operation! I never discussed the article with anyone. It was after reading the article that the implications were clearer to me of contracting the disease. I dismissed as ridiculous the part in the article about the operation, but I know that I stored it away in the back of my mind.

My mother had a radical mastectomy when she was 42 years old. As a result of the operation she was left with fluid in her right arm, which caused severe infections where she was bedridden for days. She had bouts of ill health for years but in-between she was a determined lady who never complained. She had a second mastectomy 13 years later followed by various operations and bouts of ill health. After a benign tumour was removed from her liver when she was 58, her consultant warned my brother and me that 'cancer will get her sooner rather than later'. Her ultimate illness was when she was 66 years old, short and sharp – cancer of the spine – paralysis – painful death – even now, 7 years later, I cannot think of this period without immense pain.

My mother's younger sister developed breast cancer when she was 46, and after numerous operations and great pain died two years later when 48 years old. This was prior to the days of the hospice (where my mother died) and so my mother looked after her, but the pain was not well controlled.

My other aunt died when I was only 7 years old. My mother told me she had breast cancer in her early 40s, but also had a heart condition from which she died in her mid-40s.

> ACTIVITY: Most clinical geneticists agree that genetic testing must be preceded and followed by counselling. Should such counselling be compulsory? Or, do you think that those who wish to take a genetic test ought to be able to do so freely, whether or not they want to have counselling? What are the ethical implications of this?
>
> It is worth stopping here for a moment and asking whether June would have been better off if she had had the opportunity to take a genetic test when she was in her 20s rather than coming across the information in a magazine as she did. One of the advantages of a negative test, obviously, is that it can provide tremendous relief from this kind of worry.

After finding out that breast cancer can be hereditary, I read everything I could get my hands on. Only once when in my mid-20s I attempted to bring up the subject with my mother, as I felt perhaps she could get advice for me from her specialist. But she just dismissed it and refused to discuss it. I never attempted to mention it again. My husband, however, got to know of my fears because I often imagined I felt a lump in my breast. Then I became depressed, lay awake at night imagining all sorts of things and, having two young children, I naturally worried about the children – what would happen if I weren't around for them? Throughout the years, I only ever went to the doctor twice when the 'lump' didn't seem to disappear and I was literally going round the bend. Even when at the doctor's I managed to conceal my true feelings, was very matter of fact, and he was never aware of the family history as I didn't tell him.

My mother died 7 years ago, when I was 37 years old. Within a few weeks of her death, I realized that I had to do something about my fears and get them out in the open. It was almost as though with her death this released me to discuss my fears out in the open. I wrote to my mother's oncologist detailing the family history and asking whether there was anything else I should be doing apart from self-examination.

This resulted in me being referred to an oncology clinic for regular monitoring, initially 6-monthly, then annually. These visits to the clinic I can only describe as horrendous. First of all there was the waiting area where females of all ages (many surprisingly young) were waiting to find out whether they had breast cancer or because they already had it. Then, in the cubicles while waiting to be examined, you could hear the registrar in the next cubicle talking to the patient and I knew from the conversation that all was not well. By the time I was due to be examined, I would be a wreck – then the mammogram; then the waiting a week for the result. After the result I would be elated, my first thought would be thank God, I will be around for another year. I would immediately calculate all my children's ages. This was what was of prime importance for me – I wanted to be around to see them into adulthood.

As I neared the age when my mother developed her first breast cancer, I became more fearful. Over the years I had read many articles and I did not feel that treatments were any more effective today than years ago, even if it were detected at an earlier stage. I felt that I would get breast cancer as my body was similar to my mother's in many ways – she had fibroids and a hysterectomy – she had gall stones and had her gall bladder removed. I have had both these operations by my late 30s.

My mind kept casting back to the article I'd read all those years ago about the 19-year-old who had both breasts removed as a preventative measure. I had never read of this again but decided it was time to pursue it further.

In the summer of 1991 I wrote to my oncologist asking if such an operation were possible. His answer took a fairly long time coming, mainly due to administrative procedures. While I waited for the reply, I was on tenterhooks: my feelings were that I would be told that I was crazy, that this operation could be done only in America.

Eventually when his letter arrived stating that yes, I could have this operation – I literally couldn't believe it – I read the letter over and over for days. Then I wrote another long letter with lots of questions. There followed several letters to and fro: a referral to a plastic surgeon to discuss reconstruction and a referral to a specialist cancer geneticist to discuss the genetic side of things.

It took me months to make up my mind definitely. After the second letter from the oncologist, I told my husband what I was investigating and he was horror-struck. He just could not understand why I should have both breasts removed when they were perfectly healthy. To him the logical thing was to wait and, if the cancer appeared, then it will have been caught early, then I should have a mastectomy. He didn't understand that, the way I saw it, it was too late by then. At this stage, however, I hadn't made up my mind and in fact because of my husband's attitude I put things on hold for several weeks. One day however, I woke up early feeling such anger and resentment towards him – he and I had always until now agreed on major issues.

I discussed it with him again. This time I had a different attitude: he had made me feel selfish contemplating such an operation but what I said to him was: What about me, my fears; this is my life and who's going to look after me if I get cancer – will he nurse me? At the same time I said I hadn't yet made up my mind but I was going to continue my investigations whether he liked it or not. He listened and said he'd like to come with me when I next had a consultation with either the oncologist or the plastic surgeon. I refused as I knew he was still against it but said I'd tell him everything they said.

Some days I would wake up and say, 'I'm definitely having it done'. Other days I'd think I was crazy – I tried to imagine what it would be like without breasts, although there was the chance of reconstruction.

Gradually my husband came round to my way of things. The more information I gathered the more he understood what I could be facing. One day I said, 'I don't think I'll have it done', and then

to my surprise he said, 'You should go ahead – I'd rather have you alive and well with no breasts.'

In April 1992 I made the decision to have the operation. Throughout the 6 months it took me to come to this decision I had several consultations with the three specialists. The clinical geneticist put me in touch with another lady who had had a similar operation. She had an almost identical family history to mine. I had a long discussion with her on the phone. It was invaluable to talk to someone who had been in my situation. She and her sister had had the operation and were greatly relieved that the chance of breast cancer had been removed.

The only people who knew about it were my husband, my two children and two friends, one of whom had a medical background and the other was a cousin to whom I'm very close and with whom I'd often discussed the 'family history'. I instinctively knew from the beginning that I didn't want anyone's advice on the matter, I wanted facts on which I could base my decision. The professionals were wonderful. Everyone was patient, answered my questions, was quietly supportive and never offered advice on what I should do. There's no way the outcome would have been as successful without their help and support. I should also point out that they were all males.

At the time my daughter was 18 years old and my son 16. They knew what was happening but my daughter could not understand my contemplating such an operation, so I didn't discuss it with her, and my son couldn't deal with it at all – perhaps due to his age and sexuality.

The plastic surgeon had discussed the breast reconstruction he would be performing, which involved a lengthy operation. At the same time as performing the mastectomies, he would remove fat and muscle from my stomach and use this to form new breasts. It was a complicated procedure and there was also a chance that it wouldn't work. I asked myself, could I cope with having no breasts? I'd decided not to have silicon implants because of recent bad publicity. I concluded that disfigurement was of secondary importance to the certainty of not getting breast cancer. Since 12 years of age I'd been surrounded by this disease and here was a way to get rid of it.

From the time of making my decision in April 1992 I never looked back once. Now I had to decide when to tell people because I'd be in hospital for 2 weeks and off work for a couple of months. I had lunch with a close friend and started to tell her. She was so aghast that I didn't finish telling her about the reconstruction. I couldn't wait to get away from her. She just couldn't hide her feelings. After this I told a few more people but got more or less the same reaction. I was furious and upset. The way I saw it I had made a very difficult decision and these supposed close friends were completely unsympathetic. They made comments like 'Do you know what you are doing?' or 'Why remove your breasts when you haven't got cancer?'

I told my doctor friend who had known from the beginning and she said, 'They're so busy trying to deal with their own feelings that they can't focus on you and provide support for you.' I realized just what a threat this seemed to be to other women – to have one's breasts removed. I told my husband I couldn't tell anyone else so he said to make a list and he would sit down and phone them. I gave him half a dozen names and he did it immediately as I didn't want these people to find out from others. Needless to say I received a few phone calls from people we'd not told, to say that they'd heard about it; again they were very unsupportive. Despite the lack of help I never faltered.

The operation was performed in September 1992. I was really quite ill, which was to be expected. The plastic surgeon was so attentive and kind that somehow, even though I felt very ill, so long as he was looking after me I knew everything would be OK. I was fortunate in that the reconstruction was successful. While lying in hospital I became obsessed with the imminent pathology result of both breasts. What if I'm too late and the cancer was already there? Prior to the operation I remember saying to the surgeon, 'Please cut everything out.' I didn't want any chances taken. It took about 10 days for the pathology results and when I was told that everything was OK, I just couldn't take it in.

After the operation people's attitude was how brave I'd been to have such an operation, but I didn't see it like that at all. I'd had the operation done through fear – fear of getting breast cancer.

I've never looked back since the operation. It's the best decision I made in my life or am likely to ever make.

This may sound odd, but it took about 6–12 months after the operation for the full psychological effects to be felt. I now read articles about breast cancer and watch programmes on TV without dread and despair. Something else that also became apparent was that prior to the operation I had never made any serious plans for the future – subconsciously I had thought I would die at a relatively early age from breast cancer. Now this inevitability had been removed along with my breasts. I now felt a person given their freedom, with a whole new quality of life.

Once the decision to proceed with the operation was made, my husband's support was invaluable. He is delighted that I will never get breast cancer, the bonus being that the reconstruction was successful.

With the advances in genetic knowledge, more women are going to be identified as having a high risk of contracting breast cancer. The dilemma that I faced will be much more common. I can only say that the radical surgery I decided on was for me by far the lesser of two evils.

ACTIVITY: In the light of this reading and of the list you made earlier of the benefits and harms of the availability of genetic tests for the BRCA1 gene, what are the arguments for and those against the availability of genetic testing? Although June herself didn't have a genetic test, her experience offers insight into the effect such information can have and the difficulties involved in coming to terms with it emotionally as well as those involved in interpreting it to make a decision.

The ethical questions raised by genetic testing are particularly difficult both because of the interpersonal/intergenerational nature of the information provided and also because in many cases, as in the case of the BRCA1 gene, the information is statistical and not easy to translate into action. Not all genetic tests are like this, however. In the case of the Huntington's disease gene, a positive test does mean that the test subject will develop the condition at some point and that their children will have a 50 per cent chance of inheriting the gene. As we will be going on to see in the next section, such tests raise ethical questions of their own.

ACTIVITY: In 1994 a poll by *Time* magazine and CNN asked people to imagine a situation in which a genetic test were available which could tell them all the diseases they were likely to suffer in later life. They were then asked whether they would take such a test if offered it. 49 per cent said they would not, 50 per cent said they would. As we come to the end of this section, consider for a moment whether you would take such a test? What are your reasons?

Do you think such a test should be developed and made available for those who would like it?

Before you go on to the next section, take a few moments at this point to make a short list of the main, key points, raised in this section.

Section 2: Living with certainty

A CASE OF THE RIGHT NOT TO KNOW

Mr H, a 73-year-old man, was diagnosed with depression and then with atypical Alzheimer's disease. But Mr H's symptoms were still not fully explained, and his dementia was now so severe that communication with him was effectively impossible. The H family history, however, included members who had manifested jerky movements or dementia late in life. This suggested a possible genetic link.

In conversation with a researcher from a project on memory and ageing, the psychiatric senior registrar involved in Mr H's care learned that a new testing procedure could determine accurately whether Mr H might have Huntington's disease (HD), an incurable progressive disease of the central nervous system. The testing procedure, based on the number of repeats of the gene for HD, would only be available if Mr H was enrolled on the research project. Mr H's clinical team decided to request consent from his family to use the newly available genetic test and to enrol him in the research project. The family agreed, and Mr H tested positive for Huntington's disease 10 days before his death.

But it turned out that Mr H's family hadn't really understood the implications for themselves of allowing him to be tested. Huntington's is an autosomal dominant condition, meaning that Mr H's children would have roughly 50–50 chances of developing the condition themselves. Mr H's wife now wanted everyone in the family to be tested for HD, including her grandchildren (who would have a 1 in 4 chance of developing HD). Mr H's daughter was willing to be tested herself, but refused to allow her teenage daughters to be tested. Mr H's son was adamantly against finding out his genetic status or allowing his own wife to learn about Mr H's test results, even though he and his wife already had two young children, and intended to have more.

ACTIVITY: What are the ethical issues raised by this case?

Perhaps one of the main questions is: Do Mr H's descendants have the right to resist testing even if this denies their children important genetic information about their own health? What is the moral status of the right not to know? Ought there to be limits to this right?

We would now like you to read another case study but before you do so, take a moment to think about the differences between the ethical questions raised by tests which provide information which is less than certain and those such as the test for Huntington's in which things are clearer.

In the case above, the ethical problem was created by the right not to know combined with the intergenerational nature of the information. The following case is one which, by contrast, tests how far the right to know can be taken. As you read this case, ask yourself what are the limits to the right to know, if any?

CASE – WE WANT TO TEST OUR CHILDREN

Ann and Colin Walters have been referred by their General Practitioner to the Genetics clinic. They have recently moved to London from Leeds, where Ann underwent a pre-symptomatic test for Huntington's disease, the condition affecting her father. The test showed that Ann inherited the faulty Huntington's gene from her father, although she has no apparent clinical signs of the condition. In her letter of referral, the General Practitioner says that the couple have two children, aged 4 and 5 years, and are asking for their children to be tested for the faulty Huntington's gene. Mr and Mrs Walters come to the clinic together, without their children.

Genetic Counsellor: Good morning Mr and Mrs Walters. I'm Barbara Jones, one of the genetic counsellors here in the clinic. As you know, we had a letter from Dr Allen asking if we would see you. I understand that you have been asking about the possibility of having your children tested to see if they have inherited the faulty Huntington's gene.

Colin: Yes, that's right. Ann had the test a few months ago, and we've talked about it a lot since then, and we've decided we want the children to be tested now.

Genetic Counsellor: Right (looking at Ann). Could I just ask, how long ago did you get the results of your own test?

Ann: About 4 months ago. I had the test in Leeds, where we were living until recently. We moved last month, because of my husband's job.

Genetic Counsellor: And the test showed that you did have the faulty gene?

Ann: Yes, that's right. I got it from my father. He's now in a special nursing home.

Genetic Counsellor: And how have things been for you since then?

Ann: Fine really. Well we've been busy, what with the moving and everything. It was a bit of a shock at the time. But I've always thought I had it. So it didn't really tell me anything I didn't already know, deep down. I think it's been harder for Colin, what with my test result, and starting a new job as well as moving house. He'd always thought I'd get a good result and would be OK.

ACTIVITY: The fact that Ann has the faulty Huntington's gene means that her children have possibly also got it. What are the advantages to be gained by testing the children? What are the disadvantages? Compare this list with the one you produced for the BRCA1 gene.

Genetic Counsellor: Can I just ask about your father? You say he's being looked after in a home.

Ann: Yes. He's only been there for about a year. My stepmother couldn't cope with him any more, because of the violence. He was hitting her a lot, just lashing out for no reason. He's had the disease for about 10 years now, probably longer, although we didn't realize it at the time. My mother left him about 15 years ago, because she said he'd changed so much. He became very moody and he hit her once too. He was drinking a lot, and she thought he'd turned into an alcoholic. I was only about 12 then, but I do remember him being like that at the start.

Genetic Counsellor: Those must be very difficult memories for you.

Ann: They were, but it's a long time ago now. All in the past.

Genetic Counsellor: And can you remember when you first knew you might have inherited the faulty gene?

Ann: Well, it was just after Colin and I got married. That was in 1989. No one realized for a long time what was wrong with my father. Then he saw a specialist who said he had Huntington's disease. We got some books from the library, and we read that it could be passed on. We went to see our doctor, and he told us that I couldn't have a test then. I don't think there was a test available then. But we wanted children, so we had Helen first, and then Paul.

Colin: There didn't seem any point waiting. We wanted to have children straight away. And there weren't any tests we could have then.

Genetic Counsellor: And can I ask how old you are now?

Colin: I'm 30. But Ann's only 27.

Genetic Counsellor: (looking at Ann) And did it take a long time for you to decide to have the test?

Colin: Not really. Well, a little while. We were both busy, with my work and the children.

Ann: I'd always known that I wanted to be tested. I thought it was only fair to everyone, especially Colin, because if I got ill, then he would have the children to look after by himself, and we would need to plan for that. And that's kind of why we're here now. I now know that I am going to get ill, and there'll come a time when I won't be able to talk to the children. So we've decided that we want to have the children tested now, so that we can both prepare them for what is to come, while I'm still well enough to do so.

ACTIVITY: What do you think about this argument – that having the test will help Ann and Colin to prepare their children for what is to come?

Genetic Counsellor: Did you discuss your wish to have your children tested with the doctors you saw in Leeds?

Ann: Yes. We saw a doctor in the genetics department there. He carried out my test. I saw him once after my test result, and told him about the children. He said that they didn't test children until they were 18, so they could decide for themselves about the test when they were grown up. He said that all genetic centres would say the same. Is that true?

Genetic Counsellor: At this centre, we follow certain nationally agreed guidelines about testing for the Huntington's disease gene in healthy people. As far as children are concerned, the current guidelines are that individuals should be 18 years of age before testing takes place. There

are a number of reasons for this. As you know, having the Huntington's test, or choosing not to have it, is a very difficult and personal decision. Many people prefer not to know if they have the faulty gene, especially as we don't have a cure for Huntington's disease. If a young child is tested, that would take away his or her 'right not to know' as an adult. There has been a great deal of discussion about this, not only between doctors, and it has been felt that a child's right to make their own decision as an adult outweighs any benefits that the test may have for a child and his or her family. But I can appreciate that knowing Helen and Paul could have the gene must be a very worrying and upsetting thought for both of you.

ACTIVITY: What are the reasons for this? Should it be the parents who decide what is right for their children? What are the advantages to be had from not knowing?

Colin: Yes. But at the end of the day we are Helen and Paul's parents, and we know them best, and we know what is in their best interests. I know what you're saying. The doctor in Leeds said the same thing. But, with respect, you don't know us, and you don't know our children, or what it is like to live with the uncertainty of everything. We have to know if Helen and Paul are going to be affected. We owe it to them.

Ann: That's right. I know I'm going to get ill. I know that some people with Huntington's have problems quite early on, before they are 30. And when the disease begins, I will change, and become a different person, like my dad did. And then I won't be able to look after the children properly, or talk to them as their mother who loves them, like I can now . . . (She begins to cry).

Genetic Counsellor: That must be a very frightening thought.

Ann: Continues to cry.

ACTIVITY: Ann seems to be making quite a different argument here. She seems to be saying that denying her the test is denying her the right to take care of her children in regard to what may be the most profound difficulty they will face in their lives. What do you think of this argument? Does it convince you that the test ought to be made available to Ann and Colin?

Colin: Look. We've talked about this. We've talked and talked, and thought about it in all different ways. The children may not have inherited the faulty gene from Ann. And if they haven't, they could be spared all the worry, and Ann won't feel guilty, and she could enjoy the children more before she gets ill. And if they have got the gene, then we can gradually prepare them for what is to come, so they don't have to learn it all from a doctor who they didn't know, like Ann did.

Ann: I know you mean well, but we are Helen and Paul's parents. No amount of talking will change that. We have a right to have them tested. If I was pregnant right now, and asked for the unborn child to be tested, you would do that wouldn't you?

Genetic Counsellor: If that's what you decided you wanted, we could test the fetus.

Ann: So what's the difference? I'd know if the baby had the faulty gene or not. But Helen and Paul were born before that test. If the test had been possible then, we would have had it, and then we would have known about Helen and Paul.

ACTIVITY: Ann is asking a reasonable question here. If discrimination between two cases is to be moral, there must exist a morally significant difference between the two. Is there one here?

I don't think you can discriminate. We know our children, and how we want to bring them up. We love them, and would never harm them. We want them to be tested.

This fictional case scenario was provided by Chris Barnes of the South Thames Regional Genetics Centre in London and is copyright 1996 of the centre.

ACTIVITY: We have talked about a case where the parents are requesting a test for their child but what about the situation where the child herself asks for testing? What would be the ethical questions raised by this situation?

After you have completed this activity, go on to read the following case and commentary on just this kind of situation by Donna Dickenson. As you do so, see if all the points you listed appear. Make a note of those which don't.

THE CASE OF ALISON

As a general practitioner, you are confronted with the case of Alison, an intelligent 15-year-old girl whose father has recently tested positive for Huntington's disease. His own mother died of the condition before Alison was born. Alison wants to know whether she, too, will develop Huntington's disease. Her parents, who have accompanied her to the surgery, support her wish. Alison's mother is herself contemplating genetic testing for the BRCA1 gene implicated in some breast cancers, following the death of her own mother and her elder sister from the disease.

You know that the clinical genetics unit which serves your patients will not test young people under 18, although Alison can have counselling. You point out that even those over 18 must undergo counselling before having the test, according to the unit's careful protocol. Alison thinks this over and replies, 'I can see the point of having some talks with the counsellor first. But if I do decide I want it, do I still have to wait another 3 years before I can actually have the test?'

ACTIVITY: What should we do about children and young people who want to be tested for incurable adult-onset genetic disorders? In particular, what should a practitioner do if she or he believes the young person is competent to decide, but the regional genetics unit refuses to test anyone under 18? In the commentary which follows, Donna Dickenson explores the arguments for and against allowing the young person to be tested, in terms of good practice, case and statute law, empirical evidence, and ethical arguments.

Can children and young people consent to be tested for adult-onset genetic disorders?

Donna L. Dickenson

Although many regional genetics units are evolving policies which do take young people's requests seriously, in the wake of new policy recommendations from the royal colleges, the Nuffield Council[1] and the British Medical Association[2], it would still be unusual for a request like Alison's to be granted, where the disorder is of the magnitude of Huntington's disease. This article will argue that the situation is anomalous in the light of law giving young people under 18 the right to consent to treatment, including testing. The argument primarily concerns consent, but it is also important to note that an action in negligence could arise if Alison gave birth to an HD-positive baby which she would not have had if she had known her genetic predisposition.[3]

Professional guidelines

Professional literature and guidelines on the predictive testing of at-risk children have often focused on the situation where parents request testing on the child's behalf, rather than the scenario in which the young person herself wants to be tested. In 1989 a research group of the World Federation of Neurology declared that children should not be tested for Huntington's disease on their parents' request. The age of majority remained the touchstone in the 1994 recommendations of a joint committee of the International Huntington Association and the World Federation of Neurology Research Group on Huntington's Chorea[4], although that report added: 'It seems appropriate and even essential, however, that the child be informed of his or her at-risk status upon reaching the age of reason.'

In the same year, the Clinical Genetics Society working party[5] concluded that, although discussion and counselling could and should be offered to minors, 'formal genetic testing should generally wait until the "children" request such tests for

themselves, as autonomous adults.'[6] However, the working party did say that testing should wait either until the person affected is adult or 'is able to appreciate not only the genetic facts of the matter but also the emotional and social consequences'.

The legal position

These documents mainly focused on younger children. The argument here is that the law already allows competent older children and adolescents to consent on their own behalf. There are two strands in this syllogism:

(a) Treatment includes diagnosis,[7] and therefore consent to testing is considered under the same rubric as consent to treatment.

(b) The general legal principle that 18 is the age of majority was modified in the Family Law Reform Act 1969 to allow young persons of 16 to give consent which would be as valid and effective as an adult's. Subsequent case law undermined the ability of young people under 18 to refuse consent to a procedure: in Re W (1992)[8] the Court of Appeal held that where someone with parental responsibility gave consent to treatment on the minor's behalf, the young person could not refuse.

However, both Alison's parents and she give consent, and the young person's right to consent was reiterated in Re W. Alison is still only 15, whereas the dividing line in the Family Reform Act was 16 – also the age of the girl in Re W. But in the Gillick case[9] (involving a 15-year-old girl's consent to treatment) a function-specific, flexible test of competence was set down: whether the young person had 'sufficient understanding and intelligence to enable him or her to understand fully what is proposed'.[10] (This is assumed to be an English case, but in Scotland Alison would also probably be able to consent on the similar grounds that she had sufficient understanding of the issue to make a choice.[11]) Alison is likely to have a fuller understanding than many 15-year-olds of what genetic disorders imply. She is like the children with chronic cardiac or orthopaedic conditions studied by Alderson,[12][13] who discovered surprisingly high levels of familiarity with diagnostic procedures, cognitive sophistication about probabilities and prognosis, and strong personal values. Against 'the child's right to an open future',[14][15] we could argue that young people with a family genetic history like Alison's grow up fast.

ACTIVITY: What do you think about the empirical argument here that children who have had experiences such as Alison's tend to have a fuller understanding of the issues than their peers? To what extent do you think that this is ethically important? Is there a significant difference between understanding the issues and having the moral maturity to make a decision?

Harm, best interests and paternalism

Another legal strand is the Children Act 1989, which introduced 'the ascertainable wishes and feelings of the child concerned (considered in the light of his age and understanding)' into the 'welfare checklist' that must be used in any case affecting his upbringing.[16] The act also requires consideration of 'any harm which he has suffered or is at risk of suffering'.

Would a positive test inflict harm on Alison? Even if there is no possibility of treatment, there might be benefits in terms of control, ability to plan, and family solidarity. If this is true in Huntington's disease, where the disease is terrible, no cure is possible and onset is comparatively remote from adolescence, then it is all the more true of lesser conditions.[17]

Against findings of higher psychological morbidity in those who test positive[18], some studies of both Huntington's disease and breast cancer tests report relief of uncertainty even on learning of a high-risk test result.[19] According to another study, 'a high-risk result merely exchanges the uncertainty of whether Huntington's disease will develop for that of when it will develop'.[20] However, Brandt[21] found no greater psychological morbidity for patients informed that they had

tested positive than for those told they had negative status.

Against earlier expectations that up to three-quarters of those at risk of inheriting the Huntington's mutation would choose to be tested in order to relieve uncertainty, fewer than 10 per cent of those with a Huntington's-positive parent have chosen to have counselling about the possibility of a test. Of those, only about two-thirds actually opt for testing.[22] So Alison's wish is unconventional; but one could argue that it may therefore be all the more personal and deeply considered, an 'authentic choice' of the adult sort which many developmental psychologists believe should be honoured in adolescents.[23]

ACTIVITY: What do you think ought to be made of such confusing and contradictory research? If it is not possible to decide on the basis of this evidence, how ought we to decide? Can ethics help us? Or the law?

Autonomy and paternalism

The Children Act also leaves scope for courts to find that the child's expressed wishes are not his 'true wishes', those that serve his best interests.'[24] Possibly Alison's expressed wishes are not really her true wishes, but here is a risk of paternalistic condescension.[25] Paternalism usually favours treatment on the grounds of best interests, even in the absence of the patient's consent. Yet the paternalistic thing to do in Alison's case is not to override her refusal and impose treatment, but to override her consent and withhold the test.

Alison may seem too vulnerable to request testing, because of the very fact that she has recently learned that she is at risk for HD. But we are all by definition vulnerable at the time we are asked to consent to treatment: generally we are ill, or facing uncertain results about a possible diagnosis. Another argument against allowing adolescents to be tested is that they are subject to family influence: 14- and 15-year-olds asked to make hypothetical medical decisions frequently deferred to what they saw as their parents' wishes.[26] But studies of adults might equally well show that they did what they thought their spouses or children would want. In Alison's case, where both the young person and the family agree, we must be particularly careful not to impose a conflictual, individualistic model based on the premise that individual and family interests necessarily collide.

If the young person's values and identity seem reasonably coherent and secure, then her consent should be honoured. Conversely, identity only comes with making choices and having them enacted.[27]

Key messages

(a) Existing case law almost certainly allows competent young people under 18 to consent to testing for adult-onset genetic disorders; but many clinical genetics units operate a bar at 18.

(b) Rather than relying on an age-specific test of competence, genetics units, and referring general practitioners, need to think whether they are being paternalistic in denying the test to a competent minor.

(c) Good practice suggests that each case should be considered on its own merits, taking into account the seriousness of the disorder and balancing that against the emotional and cognitive competence of the young person. This is consistent with new guidelines.

ACTIVITY: Go back through Dickenson's paper and write down the various stages in her argument. Is the argument valid? If there are any weak points in it, where are they? In the light of your reading, have you changed your views on the availability of testing for young people? If so, what made the difference?

In a moment we would like you to go on to the next section. Before you do so, take a few moments to write down what you consider the key points to be learned from this section.

Section 3: Genetics and reproductive choice

The availability of prenatal testing for genetically related disorders and other genetically influenced characteristics will increasingly raise difficult ethical questions in reproduction. In this section we will begin to explore some of these questions. Once again we start with a case.

A CASE OF SEX SELECTION

A geneticist saw a young woman with a family history of Duchenne muscular dystrophy. Her risk of being a carrier was estimated as 0.7 per cent. She requested prenatal diagnosis, despite the fact that she was aware of her low risk of being a carrier. Geneticists have come to terms with the difficult issues of terminations of all males in Duchenne carriers when they know that half of those males will be normal, but at what level of risk does it become unethical to terminate pregnancy on the grounds of fetal abnormality? If we accept termination of a male fetus which has less than 1 per cent chance of developing Duchenne muscular dystrophy, it is difficult to say why we should not terminate any male pregnancy on request (Royal College of Physicians, 1991).

ACTIVITY: What are the ethical arguments in favour and against allowing the genetic test to go ahead? How are we to assess the ethical significance of risks as low as this? If you think that this risk is too low to justify termination of the pregnancy, what constitutes a high risk for you? Why is this risk morally significant?

Bearing these issues in mind, read the following paper by Julian Savulescu, a medically trained ethicist who works in the Murdoch Genetics Institute in Melbourne.

Sex selection: the case for

Julian Savulescu

Introduction

Various methods now exist for attempting to choose to have a baby of a desired sex. With the recent advent of flow cytometric separation of X and Y sperm and preimplantation genetic diagnosis (PGD), couples no longer have to employ abortion to select sex. Sex selection may therefore become more acceptable to some couples, and requests for clinics to provide it may become more common. In Australia, requests for medically assisted sex selection are not common; for example, one in-vitro fertilization (IVF) clinic in Australia receives about 15–20 requests for sex selection each year (L. Wilton, Consultant, Melbourne IVF, personal communication).

Medically assisted sex selection for non-medical reasons is banned in the United Kingdom and Canada.[28] In Australia, sex selection employing artificial insemination or IVF is banned explicitly in Victoria by Section 50 of the Infertility Treatment Act 1995. In South Australia, Section 13 of the Reproductive Technology Act 1988 requires that artificial fertilization only be used for the treatment of infertility. Both Acts provide exceptions to avoid the risk of transmission of a genetic defect (assisted reproduction for medical reasons).

In Australia, IVF clinics now offer PGD. One centre performs sex selection for non-medical reasons using IVF and PGD. This has been provided for fertile couples, but has been fully funded privately, costing couples around $10 000. So far, two boys and two girls have been born after sex selection for non-medical reasons (R. Jansen, Medical Director, Sydney IVF, personal communication). In Victoria and South Australia, where it is illegal to perform PGD for sex selection, PGD to exclude aneuploidy may reveal the sex of embryos. Couples might in the future request 'healthy' embryos of a desired sex — 'incidental sex selection'. The legality of transferring embryos of a desired sex in this circumstance is not clear.

> ACTIVITY: Stop here for a moment and consider the ethical arguments against sex selection. Make a list of as many as you can think of. Then carry on with your reading of the paper in which Savulescu goes on to outline the arguments in favour.

Although many jurisdictions ban sex selection for non-medical reasons, there are a number of arguments in favour of allowing it.

Inconsistency

Paradoxically, it is legal to attempt periconceptual sex selection by 'natural' means, even if these employ technology developed specifically for that purpose.[29] Prenatal testing and termination of undesired-sex pregnancies is also accepted practice in some centres. It is inconsistent to provide couples with information from prenatal testing which allows them to select sex and not allow them to select sex by means which are more acceptable to them.

Harm

Harm to the child

The mutagenic risks of the sex selection procedure to children born must be evaluated.[30] Many of the methods use well established procedures (such as IVF), though the long-term consequences of some are not certain: these include PGD, intracytoplasmic sperm injection,[31, 32] and cryopreservation.[33, 34] Despite encouraging data from animal studies and existing human experience,[35] there is a theoretical mutagenic risk associated with ultraviolet light and bisbenzimide used in sperm separation. Concerns about these risks should be addressed by scientific investigation and by ensuring that consent is properly informed, not by banning the procedure.

Sex selection might also cause psychological harm if the procedure does not produce a child of the desired sex. However, parents inevitably have hopes and expectations for their children which are deflated every day. Most parents come to accept and love the child they have, even if that child has a serious disease or disability. Some parents want their children to be great musicians. Sometimes this desire becomes overbearing, as depicted in the film Shine. But the answer is not to ban music schools. The solution is to help parents to be more tolerant and accepting.

Sex selection may be beneficial to the child born if parents will treat a child of that sex more favourably. However, it might be argued that the desire to select sex itself reflects a dysfunctional psychology. Furthermore, sex selection may allow people who are 'unsuitable' to be parents to believe that they could cope with a child of a particular sex. It is dangerous to make such judgements about the 'suitability' and the 'functionality' of people as parents in the absence of any good evidence — society is now rightly loath to enquire into people's fitness to parent. Moreover, preventing sex selection is no guarantee that such people, even if dysfunctional, will not have children.

One objection in bioethics is that sex selection represents a violation of Kant's dictum never to use a person as a means, but always to treat him or her as an end. According to this argument, by selecting sex parents use their child to fulfil their own desires and fail to respect the child as a person. In one way this objection is fanciful. Parents have many desires related to their children: perhaps to have a companion, to have a friend to the first child, or to hold a marriage together. It is unlikely that any parent ever desires a child solely as an end in itself. Moreover, Kant's dictum is actually never to use a person solely as a means.[36] Provided that parents love their child as an end in itself, there is no problem with the child's life also fulfilling some of the parents' desires for their own lives.

Most importantly, without sex selection, without a unique sperm and egg uniting, that particular child would not have existed. Even if the child is disadvantaged psychologically, this is only wrong from the child's perspective if its life is so bad that it is not worth living. It is difficult to point to any life which can be judged from the outside to be not worth living (possible examples might include Lesch–Nyhan or Sanfilippo syndrome).

Harm to other family members

It is hard to see how sex selection harms parents if they have a child of the desired sex; they may even benefit. If a parent will not be able to accept a child of a certain sex (say, a woman was sexually abused as a child and wants to have a girl), then it may be better for both parent and child if the parent selects sex. Another example might be parents who have one autistic boy. Autism is more common in boys but is not sex linked.[37] Such parents might be happier with a girl.

Could other siblings of the undesired sex be mistreated? Firstly, choosing to have a child of a certain sex does not imply that the other sex is undesired in other children. Secondly, treatment of children of the other sex will be largely determined by the pre-existing belief structure of parents.

Social harm

Does sex selection represent a slide to eugenics and the creation of 'designer babies'? We already allow parents to select the kind of children they have. Parents have enormous power (often unconscious) in shaping the kind of people their children become. Parents have the right to choose the environment according to what they believe is best for their child. Moreover, they are already allowed to choose what they believe will be the best children. Parents are allowed to use prenatal testing for disability – even repairable disability such as cleft palate – because they are allowed to decide whether they can accept that child. If parents can decide whether they can accept a child with cleft palate, they should be allowed to decide whether they can accept a child of a given sex.

Are women harmed by sex selection? Some critics claim that allowing sex selection implies that, in general, one sex is superior to the other[38] — to do so is sexist.[39] According to Tonti-Filippini, it 'devalues girls'.[40] However, it does not, any more than choosing to play Australian Rules football rather than soccer implies the former is 'better' in some general sense. Boys and girls are different, and this difference matters to different families in different ways.

Sex selection is more likely to harm women in Asia. There, sex selection is already common. The male-to-female ratio has risen to close to 1.2 in China[41] and in some urban parts of India.[42] This situation has worsened since the advent of prenatal sex determination.[43] It was estimated in 1990 that, globally, there are 100 million women 'missing' (died prematurely) as a result of various forms of discrimination.[44] It has been claimed that sex selection would 'foster the already existing bias against the female child'.[43]

Yet, even in Asia, it is not clear that sex selection should be banned.[45] Disturbed sex ratios may not be a bad thing.[46] Advantages which have been postulated include increase in influence of the rarer sex, reduced population growth and interbreeding of different populations.[47] Most importantly, a false belief in the inferiority of women is not a product of sex selection – sex selection is the product of that belief. Education and improving social and employment arrangements for women are more important in correcting these false beliefs than preventing sex selection.

Consider an analogous argument: some disability advocates argue disability is a social construct; the lives of such people are made worse by the discriminatory attitudes of others.[48] They argue prenatal testing serves to reinforce these attitudes and question whether it should be available for conditions like spina bifida.[49, 50] The community accepts that parents should be allowed to employ prenatal testing and selective termination to have a child without a disability, even if having a child with a disability would improve the plight of the disabled. By analogy, parents should be able to choose the sex of their child, even if not being able to choose the sex of their child would improve the plight of women.

ACTIVITY: As part of his argument in favour of sex selection, Savulescu has set out an extensive list of the potential harms of banning it. What are the potential harms of allowing sex selection to be available? How might these positive and negative consequences be balanced in order to make a decision?

Procreative autonomy

'Procreative autonomy' is the liberty to decide when and how to have children according to what parents judge is best.[51] Parents know best their own circumstances, and ultimately it is parents who must live with and make sacrifices for their children. Procreative autonomy should not be sacrificed to correct social inequality. It is totalitarian for the State to dictate which children parents should have and rear.

In the US, 90 per cent of couples wanting sex selection wished to balance sex within the family. Parents were in their mid thirties, had two or three children and only wanted one more. In both the US and UK, just over half of couples choose a girl.[52, 53] Sex selection for family balancing would prevent, rather than contribute to, a disturbed sex ratio and harm to women. There is no risk of psychological harm to anyone with this kind of sex selection.

Playing God

Is selecting sex playing God? People have been playing God ever since they first decided to control which children they would have by abortion or by contraceptive use or abstinence. The fundamental question is: to what degree should parents be allowed to decide which children they will bear?

Conclusion

I have considered objections that sex selection might harm the child, other members of the family or society. Although, in a few cases, these objections may be valid, none is necessarily compelling in a country like Australia, where there will not be a systematic bias in favour of one sex across the whole community. The harm that might arise from sex selection is not of a degree sufficient to warrant State infringement of liberty. In my view, legislation in Victoria and South Australia should be changed to permit sex selection for balancing family sex.

ACTIVITY: Putting the arguments you listed against those set out by Julian Savulescu, what would you decide? Why? Give your reasons.

Before you move on to the final section of this chapter, take a few moments to list the key points made in this section.

Section 4: The use of genetic information

In many ways all of the preceding sections of this chapter have been concerned with the ethical implications of genetic information and how it is used. We have tended, however, to focus on the issues for practitioners, for families and for individuals themselves. There are also ethical issues relating to the use of genetic information which need to be addressed at a broader social or political level however and in this final section we want to begin the process of thinking about these issues. We say 'begin' because, as with much else in genetics, the ethical issues are emerging with the development of the technology itself. Nevertheless, it is clear that the storing of genetic and other information and the linking of databases containing such information will, in the near future, create some of the most pressing ethical questions in medicine, requiring as it does a balancing of the ethical obligation to operate in the public interest and to respect the confidentiality and informed consent of individual patients and their relatives.

ACTIVITY: This section will take the form of a reading exercise around a report which appeared in the *British Medical Journal* in 1999 concerning the establishment of a national database of genetic and other information in Iceland. As you read it, we would like you to reflect on the other possible developments which might come about as a result of record linkage, genetics . . .

The Icelandic database: do modern times need modern sagas?

Ruth Chadwick

On 17 December 1998, as a result of legislation instigated by deCODE genetics, a Delaware bio-technology company working in Reykjavik, the Icelandic parliament adopted a law making it legal for a private company to construct an electronic database of the country's health records (Ministry of Health, 1998a). deCODE has received an exclusive licence to build a database of Iceland's medical records (including diagnoses and test results, treatments and side effects) and will be able to combine and analyse these with genetic and genealogical data. The act also grants deCODE exclusive rights to commercial exploitation of the database for 12 years. Accordingly, deCODE has entered into a (non-exclusive) arrangement with Hoffmann–La Roche, which gives the latter company access to the database for the purpose of researching the genetic origins of 12 common diseases.

Summary points

The government of Iceland has granted an exclusive licence to deCODE genetics to construct a database of the country's health records. Debate about issues of informed consent, privacy, scientific freedom, benefit, and commercial monopoly is vigorous. The question at issue is whether the rules being applied to the database can deal with the issues raised. A debate that focuses on traditional principles risks ignoring new challenges brought about by advances in medical technology. If the role of commercialism is to be assessed and defined appropriately, benefits to the individual and to public health need to be articulated clearly, are the rules out of date?

The debate before and after the bill on Iceland's proposed database has been vigorous. Sigurdur Gudmundsson, Iceland's surgeon general, was quoted in the *New Yorker* as saying, 'I don't think this country can just sit here and say, "Nope, sorry, we are going to stand on rules that existed in a different era for a different world."' (Mannvernd, 1999). But are the rules being applied to the database able to address adequately the issues that have been raised? It is striking that both proponents and opponents have classified the ethical and human rights issues similarly, into five main areas: informed consent, privacy, scientific freedom, benefit to Iceland, and commercial monopoly (sometimes included under scientific freedom or benefit) (deCode, 1999; Specter, 1999). These concerns can be grouped under two broad headings: matters of medical ethics and the question of scientific freedom vs. commercial interests. The ethical issues are clearly important and relevant to international conventions and to policies concerned with human rights. However, the way we categorize issues in a debate can sometimes obscure other aspects that need to be considered and prevent us from questioning whether traditional distinctions need to be revised.

ACTIVITY: Before going on with your reading, stop here for a moment and consider the ethical issues raised by the commercial availability and use of genetic information. What are the main ethical problems? Would these problems be avoided if the project were not a commercial venture? What are the ethical plusses of the project?

Better, cheaper healthcare?

The database will not help directly any individual patient with the management of his or her condition, say those who are in favour of the database. Rather, it will be a tool in the development of new or improved methods of achieving better health, prediction, diagnosis, and treatment of disease and in establishing more cost efficient ways of operating health services (Council of Europe Steering Committee on Bioethics, 1999). The database can help to achieve the first aim by providing information for example, on genetic and environmental risk factors in common diseases and statistical data on disease and treatment. The health economics aim is a secondary one, but it is still

important. Although the average health status and the life expectancy of the population are high, Iceland's health insurance system is sixth in the Organization for Economic Cooperation and Development's league table of expenditure on health care in relation to gross national product (Council of Europe Steering Committee, 1999).

Making use of a valuable asset Iceland's population of approximately 270 000 has a genetic history that makes it particularly valuable for genetic research into common diseases (Mannvernd, 1999). Furthermore, the extent to which the new genetics will affect the delivery of healthcare remains unclear, and Iceland, say the proponents of the database, provides a unique opportunity for testing this. It has also been argued that, since the data in the records have been paid for out of public funds, they are not owned by individuals or institutions and should be used for the public benefit (Council of Europe Steering Committee on Bioethics, 1999; Ministry of Health, 1998b).

Importance of the Icelandic database

Meticulous medical records on every Icelander have been kept since the Second World War. Since the Second World War, tissue samples have been taken from a large proportion of the population and have been stored. Family trees have been drawn up for most of the population. There has been no immigration for a thousand years. The population's standard of living is uniformly good.

There will, of course, also be 'spin offs' in terms of advantages for particular people or organizations. The pharmaceutical companies who deal with deCODE will be able to develop and test new products. It is the position of the licensee and the licensee's arrangement with Hoffmann–La Roche that have given rise to some of the major criticisms. The fear is that these companies will benefit, while Icelanders as a whole, and scientists in particular, may be subject to 'harm'.

Sources of possible harm

Privacy and confidentiality

The main concern is the threat to privacy and confidentiality. Although privacy and confidentiality are different concepts, the issues have not been clearly distinguished in the debate. The central issue is the security of the information in the database. There is concern that information identifying individuals could fall into the hands of groups who might use it for their own purposes: insurers or employers, for example, might use the information to discriminate against some people. Two aspects of this issue need to be addressed – the extent (if any) to which a trade-off between privacy and other benefits is reasonable, and whether the security measures adopted by the Icelandic database afford adequate protection to individuals.

From an ethical point of view, the balancing of privacy and confidentiality against other considerations is not new. The security of data on identifiable parties has long been one consideration, and public health interests form another, though more controversial, issue. These days individual privacy is under attack on many fronts – not only in health care – and widespread surveillance of people's lives is as common in Iceland as elsewhere. However, the dangers inherent in modern technology and science are judged to be considerable (Council of Europe Steering Committee on Bioethics, 1999) and this has led to attempts to ensure protection through various international policy documents and legislation (Council of Europe, 1981; Council of Europe, 1997c; European Parliament, 1995; Council of Europe, 1997b).

One view is that the aims of genetic research, in particular, should not prevail over respect for the rights of individuals (UNESCO, 1997). Whether the database is compatible with such rights as are protected by Council of Europe Conventions has been examined by the council's steering committee on bioethics (Council of Europe, 1999). In considering what is reasonable, this body concluded that identification of the Iceland data 'cannot be regarded as reasonably possible without substan-

tial effort' and that the data are therefore anonymous according to the criteria of international law. This is so despite the inclusion of genetic information in the database and the controversy over whether genetic information should be regarded in the same way as other medical data. The act includes measures 'to ensure protection of confidentiality in connecting information from the health sector database with the databases of genealogical and genetic information' (Article 10). Though the original bill allowed for a decoding key, this was removed in the final version. Article 11 further provides that employees of the licensee must sign an oath of confidentiality.

Although the Council of Europe Steering Committee on Bioethics considers that the database is acceptable from the perspective of international law, the critics are not reassured about the protection afforded. With regard to the dangers to privacy, at least, they are concerned to have an absolute guarantee rather than one based on a criterion of reasonableness such as is used by the Committee (McInnis, 1999).

> **ACTIVITY: Chadwick here raises the difficult ethical question of how to balance privacy/ confidentiality against the public interest. Can you think of one hypothetical situation in which you would say that the use of the database involved an unacceptable infringement of privacy? Can you think of one hypothetical situation in which the use of the database in the public interest was impeded unacceptably in the name of privacy?**

Informed consent

According to the European Directive 95/46, informed consent is necessary if personal data are to be used for purposes other than those for which they were originally gathered, but consent is not required if the data are not personal (European Parliament, 1995). Iceland chose to establish a database of information that was not personally identifiable. Icelanders have been offered the opportunity to opt out of the database and will be informed continuously about their right to withdraw from the database at any time (Ministry of Health, 1998a, b).

Do these provisions protect sufficiently the interests of individual Icelanders? Once again there are different areas of disagreement. There are concerns about the adequacy of an opting out system for rights protection, as compared with fully informed consent, which is considered to be at the heart of ethical medical practice and research. Against this, the requirement for informed consent is generally viewed to be less for epidemiological research on medical records – especially where these are anonymous (Human Genome Organization, 1996). Autonomy is upheld to some degree at least by the opting out provisions included in the Icelandic act. On the other hand, the claim that some people might be in favour of research in general, while objecting to particular kinds of research that they might be unable to foresee, has some force (Greely and King, 1999).

The debate about the rival merits of opting out and informed consent, however, is undermined by a deeper problem about understanding of what is involved. At one level it is suggested that individual Icelanders mistakenly think they will not have information about them entered on the database until they next visit the doctor (J. Eyfjord, personal communication); at another there is concern that informed consent would not even be possible in principle, because doctors are not in a position to explain the risks. Although invasion of privacy is one possible source of harm, the possible future uses of the database are potentially too broad to be foreseen and explained (McInnes, 1999). So even if a system of informed consent was seen to be implemented, it could not provide genuine protection. In fact a requirement for informed consent has not been chosen on the grounds that it would be likely to reduce participation and thus the usefulness of the database (McInnes, 1999).

In genome research, different levels of consent have been recognized (Human Genome Organization, 1996). The Council of Europe Steering Committee on Bioethics has concluded that relevant Council of Europe recommendations allow research for legitimate purposes to use personal data without obtaining informed consent, provided that the scientific research is provided for by law and constitutes a necessary measure for reasons of public health (Council of Europe Steering Committee on Bioethics, 1999). This is one of the main points at issue. The Icelandic database is considered to constitute a measure in the interest of public health – but is it 'necessary' for public health? This question needs to be answered, but if one of the justifications of the database is to test the extent to which the new genetics can deliver, it is not clear how it can be answered in the affirmative beforehand and thus provide a clear public health justification for overriding considerations of informed consent.

ACTIVITY: The argument here about informed consent is also one about balancing public interest against the protection of the individual. What do you think about the stated argument that 'a requirement for informed consent has not been chosen on the grounds that it would be likely to reduce participation'?

Scientific freedom

Scientific freedom is a more complex issue. The value of the free flow of information and the importance of free scientific inquiry is widely recognized (UNESCO, 1997; Human Genome Organization, 1996). The scientific community in Iceland has been angered by the database proposals, arguing that scientists who want to undertake genetic research will find it harder to raise research funds for their work. However, deCODE's answer is that the database will increase the research opportunities for scientists in Iceland in relation to funding, access to patients, and access to patients' records. The supporters of the database have also argued that this initiative will attract funding and scientists back to Iceland and that the amount of funding provided by deCODE is greater than the medical research funding offered by the Icelandic agency that grants research funding.

However, for scientists wishing to use the database there are necessary conditions such as not using or divulging information in a way that will adversely affect deCODE's business interests. Applications from scientists working outside the licensee's business have to be addressed to the access committee (Ministry of Health, 1998a, b). However, any research carried out in the public domain (for example, by universities) is likely to have an adverse effect on the licensee's commercial interests (Greely and King, 1999).

Once again different aspects of the debate need to be considered. One concern is the extent to which scientists will be enabled or hampered by this development. Another, more difficult, question is whether the database poses a new kind of threat to scientific freedom or whether it simply presents, under the guise of commercialisation, a new twist to an old problem. Inquiry itself is not to be prevented, but commercial interests will affect who does what. However, this is becoming a widespread feature of contemporary scientific work – for example, work on the genome. What is unclear is the specification of the principles to be defended on both sides – what counts as scientific freedom in this context, and what are the purported benefits that justify the level of control that will exist?

Defining benefit

Proponents of the database consider that it will lead to a reverse brain drain as well as the better management of Icelandic health care.[54] Sceptics argue that this benefit will accrue to only a few Icelanders, and that it will take the form of highly paid jobs. The government's annual licence fee will not prove to be a net benefit to the country as a whole.

We need to determine what is understood by the word 'benefit', and this will become increasingly important in the context of population based genetic research. Does it mean financial and health gains (for example, free medicines from Hoffmann–La Roche) or does it also include more intangible benefits such as prestige to the country?

Those who believe that the Icelandic population is being turned into a commodity criticize the definition of benefit in financial terms. Lewontin says that Iceland is carrying the 'commodification' of people 'to its final conclusion by making its entire population into a captive biomedical commodity.'[55] He points to the irony of this in the light of the individualism of the Icelandic sagas. Perhaps this is an example of the value impact of new technology: the environmental impact of technologies is frequently discussed, but a value impact assessment is also required, which would include a consideration of the ways in which we are forced to reconsider, reinterpret, or enrich our understanding of cherished values and principles.

Identifying real issues?

What is interesting about this classification of the ethical issues discussed above is the way in which it centres on very traditional issues in medical ethics (informed consent and privacy) and in scientific research (scientific freedom vs. commercial interests). What has not been highlighted so much in the ethical discussion is the relevance of genetics and the phenomenon of 'geneticization', although this is a constant background presence in the debate. deCODE says that 'it may be argued that the database will save lives, improve health, and cure disease.'[56] This is analogous to the rhetoric of progress associated with the human genome project. As in that case, it is challenged by arguments concerning another shadowy presence – the history of abuse of genetic information. Both sides of the database debate, however, seem to agree about the value of the science; they disagree about commercialization and access. The prevailing model of health here is one that makes genetics central.

In the debates about informed consent and privacy there is also widespread agreement on the value of these traditional ways of looking at things. There is little scope for considering the challenges to traditional principles that result from advances in medical technology. Are these data really individual or national resources? If they are a national resource then the logic of the case might suggest that even opting out should not be offered. The disagreements over whether and to what extent informed consent and privacy will be adequately protected have not been resolved. Whether these approaches need reconsideration or supplementation in the present context should be addressed in the context of clear criteria of what would count as a public health success.

The case for the database has so far failed to convince and this is because there has been an insufficient attempt to provide an articulation of benefit, or of what 'benefit' might mean. A sharper critique of the 'why?' as well as the 'why not?' is required. Who will benefit, and in what way? If these questions are not answered, commercialization will understandably be met with absolutist support for traditional principles and frameworks in forms that may no longer be entirely appropriate.

As we come to the end of this chapter on the ethical issues raised by genetic testing Professor Chadwick's final comments seem particularly important and relevant. As genetic techniques and the sophistication of electronic information storage and transmission continue to develop at breakneck speed this will continue to throw up important ethical questions and choice. Chadwick is surely right when she says,

A sharper critique of the 'why?' as well as the 'why not?' is required. Who will benefit, and in what way? If these questions are not answered, commercialization will understandably be met with absolutist support for traditional principles and frameworks in forms that may no longer be entirely appropriate.

At the end of this chapter on genetic testing, please take a few moments to list the key points raised by this section and combine them on a list with the others you identified earlier to create a summary of key points for this chapter:

Suggestions for further reading

British Medical Association (1998). *Human Genetics: Choice and Responsibility*. Oxford: Oxford University Press.

Clarke, A. (1994). *Genetic Counselling: Practice and Principles*. London: Routledge.

Harris, J. (1993). *Wonderwoman and Superman: The Ethics of Human Biotechnology*. Oxford: Oxford University Press.

Marteau, T. and Richards, M. (1996). *The Troubled Helix: Social and Psychological Implications of the New Human Genetics*. Cambridge: Cambridge University Press.

McInnis, M. G. (1999). The assent of a nation: genethics and Iceland. *Clinical Genetics*, **55**, 234–9.

Thompson, A. and Chadwick, R. (1999). *Genetic Information: Acquisition, Access and Control*. New York: Kluwer.

Wilkie, T. (1993). *Perilous Knowledge*. London: Faber and Faber.

The Science Museum Web site http://www.scicomm.org.uk/biosis/human/scene1.html

References and Notes

1 Nuffield Council on Bioethics (1998). *Mental Disorders and Genetics: The Ethical Context*. London.

2 British Medical Association (1998). *Human Genetics: Choice and Responsibility*, p. 68. Oxford University Press.

3 Nuffield Council on Bioethics, *Mental Disorders and Genetics*, Appendix 2, 'The use of genetic information in legal proceedings', 3.

4 IHA and WFN Guidelines for the molecular genetics predictive test in Huntington's Disease (1994). *Neurology* **44**, 1533–6.

5 See Note 1.

6 Ibid.

7 Family Law Reform Act 1969, s. 8 (2).

8 4 All ER 627.

9 *Gillick* v. W. *Norfolk and Wisbech AHA*, 3 All ER 402.

10 Ibid., 423.

11 Age of Legal Capacity [Scotland] Act 1991, s 2 (4).

12 Alderson, P. (1990). *Choosing for Children*. Oxford: Oxford University Press.

13 Alderson, P. (1993). *Children's Consent to Surgery*. Buckingham: Open University Press.

14 Davis, D.S. (1997). Genetic dilemmas and the child's right to an open future. *Hastings Center Report* **27**(2), 7–15.

15 Wertz, D.C., Fanos, J.H. and Reilly, P.R. (1997). Genetic testing for children and adolescents: who decides? *Journal of the American Medical Association*, **272**(11) 875–81, at 878.

16 S. 1 (1) (3).

17 Cohen, C. (1998). Wrestling with the future: should we test children for adult-onset genetic conditions? *Kennedy*

Institute of Ethics Journal, 8 (2), 111–30.

18 Bloch, M. Adam, S., Fuller, A. et al. (1993). Diagnosis of Huntington's disease: a model for the stages of psychological response based on experience of a predictive testing program. American Journal of Medical Genetics, 47, 368–74.

19 Wiggins, S., Whyte, P., Huggins, M. et al. (1992). The psychological consequences of predictive testing for Huntington's disease. New England Journal of Medicine, 327, 1401–5. Lynch, H.T. (1993). DNA screening for breast/ovarian cancer susceptibility based in linked markers – a family study. Archives of Internal Medicine, 153, 1979–87.

20 Scourfield, J., Soldan, J., Gray J., Houlihan, G. and Harper, P.S. (1997). Huntington's disease: psychiatric practice in molecular genetic prediction and diagnosis. British Journal of Psychiatry, 178, 144–9.

21 Brandt, J. (1994). Ethical considerations in genetic testing: an empirical study of presymptomatic diagnosis of Huntington's disease. In Medicine and Moral Reasoning, ed. K.W.M. Fulford, G. Gillett and J. Soskice, pp. 41–59. Cambridge: Cambridge University Press.

22 Richards, M. (1998). Annotation: genetic research, family life, and clinical practice. Journal of Child Psychology and Psychiatry, 39, 291.

23 Leikin, S.L. (1989). A proposal concerning decisions to forgo life-sustaining treatment for young people. Journal of Pediatrics 108, 17–22. Weir, R.F. and Peters, C. (1997). Affirming the decisions adolescents make about life and death. Hastings Center Report 27, (6) 29–40.

24 Dickenson, D.L. and Jones D.P.H. (1995). True wishes: the philosophy and developmental psychology of children's informed consent. Philosophy, Psychiatry and Psychology 2(4), 286–303, at 289.

25 Dickenson, D.L. (1994). Children's informed consent to treatment: is the law an ass? [guest editorial] Journal of Medical Ethics; 20(4), 205–6.

26 Sherer, D.G. and Repucci, N.D. (1988). Adolescents' capacities to provide voluntary informed consent. Law and Human Behaviour, 12,123–41.

27 See Note 20.

28 Jansen, R.P.S. (1998). Evidence based ethics and the regulation of reproduction. Human Reproduction 9, 2068–75.

29 Benagiano, G. and Bianchi, P. (1999). Sex preselection: an aid to couples or a threat to humanity? Human Reproduction, 14, 868–70.

30 te Velde, E.R., van Baar, A.L. and van Kooij, R.J. (1998). Concerns about assisted reproduction. Lancet 351, 1529–34.

31 Bowen, J.R., Gibson, F.L., Leslie, G.I. and Saunders, D.M. (1998). Medical and developmental outcome at 1 year for children conceived by intracytoplasmic sperm injection. Lancet, 351, 1529–34.

32 Dulioust, E., Toyama, K., Busnel, M.C., et al. (1995). Long-term effects of embryo freezing in mice. Proceedings of the National Academy of Sciences, USA 92, 589–93.

34 Wennerholm, U.B., Albertsson, W.K., Bergh, C. et al. (1998). Postnatal growth and health in children born after cryopreservation as embryos. Lancet, 351, 1085–90.

35 Simpson, J.L. and Carson, S.A. (1999). The reproductive option of sex selection. Human Reproduction, 14, 870–2.

36 Harris, J. (1997). 'Goodbye Dolly?' The ethics of human cloning. Journal of Medical Ethics, 23, 353–60.

37 Ralph, I. (1997). Autism. New England Journal of Medicine, 337, 97–104.

38 President's Commission for the Study of Ethical Problems in Medicine and Biomedical and Behavioral Research (1983). Screening and Counselling for Genetic Conditions, pp. 58–9. Washington, DC: US Government Printing Office.

39 Wertz, D.C. and Fletcher, J.C. (1989). Ethics and Human Genetics: A Cross Cultural Perspective. Heidelberg: Springer-Verlag.

40 Carter, H. (1998). Couple buy a baby girl to order. Herald Sun (Melbourne) Sept 12, 9.

41 Zeng, Y., Tu, P., Gu, B.C. et al. (1993). Causes and implications of the recent increase in the reported sex ratios at birth in China. Population and Development Review 19, 283–302.

42 Registrar General of India. (1992). Census of India 1991. Final Population Totals. Series I. India, Paper 2. New Delhi: Registrar General and Census Commissioner.

43 Benagiano, G. and Bianchi, P. (1999). Sex preselection: an aid to couples or a threat to humanity? Human Reproduction, 14, 868–70.

44 Sen, A. (1990). More than 100 million women are missing. New York Review of Books, Dec 20; 61.

45 Young, R. (1991). The ethics of selecting for fetal sex. Ballière's Clinical Obstetrics and Gynaecology, 5, 576–90.

46 Singer, P. and Wells, D. (1984). The Reproduction Revolution, p. 171 Oxford: Oxford University Press.

47 Sureau, G. (1999). Gender selection: a crime against humanity or the exercise of a fundamental right? Human Reproduction, 14, 867–8.

48 Newell, C. (1999). The social nature of disability, disease and genetics. Journal of Medical Ethics 25, 172–5.

49 Davis, A. (1989). From Where I Sit, p. 19. London: Triangle.

50 Davis, A. (1985). Yes, the baby should live. New Scientist, Oct 31, 54.

51 Op cit. Note 35.

52 Batzofin, J.H. (1987) XY. sperm separation for sex selection. Urological Clinics of North America, 14, 609–18.

53 Lui, P. and Rose, G.A. (1995). Social aspects of over 800 couples coming forward for gender selection of their children. Human Reproduction, 10, 968–71.

54 deCODE genetics. www.database.is (accessed 14 May 1999).

55 Lewontin, R.C. (1999). A human population for sale. *New York Times*, Jan 23.

56 deCODE genetics. www.database.is (accessed 14 May 1999).

Reproduction

Section 1: New reproductive technologies: benefit or burden?   **Section 2:** Fetal reduction and abortion   **Section 3:** Compliance in pregnancy   **Section 4:** A case study of high risk pregnancy

Introduction

Of all the issues in medical ethics, probably none is more frequently in the news than reproductive ethics – construed broadly to include such enduringly controversial issues as:

- abortion and selective termination of pregnancy
- sale and donation of gametes
- use of fetal tissue, for example in transplants and cloning
- surrogacy or contract motherhood
- cloning
- non-consensual use of sperm, e.g. the Diane Blood case
- rights for children born as a result of sperm donation to trace sperm donors
- sterilization of people with learning disability
- enforced caesarean sections.

Yet in terms of everyday practice – the focus of this chapter – many of these issues look exotic but irrelevant. Human reproductive cloning attracted tremendous media attention in the late 1990s, but how important was it to the average practitioner? In writing a chapter about reproductive ethics, we have thus faced a dilemma about which of the vast range of issues to include, using our criteria of direct clinical relevance to everyday practice. This chapter therefore omits some issues, such as cloning and surrogacy, which at the time of writing were unlikely to be encountered in the course of ordinary practice. Other issues, such as

abortion, are commonly encountered, but suffer from exposure fatigue: the arguments for and against have been very well rehearsed over the past 30 years. We agree that the case for and against abortion remains tremendously important, but we have chosen to view it through a filter which grounds it in practice and downplays polemic: the issue of selective fetal reduction. This topic is considered in Section 2. In that section we also look at the ethical and value judgements which clinicians commonly make about 'non-compliance' in pregnant women – another everyday issue. There our focus is on asking why this creates an ethical dilemma – just as in other chapters, one of our first concerns was to ask, 'Is this an ethical problem in the first place?'

Section 1: New reproductive technologies: benefit or burden?

Here in Section 1, we begin by looking at ethical issues before the inception of pregnancy: for example, fertility-assisted treatments such as IVF and GIFT. Please begin with the following activity.

ACTIVITY: Make a list of all the new reproductive technologies you can think of. You might like to begin with the list at the start of this section, but no doubt others will occur to you. Then rank them along a spectrum of ethical acceptability and of how controversial they are. For example, you may believe that artificial insemination by husband (AVH) is ethically unproblematic, artificial insemination by donor (AID) slightly more so. If so, why? What extra ethical issues does it raise? Perhaps the question of whether children born as a result should be entitled to know the identity of the donor. The aim of this exercise is not so much to state your own views for and against each practice as to think 'laterally' about how wide a range of ethical issues each raises. Think about the practice from the viewpoint of different religions or different ethnic communities as well.

Now look at the sorts of ethical arguments you have identified. Ask yourself, 'For whom is this a problem?' For example, we suggested above that identification of sperm donors is a problem for children born as a result. But it is also an issue for the donors themselves, of course (Daniels et al., 1998) – and, perhaps less commonly noticed, for the recipients, the mothers. Arguably it is also an issue for the government: for example, the Child Support Agency.

In the guided reading which forms the bulk of the rest of Section 1, the question of 'Benefits and burdens for whom?' is considered in greater depth. We will now ask you to begin this reading, selections from a chapter in a reader on ethical issues in maternal–fetal medicine by Professor Christine Overall of the Department of Philosophy, Queen's University, Kingston, Canada. Our aim in assigning this reading is to give you an example of the very comprehensive and balanced way in which a professional philosopher 'problematizes' the new reproductive technologies, which are commonly regarded as a technological marvel. This is not to say that they are necessarily a technological nightmare instead: rather, that they raise profound ethical and legal dilemmas which must be evaluated in terms other than those of the technology's success or failure alone.

New reproductive technologies and practices: benefits or liabilities for children?

Christine Overall

In the recent ethical and social scientific literature on new reproductive technologies (NRTs) and practices, there is not much discussion about their impact on children (e.g. Birke et al., 1990; Iglesias, 1990; Marrs, 1993; Robertson, 1994; Hartouni, 1997; Steinberg, 1997). As the final report of the Canadian Royal Commission on New Reproductive Technologies puts it,

There is a dearth of information about, for instance, the direct outcomes of being conceived through assisted reproduction. Physical outcomes are important to monitor, but there may also be emotional and psychological outcomes to being born through the use of assisted methods of conception. For instance, we know very little about the effect on a child's sense of identity and belonging of being born through assisted insemination using donor sperm or following in vitro fertilization using donated eggs (Royal Commission on New Reproductive Technologies, 1993 p. 42).

Books and anthologies written from a feminist perspective mostly emphasize the effects of NRTs on women (e.g. Rowland, 1992; Spallone, 1989). None the less, there is a connection, in reproductive issues, between the status of women and the status of children. This connection is explicitly recognized within the United Nations Declaration of the Rights of the Child, which calls for 'special care and protection' both for children and for their mothers, 'including adequate prenatal and postnatal care' (Principle 4). Hence, it can plausibly be argued that if NRTs either benefit or harm women, then their children may be comparably affected[1].

In this paper I evaluate, from a feminist perspective, a number of arguments about the direct benefits and harms of reproductive technologies and practices with respect to children. As a moral touchstone for their assessment, I employ the United Nations Declaration of the Rights of the Child, which sets forth, in a reasonably clear and uncontroversial fashion, some basic and essential moral entitlements for children everywhere, entitlements that are widely acknowledged, even if they are not always acted upon. I shall confine my discussion to the western world, since that is the context in which most of the arguments on both sides have been advanced.

ACTIVITY: Stop for a moment and think about your reaction to the two separate uses of 'feminist perspective' in Overall's work thus far. She begins by saying that work on NRTs written from a feminist perspective has mostly emphasized the effect on women; yet she says that she is likewise writing from a feminist perspective, but emphasizing the effect on children. Is this a contradiction? You might like to refer to the section on feminist ethics in the chapter of this workbook on autonomy. Then continue with your reading of Overall.

Alleged benefits of NRTs and practices

Three main benefits are repeatedly cited: existence itself; loving, motivated, prosperous parents; and the avoidance of disabilities.

(a) One prominent argument is that technologies such as IVF are a benefit to offspring since without the technologies, some children wouldn't exist – even if their existence includes physical or psychological health problems and/or disabilities. Existence itself is a benefit conferred by NRTs upon some lucky children. Thus, John Robertson, a prominent defender of the use of NRTs, argues that, however difficult the problems may be arising from a life created through reproductive technology, that life is unlikely ever to be so bad as to be not worth living (Robertson, 1994, 76). He states, 'Whatever psychological or social problems arise, they hardly rise to the level of severe handicap or disability that would make the child's very existence a net burden, and hence a wrongful life' (Robertson, 1994, p. 122).

How should we assess this argument? Thomas H. Murray points out that, if it is accepted without analysis, then virtually no 'novel method of bringing children into the world' could be morally condemned (Murray, 1996, p. 37). The argument implies that criticizing a reproductive technology requires showing that the children thus created would have been better off never having been born. Of course, it seems true that being alive is usually good; I have little doubt that most children created through NRTs and practices are glad to be alive. Still, this argument should not be allowed to trump all other evidence about possible harms generated by reproductive technologies.

For it would be a moral and conceptual mistake to assume that there are children who would have missed out on a benefit, life, if not for NRTs. It's not as if children exist in a limbo, waiting to be given the opportunity to live via NRTs. Never having existed would not make some hypothetical child worse off; there is no child to harm (Parfit, 1984, p. 487). So, even if coming into existence is a type of benefit, failing to come into existence is not a harm.

Having life is the precondition that makes all other benefits – and harms – possible. If a child suffers illness or disabilities because of the circumstances of his/her conception or prenatal existence, then we seem to have harmed him/her, in the process of benefiting him/her by causing his/her existence. It's arguable that every person has an interest in possessing a healthy, non-disabled body. If the damages incurred at conception are sufficiently great, there seems to be virtually no benefit to the child at all.

I conclude that, from a perspective before conception of a child, life is not a benefit, since there is no one to benefit; only from the perspective after conception has occurred is life arguably a benefit – and then, only if the life is not heavily damaged through the process of conception itself. Causing someone to exist is not a benefit, since there is no one to benefit; but once the person exists, s/he has life, which is usually a good thing.

ACTIVITY: Stop for a moment and try to restate this insightful argument in other terms. Think also about other contexts in which similar confusion arises.

We can think of two examples from other areas of medical ethics. One is the common argument made against IVF for postmenopausal women. It is often argued that it is better for children to be born to mothers who are young enough to 'roll with the punches' of childrearing. But the choice is actually between this child, born to this post-menopausal mother, and no child at all (Hope et al., 1995). We are not making some hypothetical child worse off by allowing it to be born to a postmenopausal mother rather than to a younger mother.

A similar confusion, one might argue, arose in the Bland decision (1992), which is also mentioned in the chapter on 'End of life decision-making'. There the House of Lords decision sometimes appeared to be arguing that there could be an interest in ceasing to exist, by taking the view that it might be in Tony Bland's best interests to allow artificial nutrition and hydration to be withdrawn. For example, Lord Browne-Wilkinson declared that doctors were only obliged to sustain life when it was in the patient's best interest to remain alive. But in whose interest? We cannot appeal to the interests of someone who will not exist as a justification for ending their existence. To put this criticism another way, the question of remaining alive is prior and necessary to the question of having a best interest. It cannot be determined in the reverse fashion, as Lord Browne-Wilkinson's statement seems to do. A better formulation was that eventually used by other judges, posing the issue in terms of whether continued life on these terms was in Tony Bland's best interests, rather than whether it could be in his best interests not to exist.

Now continue with your reading of Overall.

(b) A second alleged benefit claimed for NRTs is based on the ostensible characteristics of the parents. Prospective parents who use NRTs are often prosperous, seem to really want children, are in some instances supposedly assessed for stability, and are ready to have children. More simply, the claim is that NRTs benefit (potential) parents, who want children (Snowden and Mitchell, 1983, p. 76; Macklin, 1994, p. 56) and are pleased to have them; hence they indirectly benefit the resulting child.

This argument usually takes its most explicit form in the context of debates about so-called surrogate motherhood, or what I prefer to call contract pregnancy, where the claim is made that the children resulting from the contract receive all the benefits of life within middle class or wealthy families, which are equipped to provide the material, social, and intellectual privileges seldom attained in working class families. Thus, the American Fertility Society claims, 'Even if there are psychological risks, most infertile couples who go through with a reproduction arrangement that involves a third party do so as a last resort. In some cases, their willingness to make sacrifices to have a child may testify to their worthiness as loving parents. A child conceived through surrogate motherhood may be born into a much healthier climate than a child whose birth was unplanned' (American Fertility Society, 1990, p. 312).

However, this argument is not persuasive. Its classist bias is immediately obvious: the assumption is that life in a middle or upper class family is inevitably a greater benefit to a child than life in a working class family. This assumption worked to the disadvantage of Mary Beth Whitehead, a working class woman, when she sought custody of her biological daughter, so-called 'Baby M', whom she contracted to create for William Stern, a well-off professional.

More significantly, perhaps, the argument assumes that would-be parents who resort to NRTs and practices are especially motivated and beneficent toward their subsequent children. However, as I shall suggest later, there are also reasons to be concerned about the motives and goals of these people. And, at the very least, there is no empirical evidence that I know of to suggest that they make better parents than those who do not use technology in reproduction.

(c) A third main benefit claimed for some NRTs and practices is that they can help to reduce or eliminate disabilities in children (Tauer, 1990, p. 75). For example, Deborah Kaplan lists several possible benefits to children of prenatal diagnosis (PND) and treatment.

Firstly: Prevention or amelioration of the disability using methods such as treatment through dietary changes or supplements for the mother or infant; prenatal treatment of the fetus through pharmaceutical or surgical interventions; other forms of treatment or therapy for the infant that occur after prenatal diagnosis.

Secondly: Prevention of family disruption through prenatal preparation by family members. This can entail obtaining information about the diagnosed condition and its consequences through reading or through talking to families who have children with similar disabilities or to adults who live with the disability themselves. It may also include such means as finding out about available public or private resources or forms of assistance, purchasing equipment, or making home modifications (Kaplan, 1994, p. 50).

So, the suggestion is that the technologies of prenatal diagnosis benefit children directly through the prevention and amelioration of disabilities, and indirectly, by assisting parents. These claims seem justified.

However, it would be a mistake to accept the related claim, made by some, that NRTs produce better, or even perfect, babies (Spallone, 1989, pp. 113, 117; Snowden and Mitchell, 1983, p. 77); that, for example, babies generated by IVF or donor insemination (DI) using sperm from gifted fathers are smarter or prettier (Scutt, 1990, p. 285). There is no clear evidence to support these claims. And there are reasons to be cautious about them since . . . they betray a eugenicist agenda.

ACTIVITY: Is there a duty to produce 'as good children as we can?' This issue shades over into problems encountered during pregnancy, the subject of Section 2, rather than pre-conception matters: the subject of Section 1. Before going on to Section 2, stop now and think about whether there is a moral duty to produce the best offspring possible. What would be the consequences of such a duty? What would be its origins?

This concludes your reading of Christine Overall, and your work in Section 1. Before you go on to the next section of this chapter take a few moments at this point to make a short list of the main key points raised in this section.

Section 2: Fetal reduction and abortion

If, as Christine Overall claims, it is not a benefit to the child to be born, then neither is there an obligation to maximize the number of births.

Producing the best children we can might be one thing, producing as many children as we can is another. Of course, this view would not be accepted by some religions, and even outside of organized religion, some philosophical utilitarians (e.g. Harris, 1999a, b) also hold that we can maximize the total amount of happiness in the world by maximizing the total number of people. More narrowly, Bennett and Harris claim that we have an obligation to minimize the number of people born to suffer such a miserable life that it outweighs any pleasure gained by living (Bennett and Harris, 2001).

Let us assume, for argument's sake, that most people would accept there is no necessary obligation to produce as many children as we can, but that we ought to 'do our best' by those children we do produce. What would 'doing our best' entail, in terms of pregnancy and childbirth? You have already considered this issue in the activity above. Perhaps you identified some of the following:

- Ensuring that both parents are in maximal reproductive health at the time of conception. This sounds like common-sense, but would it mean that 'older' parents should be actively discouraged from conceiving? – since the risk of fetal abnormality increases radically with maternal age (and, to a lesser degree, with paternal age).
- Ensuring that the fetus develops in the best possible environment. This also sounds unexceptionable, but it might legitimize legal interventions against pregnant cocaine addicts, refusal to serve pregnant women liquor in bars, and all sorts of ramifications which are far from uncontroversial (Daniels, 1993).
- Ensuring that the fetus has the best possible chance of a safe delivery. This, too, sounds like something everyone would want, but in

practice it legitimizes enforced Caesarean sections, which are not presently legal in either the US or the UK – after a long struggle in both countries against legal decisions which were perceived as flawed in law, and discriminatory against pregnant women as the only class of patients on whom non-consensual procedures could be performed (*In re A.C.*, D.C. App. No. 87–609 (April 26, 1990), reversed on appeal in 573 A.2d 1235 (D.C. App. 1990); *Re S* [1992] 4 All ER 671, and the 1997 case of *MS*, which reversed the holding in Re S and firmly disallowed imposed Caesarean sections .

Once again, it seems we cannot get away from ethical controversy in maternal–fetal medicine, even without tackling the 'biggest' issue directly – abortion. The apparently uncontroversial statement that we should do the best we can by the children we do have – a position which we adopted in order to avoid the even more controversial one that says we should have as many children as possible – turns out to have all sorts of ramifications. One such consequence has not yet been identified, however, and at first it does appear to be more of a technical than an ethical matter. This is the issue of selective reduction of multiple fetuses in IVF. If the health, or indeed the life, of one fetus in multiple pregnancy requires destruction of others, how can we decide what to do? Are we obliged to do anything at all? If not, do we impose unacceptably high risks on both the pregnant woman and the fetuses, including the risk that all of the latter will die? – as in the Mandy Allwood case, an octuplet pregnancy. How do we choose which, if any, fetuses to abort when it is really a matter of 'the fewer the better?'.

We will now guide you through a reading by Mary Mahowald, a professor of medical ethics at the University of Chicago, which explores whether or not that is true. You will see that the issue of abortion does in fact surface very early. None the less, we have chosen Mahowald's article because it has a more practical, less theoretical feel to it than many of the classic texts on abortion (e.g. Thomson, 1971); it is not about hypothetical cases, but again about real clinical practice. As you read, try to relate the sample cases Mahowald offers to your own experience.

The fewer the better? Ethical issues in multiple gestation

Mary B. Mahowald

Until the last part of the twentieth century, Hellin's Law governed the predictability of multiple births: the natural occurrence of twins in the general population is 1/100, and the frequency of each higher multiple is determinable by multiplying the denominator by 100, so that the frequency of triplets is 1/10 000, the frequency of quadruplets is 1/1 000 000, and so on. Since the advent of fertility drugs in the 1960s and in vitro fertilization in the 1970s, the incidence of multiple gestations has increased markedly. By the late 1980s, the rate of multiple births had more than tripled; it appears to be rising still.[2]

With each higher order of multiples, risks to both fetus and pregnant woman escalate. For women, the risks include anemia, preterm labor, hypertension, thrombophlebitis, preterm delivery, and hemorrhage. Tocolytic therapy to avoid preterm delivery introduces further risks. For fetuses or potential children, the risks include intrauterine growth retardation, malpresentation, cord accidents, and the usual sequelae of preterm delivery, such as respiratory distress, intracranial hemorrhage, and cerebral palsy.[3]

Conflicts between the interests of pregnant women and their fetuses are not new; attempts to induce abortion and to rescue fetuses have occurred through most of human history. Although medical advances have considerably reduced the mortality and morbidity risks of childbearing for most women and their offspring, that same technology has introduced methods by which people who would not otherwise reproduce can have biologically related children. These methods are mixed blessings when the pregnancies they facilitate exacerbate the risks of gestation for women and their fetuses. They are also mixed blessings when, while providing a means to desired motherhood for some, they occasion pressures on others to undergo risks they would not otherwise encounter . . .

Obviously, prevention of multiple gestation is desirable and can probably be accomplished in most cases. As already acknowledged, however, the possibility of high multiples occurs in nature, albeit rarely, and the mortality and morbidity of these gestations for women and some of their fetuses can only effectively be reduced by terminating other fetuses. In other words, the criterion on which to base the medical prognosis for women and their potential children in multiple gestations is 'the fewer the better'. How, then, does one reduce many gestating fetuses or embryos to fewer?

An apparent, relatively easy answer occurs in the context of in vitro fertilization, when higher order multiples can be avoided by declining to transfer more than three or four embryos after fertilization, storing or disposing of extra ones in some other way. In fact, this is the usual practice of reproductive endocrinologists, who tend to consider higher order multiples a failure rather than a success. The recommendation to transfer only three or four is thought to strike a balance between the risk of multiples and the risk of not achieving a pregnancy at all. This approach does not adequately answer the question raised, however, because multiple gestations are still possible, regardless of whether fertilization occurs in vitro or in vivo. Moreover, the disposition of untransferred embryos poses additional questions, which I have addressed elsewhere.[4]

ACTIVITY: Stop a moment and think about what some of those questions might be. What guidelines are you aware of concerning the storage and disposal of unwanted embryos? (In the United Kingdom this matter is regulated by the Human Fertilization and Embryology Act 1990, s. 3; the maximum term of storage for embryos is normally 5 years (s. 14.4), except where two doctors certify that the donor or recipient has or is likely to become prematurely infertile, or to carry a genetic defect, in which case it may be extended to 10 years.)

Now continue with your reading of Mahowald.

The language used to name procedures to reduce the number of developing fetuses in an established gestation is controversial in its own right. Among the terms utilized are selective birth, selective abortion, selective reduction, fetal reduction, and multifetal pregnancy reduction.[5] Others that could be utilized are partial abortion or partial feticide. The term 'selective birth' has been used for cases of multiple gestation in which a specific fetus had been identified as anomalous and targeted for termination. (Targeting could occur for other reasons, such as sex selection.) Prenatal detection of the anomaly is not possible until weeks, sometimes months, after detection of the number of gestating fetuses. Ultrasound guided cardiac injection of the targeted fetus is then the means through which termination is accomplished. Obviously and perhaps misleadingly, the term 'selective birth' focuses on the fetuses that are not targeted. 'Selective abortion' would more accurately describe the procedure, but only if abortion is defined as termination of the fetus rather than termination of pregnancy.

'Selective reduction' is accurate if specific fetuses are targeted and if the pregnancy itself is not thought to be 'reduced'. But women, after all, are neither more nor less pregnant, regardless of the number of fetuses they are carrying. What is reduced, therefore, is the number of gestating fetuses. In situations in which selective reduction of fetuses occurs, the actual procedure is direct termination of the targeted fetus or fetuses. In these cases, 'selective termination' would be a more accurate representation of what is intended and done. If abortion is defined as termination of the fetus rather than termination of a non-viable pregnancy, 'selective abortion' would be accurate when specific fetuses are targeted and 'partial abortion' would be accurate in other cases as well.[6] If abortion is defined as termination of a (nonviable) pregnancy, terminating one fetus while maintaining the pregnancy through other(s) is not equivalent to abortion.

Years ago I used the term 'fetal reduction' to describe interventions to reduce the number of developing fetuses in multiple gestations.[7] I now consider the term 'reduction' misleading or ambiguous. It is misleading because it obscures the fact that the procedure in most cases entails direct killing of at least one fetus, and in other cases makes it impossible for some fetuses to survive, which to many is morally equivalent to killing. It is ambiguous because 'reduction' is not equivalent to 'termination'. Although 'termination' is the more honest description, a fair and adequate definition of the procedure needs to include the aim of maintaining the pregnancy by preserving some fetuses.

'Multifetal pregnancy reduction' is the term most commonly used by those who perform the procedure.[8] This terminology raises some of the same problems cited above: pregnancy is not reducible, and even if it were, the term 'reduction' mischaracterizes the intervention. To be adequate, a definition of the procedure would indicate that it involves terminating fetuses while preserving pregnancy. Awkward but accurate definitions could therefore be any of the following: fetal termination with pregnancy preservation, fetal termination and preservation in multiple gestation, reducing the number of fetuses in multiple gestation, abortion with pregnancy preservation, and partial abortion. As already suggested, the last two definitions are only accurate if abortion is defined as termination of the fetus rather than termination of pregnancy. Hereafter, I will use the first definition, which I consider simplest, clear, and accurate: fetal termination with pregnancy preservation, which I will shorten to FTPP.

ACTIVITY: Why is it important to get the terminology right, according to Mahowald? Is she just splitting hairs? In our view, what she is doing is clarifying the assumptions which often remain hidden, and exposing uncomfortable truths. 'Reduction' does camouflage what is really going on: for any single fetus, the issue is not being 'reduced' but being 'terminated'. Regardless of whether one favours or opposes the right to abortion, it is important to see that abortion is involved. Feminist bioethicists, of whom Mahowald is one, have been particularly perceptive about the ways in which language is used to decide the debate before it even starts. For example, the term 'surrogate mother' implies that the birth mother is not the 'real' mother, with the corollary that if she refuses to hand over the baby to the contracting couple, their rights rather than hers will be respected (e.g. the case of Mary Beth Whitehead, mentioned earlier by Christine Overall). Feminist bioethicists have urged instead the terms 'contract mother', or 'gestational/genetic mother', depending on whether the woman's contribution includes her own ova.

Now continue with your reading of Mahowald, moving into the section of her article which asks you to consider what differences are ethically relevant in cases with similar clinical facts.

Although fetuses are not legally persons, and their personhood is morally debatable, they are in fact living, human, and genetically distinct from the women in whom they develop. Many human fetuses have the capability of becoming persons both legally and morally. In high order multiple gestations, however, that capability is so greatly and unalterably reduced (without intervention) that the scenario is morally different from, say, a twin gestation, where the capability of both fetuses becoming legal and moral persons is high. The following cases illustrate this morally relevant difference along with other variables that influence the capabilities of individuals. Consideration of these variables is crucial to ethical decisions about whether FTPP should be requested or performed. Case 2a is one in which I was personally involved; case 3a is the well-publicized case of the McCaughey septuplets. Although the other cases are fictitious, all of the features enumerated have occurred in real cases.

Case 1a: Normal twins

During her second prenatal visit, a 36-year-old mother of five, ages 2 to 12 years, is told that she has a twin gestation. She tells her doctor that she thinks she can handle a single newborn but not two at once. 'I simply don't have time for twins,' she says. Having heard about FTPP, she asks whether this is an option for her. The alternative of adoption is suggested but rejected

Case 1b: Same case as Case 1a except that one fetus has trisomy 21 (Down's syndrome).

Case 1c: Same case as Case 1a except that one fetus has trisomy 13 (editor's note: which may produce cleft palate, atrial septal defect, inguinal hernia, and lower limb abnormalities. For children with full trisomy 13, survival beyond the first year is uncommon; however, it is rare for fetuses with this condition to go to term, so it occurs in only one of every 6000 live births.)

> ACTIVITY: What would 'producing the best children we can' suggest in each of these cases? Is this enough of a guideline, or do we need to incorporate other factors? – for example, the effect on the five other children in this case. You might want to start a grid in which you note, first, whether you would approve of FTTP (fetal reduction) in this case, and if so, why. At the end of this extended exercise, look back over the factors you identified as ethically important in making such decisions. This could be the basis of a checklist for your own practice.
>
> Now continue with your reading of Mahowald.

Case 2a: Infertility drug + twin gestation

A childless woman undergoing infertility treatment for 2 years becomes pregnant after taking per-ganol. She has been told that this drug might cause multiple gestation. At 8 weeks' gestation, ultrasound confirms the presence in utero of two fetuses, both of which appear healthy. One week later, the woman asks her physician to reduce the number of fetuses to one. Although the patient is informed that this procedure involves risk of losing the other fetus also, she persists in her request for FTPP, indicating that if this cannot be done, she will seek abortion of both fetuses, and 'try again' for another pregnancy.

Case 2b: Same case as Case 2a except that the twins are known to be male and female, and the woman asks the physician to target the female fetus.

Case 2c: Same case as Case 2a except that the woman asks the physician to target the male fetus.

Case 2d: Same case as Case 2a except that the woman has a triplet gestation and wants to have a singleton.

Case 3a: Infertility treatment and high order multiples

After having a daughter with the assistance of a fertility drug (metrodin), Bobbi McCaughey asks her doctor for similar assistance to have a second child. Six weeks later, ultrasound shows that she is carrying septuplets. Doctors present the option of FTPP as a means by which to optimize the chance of live healthy birth of at least one child. The option is rejected by the McGaugheys on grounds that it is morally equivalent to abortion.

Case 3b: Same as Case 3a except that fertilization occurs in vitro, allowing transfer of fewer embryos.

Case 3c: Same as Case 3a except that Mrs McCaughey is carrying quadruplets rather than septuplets.

> ACTIVITY: Before you go on to the next section of this chapter take a few moments at this point to make a short list of the main key points raised in this section.

Section 3: Compliance in pregnancy

In the previous section, we used fetal reduction (or as Mahowald prefers to call it, fetal termination with preservation of pregnancy) as a practical sort of prism through which to view abortion, fetal and maternal rights, and the other 'big issues' of reproductive ethics. We hope that the exercises in the final activity will have helped you analyse your own views on these subjects in varying contexts. However, it has to be recognized that fetal reduction is only an issue in a small minority of pregnancies, as indeed is IVF itself. You may have noted such issues as enforced

ACTIVITY: What about 'ordinary' pregnancies? Do they also present ethical problems, and if so, what? Stop a moment to jot down the ethical dilemmas which may face clinicians dealing with 'normal' pregnancy.

Caesarean section, imposed by clinicians, or conversely, the mother's right to an elective Caesarean against the clinical judgement of her obstetricians. These are important issues, but only, of course, at delivery. Most of the debate on ethical and legal dilemmas surrounding pregnancy and childbirth has, in fact, tended to focus on childbirth. What we want to suggest in this section is that there is another, more everyday sort of issue throughout pregnancy: compliance. Non-compliance is the sort of problem which looks purely clinical, but actually turns out to raise more ethical dilemmas than we generally think. The first stage of solving ethical dilemmas is recognizing one when you see one, and elsewhere in this workbook we often ask you to think about the ethical aspects of what looks at first to be purely a 'technical' question: for example, in the research ethics chapter, where we begin by asking whether a research proposal is merely clinical audit, or raises issues that demand ethics committee approval.

Once again, we will ask you to undertake a guided reading activity exploring the ethical issues in compliance, by Françoise Baylis and Susan Sherwin, respectively of the School of Medicine and Department of Philosophy at Dalhousie University, Halifax, Nova Scotia. Essentially, Baylis and Sherwin argue that 'non-compliance' is a value-laden term which prejudges the issue against the pregnant woman. Rather, they assert, we should think in terms of the woman's consent to or refusal of treatment at various stages of pregnancy. We already recognize

that competent patients have the right to refuse consent at any stage of the treatment process; even once given, consent can likewise be withdrawn. This is now true in law of Caesarean section, where courts in both the US and the UK have made it clear that pregnant women enjoy the same rights in regard to treatment refusal as any other class of pregnancy. At least 'a subset' of non-compliant actions, Baylis and Sherwin argue, should also be considered legitimate treatment refusal. The task for ethically sensitive physicians to think hard about what sorts of actions are included in that subset.

As you read, think about the implications for clinical practice of Baylis and Sherwin's argument. If you disagree with their view, ask yourself, too, whether there are any limits to which women need not go in order to produce 'as good babies as we can'.

Judgements of non-compliance in pregnancy

Françoise Baylis and Susan Sherwin

Medical knowledge regarding the ways in which women can actively pursue healthy pregnancies and the birth of healthy infants covers an increasingly broad spectrum of activities before, during and after the usual 9 months of pregnancy. In fact, depending upon the clinical situation, the number and range of activities are such that, if a woman were to take all obstetrical advice seriously, she would be faced with a daunting list of instructions ranging from mere suggestions to strong professional recommendations. Few women could (or would want to) fully adapt their lives to the entire range of advice from physicians, midwives, nurses, nutritionists, physiotherapists, and childbirth educators, and generally this is not a problem. In principle, professional advice is something that patients can choose to follow or not – this is the essence of informed choice (Faden and Beauchamp, 1986). In some instances, however, failure to follow professional recommendations elicits pejorative judgements of non-compliance (Feinstein, 1990), and while these judgements are provoked by a failure to comply with specific advice, typically they are applied to the patient as a whole. Moreover, even if the patient ultimately consents to the recommended course of action, she may continue to carry the label of non-compliant because of her initial efforts to resist medical authority, and this labelling frequently has repercussions for her subsequent interactions with healthcare professionals.

[W]e suggest that a subset of the behaviours and choices that the language of non-compliance now captures are not inherently problematic. They ought not to be construed as non-compliance, but rather as informed or uninformed refusals. In our view, the only situations that are inherently problematic are those where the patient fails to comply with her own choices, which may or may not be consistent with directions from her physician. A commitment to provide respectful healthcare requires that these situations be dealt with in a way that enhances, rather than undermines, autonomy-respecting, integrity-preserving patient–physician interactions.

> ACTIVITY: As Baylis and Sherwin say in the last sentence, their argument emphasizes patient autonomy, and views the pregnant woman's autonomy as no different from that of any other patient. Think about some 'tough cases' that might test that assertion. What about the pregnant crack cocaine addict, for example? Is her autonomy limited by her addiction? Or by the risk to the fetus of being born addicted? Even if it is, are we any more entitled to intervene against her wishes than we would be with a non-pregnant addict? (See also the discussion of the Mr C case in the Mental Health chapter.) Now continue with your reading of Baylis and Sherwin.

None the less, not all divergence from physician opinion will evoke the label non-compliant. For example, the term is seldom used when the behaviour in question is within a morally contested realm such as prenatal genetic testing. In the face of public and professional debates about the

appropriateness of the genetics agenda, refusal of genetic testing is generally tolerated. Also, the label non-compliant is seldom used when patients demonstrate excessive enthusiasm for medical interventions deemed unnecessary. For example, patients who request Caesarean deliveries that their doctors do not consider medically required may have their requests refused, but they are unlikely to be seen as non-compliant. The same is true with patients who request/demand an amniocentesis in the absence of professionally accepted risk factors. Thus, it appears that failure to act in accordance with patient-specific medical advice is a necessary but not a sufficient condition for being so labelled.

> ACTIVITY: What is the legal basis for viewing patients who 'request too much' differently from patients who 'refuse too much'?

There is no entitlement for a patient to demand a particular level of treatment in English law (*ex parte Hincks*, 1979), whereas there is a common-law right not to be subjected to unwarranted bodily interventions. Treatment without the patient's consent may be a battery; no treatment, even if the patient would have given consent, is not an offence. In this respect, pregnant women are no different from any other patient. So perhaps the anomaly which Baylis and Sherwin identify about 'excessively enthusiastic' patients not being labelled non-compliant is not really surprising. You will see, however, that they would be likely to explain these legal positions in terms of power and authority, rather than just accepting it at face value.

Now continue with your reading of Baylis and Sherwin.

Some clear patterns emerge regarding judgements of compliance and non-compliance. First, these judgements not only denote the existence of a doctor–patient (or healthcare professional–patient) relationship (or formal interaction); they also reflect certain assumptions about the nature of that relationship. Specifically, the framework of patient compliance and non-compliance implies a commitment to an implicit hierarchical structure within medicine, in that these terms reflect an understanding of the doctor–patient relationship as inherently unequal. The labels compliant and non-compliant apply in cases where those with greater power have issued directives to those with less power, and these directives have either been followed or set aside. In marked contrast, those with lesser power can only make requests of those with greater authority. For example, patients who refuse to act in accordance with physicians' professional recommendations can be deemed non-compliant with medical advice. On the other hand, physicians who refuse to act in accordance with women's requests may be judged unco-operative, but not non-compliant. To be sure, it is possible for physicians to be labelled non-compliant, but in their case it is not for failure to respond to patients' demands, but rather for failure to comply with practice norms or professional guidelines, such as established protocols, prescription standards, or research criteria (Helfgott et al., 1998; Cheon-Lee and Amstey, 1998).

In addition, situating patient behaviours within a framework of compliance and non-compliance discourages development of the trust that is essential for a good doctor–patient relationship. In labelling a patient non-compliant, the physician is expressing his/her distrust in the patient's ability or motivation to make appropriate use of medical expertise. The term is pejorative and often functions as an expression of exasperation at the patient's 'irresponsible' behaviour. For her part, the patient may be sensitive to any moral judgements surrounding her behaviour. She may be wary of negative labels generally, and, in particular, worried about labelled non-compliant and abandoned by her physician if she is judged unworthy. Hence, she may feel anxious about being fully honest with her physician. Rather than bringing her questions and concerns to the forefront, she may tell the physician what she thinks he/she wants to hear and may also seek to minimize the time spent with the physician in order to hide her

'negative' behaviour and avoid disapproving lectures . . .

In sum, the framework of compliance and non-compliance trades on the unequal, hierarchical nature of the physician–patient relationship, potentially denigrates patients, undermines trust, reduces patient agency, and conflicts with goals of informed choice. Given these problematic implications, it is curious that the framework is so prominent in obstetrics and other areas of medicine.

> **ACTIVITY:** In your experience, are judgements of compliance prominent in obstetrics? More or less so than in other areas of medicine? Could the framework of non-compliance be completely jettisoned? If not, why not?

Now continue with your reading of Baylis and Sherwin, to see their answer to this question.

[E]ven though countless studies demonstrate that patients in all areas of medicine routinely diverge from medical directives and that judgements of non-compliance are common throughout medicine, these judgements take on a particular urgency in obstetrics. This is because a non-compliant patient is thought to be risking not only her own health, but also the well-being of the future child she is expected to be nurturing. Social stereotypes that demand that women be self-sacrificing for the sake of their (future) children judge women especially harshly if they fail to make all reasonable efforts to protect the health of their developing fetuses. It is one thing to be bad at caring for oneself. It is generally considered a far greater flaw for women if they are bad at caring for their (future) children. These judgements are not entirely external. Women tend to internalize the social messages of good mothering, and pregnant women may well feel guilt-laden if they suspect their own behaviour could harm their future children.

To better understand the problems that the compliance and non-compliance framework is meant to capture, and to help set the stage for an alternative approach, we review a fairly standard range of behaviours in which patients fail to follow the specific advice of their doctors. In identifying these behaviours, we are particularly interested in understanding whether patients and physicians agree about the nature of the problem. Our aim is to see if other responses might better address the perceived problem than the pejorative labelling represented by judgements of non-compliance, and to determine whether the situations might be better described according to alternative frameworks.

Deliberate refusals: value conflict

As noted above, women sometimes make a deliberate decision to reject their physicians' advice because it runs contrary to their values. For example, a woman who has undergone infertility treatment and is carrying three or more fetuses may be advised to submit to selective termination in order to increase the chance of a healthy pregnancy, uncomplicated delivery and the birth of healthy infants. If she is adamantly opposed to abortion, however, she will reject the advice out of hand, as it is in direct conflict with her deep-seated values. As long as the choices that the women are following are clear and accepted within the culture, she is unlikely to be labelled non-compliant. None the less, she may experience less support from her physician as tensions mount because of potential harms associated with her choice. In the abstract, most physicians will formally acknowledge a patient's right to make her own deliberate value choices; in practice, though, some will find it extremely difficult to demonstrate full respect for what they perceive to be poor choices.

> ACTIVITY: Whereas congratulation greeted the birth of the McGaughey septuplets in the US, following their mother's refusal on religious grounds to consider selective termination (fetal reduction, or fetal termination with pregnancy preservation), the media in the UK were very condemning of Mandy Allwood, who refused to consider selective termination of octuplets. In Allwood's case, all the fetuses died. Is the difference explained merely by hindsight, do you think? – in that Allwood's decision turned out badly. Or was it a poor choice to begin with? What might we mean by a poor choice? – clinically inadvisable? Untrue to the mother's personal values? To the clinician's values? To the best interest of the fetuses?

Now continue with your reading of Baylis and Sherwin.

Deliberate refusals: epistemological conflict

In other cases, women may agree with the values that inform the physician's recommendation (e.g. promotion of their own health and that of their fetuses), but question the medical knowledge on which that advice is based. Medical knowledge is, after all, imperfect and continually subject to revision and re-interpretation. Consider, for example, how in the past 100 years medical advice regarding morning sickness has changed. In 1899, a pregnant woman might have been advised to take cocaine for nausea (10 minims of a 3 per cent solution) and to sip champagne to prevent vomiting (*Merck's Manual of the Materia Medica*, 1899 edition). In the 1950s, tragically, thousands of women worldwide were advised to use thalidomide to control nausea in pregnancy, until the disastrous effect on the fetuses' developing limbs became evident. Current wisdom is that cream crackers and a soft drink will frequently relieve nausea (*The Merck Manual*, 1999 edition). Similarly, in recent decades advice on weight gain during pregnancy has varied dramatically: first, women were told that all weight gain was good; subsequently, they were told that weight gain should not exceed the estimated total weight of the placenta and the baby; today, most women of average weight are advised to strive for a weight gain of between twenty-five and thirty-five pounds.

Not only are there inconsistencies over time with respect to the information on which medical advice is based, there are sometimes also significant inconsistencies among physicians at any one point in time. For example, there is significant variation in rates of Caesarean deliveries, use of fetal monitors, and numbers of ultrasounds performed in different geographical centres. Not surprisingly, such differences in professional practice patterns undermine patient confidence in expert medical opinion.

A second reason for some women to doubt medical knowledge is evidence of past mistakes. In the 1950s, for example, women considered at risk for miscarriage were advised to take DES to reduce the likelihood of miscarriage, even though research failed to establish its effectiveness at this task. The tragic consequences of such marketing include an exceptionally high frequency of genital cancers among the young adults whose mothers took DES while pregnant . . .

Finally, women may also doubt medical knowledge because they 'know' better: as when their lived experience (or that of a family member or close friend) contradicts medical dicta. A woman advised to exercise during pregnancy because this will help ease her labour may deny this claim based on personal knowledge, e.g. she may have experienced a long hard labour with her last pregnancy, despite having followed medical advice in favour of exercise. Similarly, a woman informed of the need for a Caesarean delivery may remember having a successful vaginal delivery after having been told once before of the need for a Caesarean.

In addition to any doubts that women may have about the validity of particular medical knowledge, there may also be disagreement with the (problematic) epistemological assumption held by many physicians that medical knowledge is preferable to other forms of knowledge and should always be privileged. As feminist epistemologists have argued, there are multiple ways of knowing; scientific knowledge is one form among many . . . Experiential, and particularly, embodied ways of knowing provide other essential kinds of knowledge that cannot always be accessed through scientific methods. In the complex, embodied experience of pregnancy, women must depend upon both scientific and experiential forms of knowledge (Abel and Browner, 1998).

For many women an important test of whether their doctor values experiential knowledge is if the doctor is attentive to (and validates) her reports about her experiences throughout her pregnancy. To care well for their obstetrical patients, physicians need to listen carefully to women's descriptions of their bodily experiences. If this is a repeat pregnancy, for example, they should be very interested in learning what is different in this experience from that of the earlier pregnancies. Often, it is women's own reports that give the first indication of complications or difficulties in a pregnancy. Physicians who disregard women's reports or concerns about their embodied experience in favour of abstract scientific knowledge may find that their own advice is disregarded in turn because their patients do not believe it was based on all relevant information.

Deliberate refusals: distrust

Some women who intentionally reject medical advice do so not because of conflicting values, or problematic knowledge claims, but rather because of a deep-seated mistrust of physicians and the medical profession as a whole. There is some evidence, for example, that African–Americans who reject medical advice do so in part as 'a response to racially differentiated histories and sentiments concerning medical intervention and experimentation' (Rapp, 1998, p. 147). In some jurisdictions, women from ethnic-racial minorities are much more likely to be encouraged to accept sterilization as a form of contraception than are women who are part of the dominant social group (Lopez, 1998). Poor women, especially those dependent on welfare, are subject to intense monitoring and regulation by the state in many aspects of their private life, and may assume that the physician is simply one more agent of the state, intent on extending the state's control ever further into their lives. Lesbian women may sense their doctor's disapproval of their plans to raise children in a nonstandard family. And women with serious addictions, especially those with criminal records, may expect that the physician has only contempt for them and little concern for their welfare. Women from these various social groups have reason to see physicians as representing a culture that is hostile to them; hence they may distrust the physician's commitment to their well-being and that of their children. Under such pervasive conditions of distrust, it is difficult to see why women would choose to follow medical advice unless the value of doing so is made very clear to them.

> ACTIVITY: Baylis and Sherwin are writing from a North American perspective. How would distrust between doctor and patient manifest itself in other cultures? Is it equally problematic in your own practice? It is also interesting to reflect on how 'politics' enters clinical practice this way, no matter how separate one may want to keep the two. Now continue with your reading of Baylis and Sherwin.

Failure of understanding

Failure of understanding also colours many decisions regarding prenatal testing where patients who are not scientifically literate may have difficulty deciphering the language. Consider, for example, the counter-intuitive use of the medical phrase 'positive test result' to denote a negative outcome. There are also patients who will have difficulty with statistical thinking and who may forgo or accept testing having misunderstood the risk of miscarriage or the risk of carrying a fetus with a chromosomal abnormality.

Inadvertent non-compliance

Medical attention often focuses on specific behaviours without considering the full range of concerns and constraints that structure patients' lives. Consider, for example, patients whose jobs depend on working long and unpredictable shifts. They may not eat properly, get adequate exercise or be able to keep their doctors' appointments. They may appear irresponsible to doctors who do not appreciate the lack of control these women have over their time. Similarly, pregnant women who work in unhealthy environments may not be

able to change jobs and for financial reasons may not be able to quit working. They may be judged non-compliant if they have been advised that the workplace exposes the developing fetus to toxic substances. Another example of this problem is women who develop diabetes during pregnancy. They will need to learn to test their blood sugar frequently, to eat at regular intervals, to modify their diet significantly, and perhaps to administer insulin daily. They can agree with their physicians about the medical need for such adjustments, but still find that the stresses of daily life make adaptation to the recommended regimen very difficult. . . . Further, their own conflicting emotions about having such a serious disease may foster ambivalent attitudes about fully acknowledging and addressing their state.

For other women, apprehension (possibly engendered by a failure of understanding) is another reason for diverging from recommended actions. For example, fear of amniocentesis, chorionic villus sampling and percutaneous umbilical cord sampling is often the reason for missed prenatal diagnosis appointments . . . In yet other cases, patients have difficulty explaining, even to themselves, the reasons for their failure to follow medical advice and feel very confused about their competence as future mothers. The underlying assumption with compliance and non-compliance judgements is that patients are purely rational beings who will follow medical advice if it is fully explained to them and they understand the likely consequences of their behaviour. Yet human beings are more complex than this simplistic picture suggests. Our actions reflect both conscious and unconscious motivations, and our reasons for action are not always transparent to us. The biomedical model suggests that experiences should all be subject to rational evaluation and control, but daily life makes it evident that the experience of pregnancy cannot be reduced to this model without losing important dimensions. Emotional and physical experience – yes, even 'intuitions' – need to be acknowledged as part of a patient's motivational structure.

Judgements of non-compliance in review

In this schema, there is no place for the language of compliance and non-compliance – language that is imbued with the hierarchy of medicine and thus is fundamentally at odds with the commitment to promote agency and respect the autonomous choices of patients. Such language inappropriately obscures that which is important, namely the context within which, and the reason(s) why, a patient does not conform with medical advice. To fashion an ethically acceptable response to situations where patients do not follow medical advice, it is necessary to understand the patient's motivations and life setting, the legitimacy of goals other than the pursuit of health, and the limits of individual physicians and of medicine more generally. Seeking appropriate targets for blame inhibits rather than facilitates this task. Enhancing the patient's sense of agency and control is more consistent with a commitment to respectful patient care and, moreover, helps to support the patient's own desires for achieving a healthy pregnancy.

ACTIVITY: As your final activity for this guided reading, make a list of the 'big' philosophical and ethical concepts and dilemmas which have been raised in what may seem the rather everyday, non-ethically charged area of non-compliance in pregnancy. For example, the question of the relationship between rationality and reasons for action arises toward the end of Baylis and Sherwin's article. Social justice, too, is an issue in judgements of non-compliance, as are autonomy and paternalism. Underlying many of the other issues, one might argue, is the question of why pregnant women appear to be labelled non-compliant so easily, perhaps more so than other patients. Does this itself raise issues about justice and fairness? Why is it so, if it is so?

ACTIVITY: Before you go on to the next section of this chapter take a few moments at this point to make a short list of the main key points raised in this section.

Section 4: A case study of high-risk pregnancy

So far in this chapter, as in the rest of the *Cambridge Medical Ethics Workbook*, we have concentrated on 'everyday' ethical issues in preference to hypothetical situations or rare clinical events. Our reasoning here has been twofold:

- We think it is important for you to see that there are ethical issues in what may look like routine decisions that can be made on a purely clinical basis. Thus we frequently begin by asking you to think about what might be ethically problematic in what looks ethically problem-free. For example, the extended case study in the research ethics chapter begins by asking, 'Why isn't this just a matter of clinical audit? Where does ethics come in anyway?'
- We prefer 'real-life' situations to the hypothetical cases beloved of many philosophers. For example, in the area of abortion, instead of fetal reduction, we could have used Judith Jarvis Thomson's famous 'violinist' hypothetical (Thomson, 1971), in which you are asked to imagine that you wake to find a famous violinist plugged into your circulatory system for nine months. Although Thomson's compelling hypothetical case has generated an enormous literature, it leaves out childbirth in favour of pregnancy itself, and in our opinion this is a fatal omission (Dickenson, 1997). It is easier not to forget the full realities of the situation if one uses 'real-life' cases.

However, it is important to remember that there are plenty of real-life situations which are far from routine. In the final part of this section on pregnancy and childbirth, we look at an anonymized case study illustrating the ethical problems of paternalism and autonomy which arose during a high-risk IVF pregnancy. The case study was written by Gillian Lockwood, an infertility specialist with an interest in ethical issues. It has the great merit of bringing together your earlier work on assisted reproductive technologies (Overall and Mahowald) with the issues about management of pregnancy and non-compliance raised by

Baylis and Sherwin. Again, this section is designed as a guided reading exercise. As you read, we would like you to keep a 'log' of the ethical problems you identify at each stage of the clinical situation, and what you would advise the clinician to do at this stage. Ask yourself, too, whether the clinical team handled this patient's quite profound 'non-compliance' in the right way, refusing to view it judgementally as non-compliance but none the less setting limits to what they, as clinicians, felt called upon to do.

Problems of paternalism and autonomy in a 'high-risk' pregnancy

Gillian M. Lockwood

Introduction

Renal transplantation, the treatment of choice for patients with end-stage renal failure, can correct the infertility due to chronic ill-health, anaemia and tubal damage generally encountered when these patients are managed by renal dialysis. Currently only one in fifty women of child-bearing age becomes pregnant following a renal transplant, and it may be that many more would welcome the chance of biological parenthood if their fertility problems could be overcome. The first successful pregnancy, conceived in 1956 following an identical twin renal transplant, was reported in 1963 (Murray et al., 1963).

Until recently pregnancy had been thought to present considerable hazards to the transplant recipient. However, some reviews (Sturgiss and Davison, 1992; Davison, 1994) have suggested that pregnancy in the graft recipient, unlike the rare pregnancy in patients undergoing dialysis, is usually likely to lead to a live birth, and the pregnancy may have little or no adverse effect on either renal function or blood pressure in the transplant recipient. The current medical consensus is that if, prior to conception, renal function is well preserved, and the patient does not develop high blood pressure, then only a minority of trans-

plant recipients will experience a deterioration of their renal function attributable to pregnancy (Lindheimer and Katz, 1992).

It is inevitable that the rapid return to good health enjoyed by the majority of women following successful renal transplantation should encourage them to consider conception. Although only a small proportion of women with a functioning graft become spontaneously pregnant, modern Assisted Reproductive Technologies (ARTs), especially in vitro fertilization and embryo transfer (IVF–ET), could theoretically increase this proportion to near-normal levels. Pregnancy, especially if ART is required, clearly entails extra risks for the renal transplant recipient, but these are risks that, with appropriate counselling, the patient may be prepared and even eager to take.

In this paper, I shall discuss the ethical dilemmas involved in counselling renal transplant patients seeking pregnancy but requiring ART. This case concerned a couple with long-standing infertility by means of IVF–ET. The wife was a renal transplant recipient whose initial renal failure was due to severe, recurrent pre-eclampsia, a potentially life-threatening condition of late pregnancy causing raised blood pressure and renal complications, which can progress to cause fits and cerebro-vascular accidents [strokes]. It is associated with severe growth retardation of the fetus, and often, premature delivery.

A CASE OF HIGH-RISK PREGNANCY

A 34-year-old woman (Mrs A) was referred to an IVF unit following 8 years of failure to conceive after a reversal-of-sterilization operation had been performed (Lockwood et al., 1995). She had been born with only one poorly developed kidney, but this was not known until, at age 20, she was investigated for very severe pre-eclampsic toxaemia (PET), which she suffered during her first pregnancy. Her baby was born very premature at 26 weeks' gestation, and he died shortly after birth from complications of extreme prematurity.

A second pregnancy in the following year was also complicated by severe PET, renal damage, premature delivery at 26 weeks' gestation, and neonatal death. Sterilization by tubal ligation was offered and accepted under these circumstances, in view of the anticipated further deterioration of her renal function with any subsequent pregnancy. There was a significant further advance of her renal disease, necessitating the initiation of haemodialysis (a kidney machine) 2 years later, and a living, related donor renal transplant (from her mother) was subsequently performed. After the transplant, Mrs A remained well and maintained good kidney function on a combination of anti-rejection drugs, steroids and blood pressure tablets. At age 26, a reversal-of-sterilization operation was performed because she had become so distressed by her childlessness, but hysterosalpingography (a test to check for fallopian tubal patency) 2 years later, when pregnancy had not occurred, showed that both tubes had once again become blocked.

ACTIVITY: This should be the first stage of your 'log'. What ethical issues are presented at this point? For example, is it right to try to help Mrs A become pregnant, no matter how distressed she is about her childlessness, if it may harm her clinical condition? Is this part of the duties of a doctor? – conceived as responding to the patient's autonomous wishes. Or, is it actually antithetical to the duties of a doctor? – seen in terms of benefiting rather than harming patients, and with benefit primarily seen in turn as being to do with medical best interests.

You might also want to look at the autonomy chapter, and consider how reproductive ethics takes our concern beyond the patient alone. In the Lockwood case, it might be argued that patient autonomy is not the same as giving the patient what she wants – particularly because others in the family constellation also need to be considered. For example, Mrs A's mother now has only one kidney, because she has donated her other one to her daughter. Does this mean that Mrs A is in some sense not entirely free to risk the donated kidney on her high-risk pregnancy? If it gives Mrs A's mother some say, exactly how much and what kind of say?
Now continue with your reading of the case.

At the time that Mr and Mrs A were referred to the IVF unit, there were no case reports of successful IVF in women with renal transplants, but specialists were becoming increasingly reluctant to advise women with transplants against trying for a baby, as medical care for 'high-risk' pregnancies was improving dramatically. Following discussion with the Transplantation Unit and the high-risk pregnancy specialists, the IVF unit felt that an IVF treatment cycle could be offered to Mr and Mrs A as long as the risks of IVF-ET, over and above those attendant upon a spontaneous pregnancy in these circumstances, were understood and accepted by the couple and minimized as far as possible, by the IVF team.

ACTIVITY: How would you characterize the solution taken by the IVF team to the dilemma identified in the last activity? One way to see it is in terms of informed consent to treatment. The IVF team seem to take the view that provided consent to treatment is genuinely informed, and that all risks are fully communicated to the couple, it is really up to the couple to decide. This is consistent with the view of the function of informed consent which one of us has argued for elsewhere (Dickenson, 1991), as transferring responsibility for ill-luck in outcomes from clinician to patient. (Of course, the team also view their duty as including maintaining good medical standards and minimizing risk; it would not be sufficient to say the couple had consented if the procedure was then performed negligently, in effect increasing the risks beyond the level to which they had given consent.)
Now continue with your reading of the case.

An IVF treatment cycle was started using the normal drug regimen, but the patient was given a much lower dose than usual, with the aim of minimizing the effect of the hormone stimulation on the transplanted kidney. Two oocytes (eggs) were obtained, which fertilized normally in vitro, and the two embryos were transferred to the uterus (womb) 54 hours later. Mrs A's pregnancy test was positive 13 days after embryo transfer, and an ultrasound scan performed at 8 weeks' gestation showed a viable twin pregnancy.

Throughout the treatment cycle and during pregnancy, the patient's antirejection drugs (azathioprine and prednisolone) were continued at maintenance doses. Renal function was monitored closely throughout the treatment cycle and during pregnancy, remaining remarkably stable.

The pregnancy was complicated at 20 weeks' gestation by a right deep vein thrombosis, affecting the femoral and external iliac veins, and anticoagulation with heparin and warfarin was required. Spontaneous rupture of the membranes, leading to premature delivery, occurred at 29 weeks' gestation; the twins were delivered vaginally and in good condition three hours later. The twin girls were small for dates (at 1.48 and 1.19 kg) but were otherwise well, requiring only minimal resuscitation and respiratory support. After delivery of her babies, Mrs A remained well and her renal graft continued to function normally, with no change in immunosuppressive or antihypertensive (blood pressure) medication required.

ACTIVITY: Stop again to make another entry in your log. Does the favourable outcome indicate that the decision to treat Mrs A was ethically correct? Or is this judgement from hindsight? Consider some further evidence of the risks to health of both mother and child, presented by Lockwood.

Risks to the mother, the fetus and the neonate

Severe pre-eclampsia and eclampsia can result in irreversible damage to the maternal kidney, particularly due to acute renal cortical necrosis. Women who have recurrent pre-eclampsia in several pregnancies or blood pressures that remain elevated in the period following delivery (the puerperium), especially if they have pre-existing renal disease and/or hypertension, have a higher incidence of later cardiovascular disorders and a reduced life expectancy (Chesley et al., 1989). Pregnancy is recognized to be a privileged immunological state, and therefore episodes of rejection during pregnancy might be expected to be lower than for non-pregnant transplant recipients. Nevertheless, rejection episodes occur in 9 per cent of pregnant

women, occasionally in women who have had years of stable renal functioning prior to conception. More rarely, rejection episodes occur in the puerperium, when they may represent a rebound effect from the altered immunosuppressiveness of pregnancy.

Immunosuppressive (antirejection) drugs are theoretically toxic to the developing fetus; however, maternal health and graft function require continuation of maintenance immunosuppression. Women with impaired renal function are recognized to be at risk of giving birth prematurely, often to growth-retarded or small-for-dates babies. A large French study of women with pre-existing renal damage reported a prematurity rate of 17 per cent and a spontaneous abortion rate (miscarriage) of 20 per cent, as compared to prematurity and spontaneous abortion rates of 8 and 12 per cent, respectively, in the normal population (Jungers et al., 1986). However, the long-term health effect of events in utero for the offspring of transplanted mothers is harder to quantify. There is animal evidence of delayed effects of immunosuppressive therapies and intrauterine growth retardation.

ACTIVITY: At this point, review your log of the ethical issues in the case, before reading Lockwood's discussion of them. As you read her analysis, you may wish to add other considerations, or perhaps her discussion may suggest counter-arguments to your own views, which you might want to consider. When you have finished, you should have a matched list of arguments for treatment, and corresponding counter-arguments against, together with an overall conclusion weighing up both pros and cons. Lockwood puts her analysis primarily in terms of paternalism and autonomy, but your arguments and counter-arguments may be structured differently. For example, having just read Baylis and Sherwin's discussion, you may be asking yourself whether Mrs A's decision to request IVF was in a sense 'non-compliant' with medical advice concerning her kidney condition. You will see that there is also a link to multiple embryo transfer for successful pregnancy in kidney recipients, so that your reading of Mahowald should have alerted you to the ethical complications here. You will probably also want to ask Overall's question, in a slightly different context: is it clear that IVF in this case would benefit the children who might be born as a result? Given that the babies were born at rather dangerously low birthweights, and that two previous pregnancies had resulted in stillbirths, this is a very real question.

Case discussion

The decision to accept the couple for IVF treatment posed significant dilemmas of both a technical (obstetric and renal) and an ethical nature. Severe pre-eclampsia can present as a progressive condition, tending to occur with greater virulence in successive pregnancies (Campbell and MacGillivray, 1985). This, after all, had been the rationale behind the original decision to sterilise the patient after the death of her second baby, precipitated by pre-eclampsia and extreme prematurity. The successfully functioning transplanted kidney had been donated by the patient's mother and therefore, as an organ, was thirty years older than the patient herself. Hence there were real concerns that the transplanted kidney could be jeopardised by the strain of a normal pregnancy. The use of donated oocytes, which can permit postmenopausal women of 50+ years to become pregnant through IVF–ET, has demonstrated a significant incidence of pregnancy-associated hypertension and frank pre-eclampsia, suggesting that the aged kidney is less able to withstand the stress of pregnancy.

An editorial review (Davison and Redman, 1997) reported that 35 per cent of all conceptions in renal transplant patients failed to progress beyond the first trimester because of therapeutic (approximately 20 per cent) and spontaneous (approximately 14 per cent) abortions. Problems occur some time after delivery in 11 per cent of all women with transplants, unless the pregnancy was complicated prior to 28 weeks' gestation, in which case remote problems can occur in 24 per

cent of pregnancies. However, of the conceptions that continue beyond the first trimester, 94 per cent end successfully, in spite of a 30 per cent chance of developing hypertension, pre-eclampsia, or both. Distinguishing between time-dependent and pregnancy-induced problems is clearly difficult, however. Davison (1992) cites registry data indicating that 10 per cent of mothers who are transplant recipients die within 1 to 7 years of childbirth.

The technique of IVF–ET also poses additional problems for the renal transplant patient. The hormone drug regime involves supraphysiological levels of estradiol, which are associated with a higher risk of thrombotic (blood-clotting) episodes than in normal pregnancy. Access to the ovaries may be compounded by the positioning of the transplanted kidney in the pelvis, although ultrasound screening does permit the kidney to be readily visualised. Successful pregnancy rates per embryo transfer in IVF–ET have tended to depend on multiple embryos, but a multiple pregnancy (seen in 25 per cent of all IVF pregnancies following a three-embryo transfer) would exert even greater strain on the kidney than a singleton; is more likely to be associated with the development of pre-eclampsia; and carries increased risk of premature delivery of the babies.

In an attempt to mitigate all these medical factors, the IVF unit embarked on a very low-dose stimulation regime and was content with a lower than usual harvest of eggs at retrieval. It was agreed that only two embryos would be transferred, and minimal post-transfer hormone support was given to minimize the risks.

The ethical aspects of undertaking IVF and embryo transfer in these circumstances are possibly harder to quantify and yet more contentious. It is recognized that even under optimum circumstances, at the most effective units, the probability of a successful pregnancy with a single treatment cycle of IVF–ET is only about 25 per cent. Was it acceptable to expose Mrs A to all the risks of an IVF cycle that was four times as likely to fail as to succeed? Even where the IVF is successful in establishing a pregnancy, there is still the non-negligible risk that renal function may deteriorate. The patient may be safely delivered, but again become dependent upon renal dialysis. The Human Fertilization and Embryology Act 1990 laid great stress of the importance of obtaining true informed consent from patients undertaking procedures such as IVF; it was particularly important that the patient and her husband were made aware of the risks associated not only with the failure of IVF–ET but also with its success.

Arguments that could be advanced against offering fertility treatment to renal transplant recipients, such as whether it is in the best interests of the patient to be helped to achieve a state as a result of which she may suffer chronic ill-health or even early death, have also been advanced against permitting 'old', i.e. post-menopausal, women to become pregnant through the technique of egg-donation IVF. In both instances, one could argue that as long as the risks associated with fertility treatment and pregnancy were thoroughly explained to and accepted by the woman (and her partner), then to refuse treatment on the sole ground that her health may deteriorate is unacceptably paternalistic on the part of the clinicians involved. Mrs A stated that if she had not agreed to the sterilization (which she claimed she had been placed under undue pressure to accept at the time she was diagnosed with renal failure), then she would not only have been able to, but definitely would have tried to, achieve a further pregnancy, as she did after the reversal of sterilization was performed.

The Human Fertilization and Embryology Act 1990 also places great emphasis on the 'interests of the child' who may be born as a result of procedures such as IVF–ET. This emphasis has been interpreted by some authorities as encouraging fertility units to feel justified in refusing treatment to women with significant health problems (or to post-menopausal women) as it would, so they claim, not be in the 'interests of the child' to be born to a mother with reduced life expectancy due to chronic ill health or comparatively advanced age. Apart from the obvious rejoinders that society happily countenances men becoming fathers at an age when their life expectancy is reduced, and the medical profession's heroic efforts to assist women with serious health problems who become pregnant spontaneously, it is unquestionably in the interests of the child. After all, the child will only be born if his transplanted mother is offered fertility treatment, that she should be offered such treatment even if he loses his mother at an early age or has to deal with the consequences of her ill-health, as otherwise he won't exist!

> ACTIVITY: Compare the stances taken by Lockwood and Overall on the prospective child's interests. How do they differ? How would Lockwood's view affect her opinion of whether IVF treatment was right in this case?

Our answer is that Lockwood, who has elsewhere described herself as an ethical consequentialist, like Harris, appears to believe that it is 'unquestionably' in the child's interest to be born. This would presumably be an argument in favour of IVF, although it assumes that existence is a benefit – a view with which many religions and world views, Buddhism for example, or the Greek tragic authors – would emphatically not agree. Overall, on the other hand, views the question of the child's best interests as a nonsense, because there is no entity which can have best interests if the child is not born.

Your comparison of Lockwood and Overall has brought this chapter full circle. We hope that you have enjoyed working through a small but, we hope, paradigmatic selection of some of the highly charged issues in reproductive ethics.

> ACTIVITY: As we come to the end of this chapter take a few moments at this point to make a short list of the main key points raised in this section and then to combine them with the points from the other sections to produce a summary of Key points from this chapter:

Suggestions for further reading

Callahan, J. (1995). *Reproduction, Ethics and the Law: Feminist Perspectives*. Indiana University Press.

Chadwick, R. (1987). *Ethics, Reproduction and Genetic Control*. London: Routledge.

Dickenson, D. (ed.) (2001). *Ethical Issues in Maternal–Fetal Medicine*. Cambridge: Cambridge University Press.

Thomson, J.J. (1971). A defense of abortion. In *Philosophy and Public Affairs*, 1: 1 (Fall 1971) pp. 47–66

Warren, M. (1991). Abortion. In *Companion to Ethics*, ed. P. A. Singer. Oxford: Blackwell.

References and notes

1 For example, the criminalization of maternal substance abuse indirectly threatens the well-being of children, since the threat of criminal prosecution may deter pregnant women from seeking medical care (Blank and Merrick, 1995: 165).

2 Hammon, K.R. (1998). 'Multifetal pregnancy reduction,' *Journal of Obstetric, Gynecologic and Neonatal Nursing*, **27**, (3) (May/June 1998): 338.

3 Hammon, p. 339.

4 See Mahowald, M.B. *Genes, Women, Equality*, ch. 12.

5 Berkowitz, R.L., Lynch, L. Stone, J. and Alvarez, M. (1996). 'The current status of multifetal pregnancy reduction,' *American Journal of Obstetrics and Gynecology*, **174** (4) 1265–66.

6 Clinical texts usually define abortion as termination of a non-viable pregnancy; popular understandings tend to identify it with termination of fetuses; cf. Mary B. Mahowald, 'concepts of abortion and their relevance to the abortion debate,' *Southern Journal of Philosophy* XX (1982): 195–207.

7 Mahowald, M.B. (1993). *Women and Children in Health Care: An Unequal Majority,* pp. 87–90. New York: Oxford University Press.

8 E.g., Berkowitz et al., p. 1265, Evans et al., p. 771, and the American College of Obstetricians and Gynecologists; cf. Rorty, M.V. and Pinkerton, J.V. (1996). 'Elective fetal reduction: the ultimate elective surgery,' *Journal of Contemporary Health Law and Policy*, **13**, 55.

Medical research

Introduction

During the Second World War, Nazi doctors conducted some of the most horrific experiments imaginable in the name of medical research. An example is the experiment in which healthy people were thrown into freezing cold water in an attempt to see how long pilots who bailed out of aeroplanes into the sea could be expected to survive.

After the war, the international community responded to these and other atrocities carried out in the name of medicine by creating the Nuremberg Code, which you will find reproduced at the end of this chapter. This was the first internationally agreed ethical code concerning the conduct of clinical trials. The code has since been superseded to some extent by the World Medical Association's Helsinki Declaration (first drawn up in 1964 and revised several times since) and, to some extent, in relation to research in developing countries, by the guidelines of the Council of Medical Organizations of Medical Sciences (CIOMS) and the World Health Organization (WHO). It remains none the less an extremely powerful reminder of the horrors which have been and could be carried out in the name of medical advance.

Notwithstanding the actual and possible harmful abuses of medical research, it remains the case that advances in medicine and the knowledge gained through medical research have been at the heart of many of the most significant developments in the improvement of the human condition. Medical research and the advance of medical understanding represents what is best about human endeavour and has been directly responsible for some of the most profound improvements in human well-being, particularly in the past two centuries. It seems certain that medical research will play an increasingly important role in the improvement of human wellbeing in the future too.

Such actual and possible benefits to the lives of real human beings should not be forgotten in any account of the ethics of medical research. What the Nazi experiments and the Nuremberg Code remind us, however, is that such benefits ought not be bought at any price, that the advance of human well-being through the understanding of particular medical conditions is not in itself sufficient justification for medical experimentation to be considered ethical. In this chapter we shall be exploring the ethics of medical research in a range of different settings by means of the following unifying activity.

ACTIVITY: As you read through this chapter, we would like you to build up your own research ethics checklist, which will provide a useful tool for the identification of the ethical questions raised by a particular piece of medical research. In order to do so, we would like you, as you work your way through the

Section 1: What counts as medical research?

It may seem strange to start off by asking what is medical research. The distinction between research and clinical practice, however, is becoming increasingly narrow. On the one hand, the growing importance of Evidence-based Medicine means that, increasingly, clinicians, even those who are not trained researchers, are expected to carry out research of one kind or another or to assess the clinical implications of research carried out by others. On the other hand, the increasing importance of clinical audit and of clinical governance is leading to a proliferation of research-like activities in everyday medicine, many of which are difficult to distinguish from what is usually thought of as medical research. The blurred line between these activities inevitably raises the question: to what extent ought these activities be subject to ethical review? What are their ethical implications? Just what is the difference then between research and clinical audit? How, if at all, are the ethical questions raised by medical research different from those that occur in everyday clinical practice? All of this, taken together, means that any consideration of research ethics must address the question of what counts as medical research?

This is not an entirely new question and neither is it of merely academic interest. When the need for the ethical review of research first began to be acknowledged in the UK in the 1960s, there was a vigorous debate about precisely how research might be distinguished from ordinary clinical practice. This was motivated by two concerns. First, it was feared that an unduly restrictive approach to clinical work would restrict therapeutic freedom and inhibit innovation. This concern remains with us today, though now more closely associated with the way in which evidence-based guidelines may be allowed to 'trump' individual clinical experience. The second concern was that too broad a definition of research might result in Research Ethics Committees being overwhelmed with applications.

In the first section of this chapter we shall be exploring what counts as medical research by investigating the relationship between medical research and clinical audit in a real case. The case, which starts below, is based on the correspondence between the director of a Health Trust and the chair of a Local Research Ethics Committee (LREC). The case itself was provided by Professor K. W. M. Fulford who is a British psychiatrist and Director of the University of Warwick Distance Learning Masters Programme in the Philosophy and Ethics of Mental Health. One of the aims of this section is to give you a sense of what is involved in reading and carrying out an ethical review of a real research proposal.

A CASE OF AUDIT OR RESEARCH

Dear Mr Smith

re: Primary Care Mental Health Evaluation Project

Following our conversation before Christmas I am pleased to enclose an outline of the nature and objectives of this project.

Our aim is to compare the cost-effectiveness of two ways of providing mental health services in the community, one based on community Mental Health Teams, the other based on General Practices (family doctor teams). We have approached the Jonsen Centre for Mental Health who have a well-established reputation for evaluation of mental health services to assist us in the task of evaluating our preferred model of community-based mental health services alongside a general practice-based model. They have proposed a two-stage study, the first stage involving an audit of mental health needs and how they are being met in the two models, the second stage involving semi-structured interviews of key informants (including users of services). We have obtained financial assistance from West Fenland Health to meet the cost of the project.

I should make it clear that, at this stage, what I am seeking is your opinion as to whether this evaluation of mental health services in Erehwon should be referred to your full Committee for approval. If it is your conclusion it should be, I am assuming you would wish to see copies of the protocols to be used for the 'semi-structured interviews' in the second stage of the project, which have yet to be finalized.

I hope this is helpful. If you do require any further information, please do not hesitate to contact me.

Yours sincerely

Christine Ready
Director of Primary Care and Commissioning
Erewhon Health Care

> **ACTIVITY: Stop here for a moment and consider whether, at this stage, you would see the proposal as research or audit? Can you identify any ethical issues arising from this letter and from the proposed study? If so make a note of them. You may of course feel that there are none.**
>
> **Before you go on to read the rest of the correspondence between the Trust and the LREC, we would like you to read the following commentary on the above letter by K.W.M.Fulford himself.**

Is this research?

K.W.M.Fulford

[. . .] Christine Ready's letter emphasizes that she is not actually making an application for ethical review but only requesting an opinion as to whether such a review is necessary. Moreover, she implies that it is only for Stage 2 of the project that the question arises at all, this being the stage at which patients (and others) will be approached in person to be interviewed (note her offer to supply the interview protocols if required). If the study had been limited to the first stage, which is just an audit, then the Research Ethics Committee would not have been approached at all.

Christine Ready's implied distinction between audit and research, is consistent with one strand of thought in the research ethics literature. This is to the effect that audit, being 'routine', non-invasive, and therapeutic (in the broad sense of being aimed at identifying best practice for the conditions from which the patients involved in the audit are suffering), is not ethically sensitive. Moreover, as in earlier debates about the distinction between clinical work and research, it is argued that to include audit within the remit of the Research Ethics Committees, would both inhibit the proper monitoring and review of services, and lead to an overload of the Committees themselves.

A number of attempts have been made to distinguish audit from research in terms of the procedures involved. At best, however, this approach helps to draw out certain differences of emphasis or degree between audit and some kinds of scientific research, notably research based on laboratory rather than field work.

Opinion in the UK is currently swinging towards the view that audit should be included in ethical review: the Association of Local Research Ethics Committees, for example, has come down firmly on this side. If more resources are needed, well, so be it. Audit need not, however, be resource intensive: what is required, after all, is a review of audit *procedures* rather than review of each and every audit. More importantly, though, audit shares with research the key shift of intention, from the best interests of the person who is the subject of the research (or audit), to the intention of advancing knowledge. It is this shift of intention which is at the heart of the greater ethical sensitivity of research, and, by extension of audit. In both cases, the shift implies an inherent conflict of interest and, hence, the need for external monitoring. Moreover, just as ethical review should facilitate good practice rather than inhibiting the advance of knowledge, so too should the ethical review of audit.

> ACTIVITY: What do you think about the attempt to make a distinction between research and audit? Do you think it is possible to make such a distinction conceptually? If so, how? In his commentary Fulford argues against the distinction and argues that both audit and research can be distinguished from other forms of clinical practice by means of the notion of 'intention', where the research/audit intention is oriented towards the advance of knowledge and is to be contrasted with the therapeutic intention of clinical practice. Do you think that this is a workable definition of medical research? Can you think of any examples of medical research or of clinical practice which would challenge this distinction? Is it possible to separate the intention to advance knowledge from the therapeutic intention? Now continue with your reading of the case.

On receipt of the letter you have just read, the Chair of the Local Research Ethics Committee, Mr Smith, was in no doubt that both stages of the proposed evaluation should be subject to review and he wrote back requesting full details. He later received a copy of the Jonsen proposals. They began with a brief resumé of the shift in GP (General Practice) referral patterns for mental health problems from hospital specialists (i.e. psychiatrists working in inpatient or outpatient settings) to community psychiatric nurses (CPNs) and counsellors. They continued as follows:

A CASE OF RESEARCH OR AUDIT
(cont.)

The Proposal

There is evidence that the number of people using mental health services can increase threefold when the service becomes community orientated (Gater and Goldberg, 1991). The vast majority of this increased demand comes from people with non-severe mental illness. As resources do not increase at the same rate, this puts pressure on Community Mental Health Teams (CMHTs) in terms of the sheer number of referrals and the difficulty they then have prioritizing people with serious mental illness.

How then can mental health services have a close working relationship with primary health care without being over-burdened and while still prioritizing people with severe mental illness? Erehwon Health have developed two models of service provision. In one, a CPN [community psychiatric nurse] is purchased by the Health Agency to serve a consortium of GPs as a member of the Community Mental Health Team: in the other, a CPN is purchased direct by a GP fund-holder or Primary Care Group and becomes a member of the local Primary Health Care Team.

Expected benefits

As a result of this evaluation, the following key issues will be addressed:

- What are the needs of people with mental health problems attending primary healthcare?
- What is the role of the CPN working as part of the primary health care team?
- Do different models of specialist mental health-care provision lead to different numbers of referrals from primary healthcare?
- What mental health services do people referred go on to receive?
- What is the match between people's needs and the resources they receive?
- Are GPs more satisfied with some models of mental health provision than others?

- How do service users view mental health services?
- What are the clinical outcomes for service users?
- How cost-effective are the different models?

Mental health needs in primary healthcare

The first stage of developing mental health services is an assessment of need. The aim here will be to assess the needs of people using primary healthcare. To enable a comparison throughout all components of this evaluation, a third GP practice that will not initially receive the pilot service will be recruited. The CMHT, psychiatrists, in-patient wards and day services will be asked to identify all people using mental health services who are under the care of the three practices (total population 42 000). GPs within the practices will then be asked to augment these lists with anybody else whom they feel should receive mental health services. Mental health services, or GPs, as appropriate will be asked to rate whether each individual person meets severity criteria as used by the Audit Commission. In addition, they will be asked to give socio-demographic details, mental health history and to complete a Health of the Nation Outcome Scale (HoNOS). A similar needs assessment method has been successfully employed by the Jonsen Centre in a previous study carried out at the secondary level. Estimate 3 months' work for a full-time junior researcher with support from senior evaluation staff (13 days).

Role of the primary healthcare and CMHT mental health nurse

On the basis of needs identified, the Jonsen Centre will carry out key informant interviews, e.g. with service users, GPs, CPNs, Consultant Psychiatrists, Social Workers, trust managers and purchasers. The results of the needs assessment, key informant interviews and expertise gained from other evaluations and research will be presented by the Jonsen Centre as advice to a

decision-making steering group. Estimate 2 month junior researcher plus high level of input from senior staff (10 days).

The proposals then continued with three pages of details of the comparative analyses to be carried out. A final statement was given of The Jonsen Centre's policy on dissemination.

Dissemination

The Jonsen Centre would like to report at regular intervals to a steering group with local purchasers in the lead. An interim written report will be provided after the needs assessment. A final report will be produced after the impact stages. Findings will also be presented to study participants such as the primary healthcare teams and CMHT.

Our usual policy is as follows:

The Jonsen Centre undertakes work of this nature so as to inform the national mental health field of progressive developments. Publication will therefore be sought by the Jonsen Centre. No individual service user or member of staff will be identifiable in any report or publication, without their express consent. Organizations will be given copies of intended publications in advance so that they may comment.

The Jonsen Centre takes pride in the quality and independence of its evaluations. Evaluation commissioners should be aware that study findings may not be seen as positive by all interested parties.

After careful consideration of the proposal, the Committee asked the Chair to write to The Jonsen Centre for clarification as follows,

ACTIVITY: What would be your assessment of the ethical implications of this research? Would you allow it to proceed at this stage or would you require more information about the nature of the research? If you were the chair of the ethics committee, what questions would you want to ask the researcher at this stage?

A CASE OF RESEARCH OR AUDIT
(cont.)

John Jones
Head of Service Evaluation
The Jonsen Centre for Mental Health

Dear Mr Jones

re: Evaluation of primary mental healthcare project

Many thanks for sending me these proposals which were considered by the Erehwon Research Ethics Committee yesterday.

The Committee have asked me to thank you for the clear and detailed information you supplied. They recognize the importance of the project, the need to complete it as soon as possible, and the central place you give to obtaining the views of those with serious mental illnesses.

They have asked for:

(a) Further information on the process by which consent will be obtained at Stage 2, including sight of the patient information sheet and consent form.

(b) Your comments on the absence of consent for Stage 1. Their concern here is that releasing information to your researcher in the form described could amount to a serious breach of confidentiality.

Yours sincerely

Mr L. R. Smith
Chair
Erehwon Research Ethics Committee

John Jones replied . . .

Mr L. R. Smith
Chair
Erehwon Research Ethics Committee

Dear Mr Smith

I hope the following notes will provide you with enough information on how we intend to approach service users and store data.

(a) Mental health needs in primary care

All primary and secondary services will be asked to identify all people who use, or should be using, mental health services. Names of individuals along with basic socio-demographic details, diagnosis and professional's Health of the Nation Outcome Scale Rating will be collected. The use of names is essential so that 'doubles', i.e. people who use more than one service, can be identified.

Based on our work elsewhere we would estimate that there will be five to ten people per 1000 population in contact with services. At the top end there may therefore be 420 people identified, and it would not be feasible to ask each individual for consent to include them in this very limited needs assessment. As soon as all 'doubles' have been identified all individual identifiers will be stripped from the database.

Raw data will only be available to Jonsen Centre research staff and will only be used for research purposes. The Jonsen Centre is registered under the Data Protection Act. All reports based on this data will be summary in nature and it will not be possible to identify any individual service user. All paper records will be kept in a locked cupboard and only the local researcher will have access. These records will then be transferred to the Jonsen Centre's locked store. Once the needs assessment reports have been accepted, all original paper records will be shredded.

(b) Role of primary healthcare and the CMHT mental health nurse

A small number of service users will be approached to participate in a more qualitative semi-structured interview. Consent will be obtained in advance on all occasions. Confidentiality will be assured and no individual will be identified in any report.

Patients will be approached initially through their General Practitioner who will send them the attached Information Sheet and Consent Form. If they return the form, an appointment will be made for them with the Jonsen Centre researcher, Rebecca Smith, to be seen at Erehwon Health. The latter have agreed to provide a room for the interviews in which participants can talk freely without fear of being overheard. Rebecca Smith is a former psychiatric social worker and has considerable experience working with people with severe mental illness. The Study has been costed to allow her sufficient time to explain the aims of the study to participants and to answer any questions they may have. If they are still happy to proceed she will then continue with the interview.

Our intentions with this study are to provide a feasible way of making the best use of information that is already collected. The only additional data for part 1 is the HoNOS, which is set to become part of the Department of Health's minimum data set requirement for all providers. Where users are to be interviewed, in Part 2, prior consent will be obtained.

Please do get back to me if you require further details.

With best wishes.

Yours sincerely,

John Jones
Head of Service Evaluation

ACTIVITY: A copy of the proposed Patient Information Sheet and Consent Form were attached to the letter. Before you read the Patient Information Sheet take a few moments to make a short list of all the qualities you consider essential to a Patient Information Sheet and Consent Form. Then check the following example to see if it meets these standards. Perhaps, in the light of your reading, you will feel you should add further items to your list.

The Jonsen Centre for Mental Health

Evaluation of Mental Health Services' response to needs identified in Primary Care

Patient information sheet and consent form

The Jonsen Centre for Mental Health is an independent charity which specializes in developing services and in carrying out research into issues around mental health. The Jonsen Centre has been commissioned by Erehwon Health Authority to carry out this piece of research, which focuses on the role of community psychiatric nurses (CPNs) who work in primary healthcare teams (GP practices) and in the community mental health team.

One way of finding out about the different work and role of CPNs working in primary healthcare teams and in the community mental health team is to gain the views of people who use these/their services. Your opinions are therefore extremely important in helping to find out how CPNs work in different settings.

The interviews, which will last on average 40 minutes, will be conducted by Rebecca Smith, a researcher from The Jonsen Centre, who is based at the Health Authority. The information that you give will only be available to the researcher and a statistician at the Jonsen Centre (who will help in analysing the information) and nobody providing your care, including your GP or any health professional, will have access to your answers. You can withdraw from the study at any time and this will not affect the services that you receive. All the information is confidential and will be kept securely. Serial numbers will be allocated to ensure anonymity and confidentiality will be respected at all times. In order to participate in the study, please complete the consent form below and return it to your GP.

I agree to participate in the study being conducted by The Jonsen Centre and agree to be interviewed by Rebecca Smith.

Name ....

Signed ....

Date ....

> **ACTIVITY:** Now read the following account of how the review process proceeded to a conclusion. After you have read it through, take a few moments to consider the process as a whole from start to finish. Do you think that this was a good example of ethical review? What would be the qualities essential to an effective and ethical process of ethical review? Add these to your checklist.

The Committee's response

L. R. Smith reviewed all this new information under 'Chair's action'. He felt that the consent procedures proposed for Stage 2 would be acceptable to the Committee. The form made clear in particular, (a) who was doing the research, (b) who had commissioned it, (c) its aims and why the views of participants were important, (d) the name of the researcher, (e) that confidentiality would be ensured (in particular in respect of those on whom the patient depended for services), and (f) that subjects could refuse to take part or withdraw at any time without prejudicing the services they receive.

All the relevant points had therefore been covered. Moreover, the process by which consent was to be obtained seemed fine. Firstly, patients would be approached initially through their own GPs. Secondly, the Information Sheet was clearly written: some of the language used seemed a little technical, e.g. 'serial numbers will be allocated to ensure anonymity...', but the main messages seemed clear. Thirdly, if patients agreed to take part, they would have an opportunity to talk through the project with a researcher, who was experienced in working with people with severe mental illness. Finally, the circumstances in which the interviews would take place (as described in John Jones's letter) were acceptable.

Methodologically, there would be some advantage in interviewing patients in the familiar environment of their own homes. But a confidential room at the offices of Erehwon Health should allow patients to talk freely about any problems they had encountered with the services they were receiving.

In relation to Stage 1, however, the further information supplied by John Jones reinforced his (L. R. Smith's) concerns. It seemed that there really would be a substantial breach of confidentiality, not only for those receiving mental health services but also for those who, in the GP's opinion, 'should be using' them. The problem was clearly recognised by The Jonsen Centre, but, if the research was to go ahead, they considered it essential that information from the GPs should be personally identified in order to avoid double counting. It was not feasible to obtain consent because of the large numbers potentially involved.

Action plan

L. R. Smith was now clear that his Committee could not approve the Jonsen Centre proposals, important as the research was, in their present form. He could have written to John Jones at the Jonsen Centre to this effect, leaving it to him and the Commissioning authority, Erehwon Health, either to come up with a revised protocol or to drop their evaluation altogether. Instead, he decided to build on the positive working relationship that had been established to suggest that John Jones might liase with a member of the Research Ethics Committee who had specialized in mental health research, to see if they could come up with a mutually acceptable plan. This could then be put to the full committee.

In the event, the solution was straightforward, though not without resource implications – it was to introduce an additional step into the data-gathering process in Stage 1 whereby the breach of confidentiality could be avoided. The lists of names produced by the GPs would be scrutinized initially by someone from Erehwon Health who was entitled to see them. This 'scrutineer' would be responsible for identifying any 'doubles', subjects would then be labelled with serial numbers. The Jonsen Centre researcher would then correlate the serial numbers with the information provided about each subject.

Erehwon Health agreed to make the additional resources available and the Committee approved the proposal on this basis at its next meeting.

Follow-up

Although the revised protocol worked up to a point, a number of difficulties were encountered. Firstly, Erehwon Health found it difficult to provide a scrutineer who could work consistently with the researchers. Hence there were a number of discontinuities and the Jonsen Centre were not fully satisfied that all doubles had been identified. Secondly, there was evidence that some 'doubles' were using different names. A single researcher with access to all the relevant information might have been able to identify these. Overall, the Jonsen Centre's conclusion was that the 'blind' method did not work.

On the other hand, there was evidence, particularly from the interviews in the second stage of the research, that a growing number of those with long-term mental health problems were seeking help through advisory groups, such as MIND, or through alternative or complementary services (including local churches and other faiths, and counsellors and psychotherapists). This appeared to be in part because of a growing concern among users about confidentiality. To this extent, then, the LREC's original concerns, notwithstanding the methodological difficulties, were justified.

Most researchers strongly support the principle of ensuring that all research, evaluation and audit should be considered by local research ethics committees. However, there is a difficult tension to manage. Individual service users' immediate interests may be best served by not releasing named information to an organization working on behalf of the health authority. But on the other hand, the health authority has a duty to act in the interest of society and the long-term interests of service users. For the health authority to carry out these obligations they must assess need and evaluate the care provided to meet these needs. To do this effectively, health authorities will require named data. They may, of course, have the resources to evaluate their own services. But this is not always satisfactory, self-assessment being peculiarly prone to bias. Social Services already have a duty to find 'Best Value' by using external agencies. Health Services may well have to follow, particularly if, as is proposed in some parts of the UK, Health and Social Services come together into single provider agencies. Faced with the additional difficulties that this will generate, it will be even more essential that commissioners of research, LRECs and researchers work together in a positive problem-solving approach.

ACTIVITY: The case we have been reading shows the importance of a good relationship between researchers and research ethics committees and shows too the importance of subjecting all research proposals to a rigorous process of ethical review. We would now like you to go on to consider the extent to which it is possible to come up with a workable set of ethical principles of medical research. We would like you to do this by means of a guided reading exercise based on a paper by K.W.M Fulford. In his paper on the 3 Rs of Medical Research, which follows, Professor Fulford discusses the problems raised by the ethical review of medical research and proposes a framework for such review. We would like you to read his paper and, as you do so, to attempt to identify any further additional questions it suggests that it might be useful to ask researchers. Add these to your checklist. Note that Fulford is principally concerned with research in psychiatry. How would these principles apply to other types of research?

The 3Rs of medical research

K.W.M. Fulford

Is this good research?

What is most important is often what is left out. What is said may be important. But what is not said, the gaps and contradictions in the proposal, are often particularly significant ethically. This is not because researchers set out to deceive themselves or others. It is because the imperatives that drive research push one to think about a given project from a particular point of view. We have found a structured framework provided by the following four principles particularly helpful in opening our eyes to aspects of a situation we had neglected.[1]

(a) Knowledge: the proposed research should be likely to produce an increase in knowledge directly or indirectly relevant to patient care.

(b) Necessity: it should be necessary for the research to be carried out with the subjects proposed rather than with some less vulnerable group.

(c) Benefits: the potential benefits arising from the research should outweigh any inherent risks of harm.

(d) Consent: research subjects should give valid (i.e. free and informed) consent to their participation.

> ACTIVITY: Fulford argues that these principles can be used to assess research in any area of medicine. As you read through the next section of his paper in which he describes the principles more fully, we would like you to attempt to apply them to the Jonsen Centre's proposals which you read earlier. Are there areas of research and ethical problems that arise in research that would not be captured by the principles approach suggested by Fulford?

(a) Knowledge: The 'corpus of knowledge' is less well established in psychiatry than in other

---

[1] The four principles were first described in Fulford and Howse (1993).

areas. This is due to scientific difficulty rather than scientific inadequacy. All the same, the lack of consensus in psychiatry is problematic. Against this, psychiatry offers the advantage that much of its research is close to the clinical coal face: the relative lack of mature theories of brain functioning means that the gap between research and clinical practice is much smaller than in, say, biochemical research on neurological disorders. Psychiatry has its theory–practice 'gaps', of course. Genetic research, in particular, leaves a whole series of intervening variables between the data and their practical applications. But the Jonsen Centre proposals fall firmly into the category of research which is directly relevant to practice: it is concerned with the needs of users and the cost-effectiveness of two models for supplying relevant services; its particular focus is those with severe mental illness; and the design proposed makes the views of users themselves central to the appraisal process.

(b) Necessity: This principle implies a rough hierarchy: that in vitro preparations be used in preference to animals, that animals be used in preference to healthy subjects, and that healthy subjects be used in preference to patients. This principle, too, presents particular problems for psychiatric research. This is essentially because many forms of psychopathology are uniquely human experiences. There are animal models for, say, some forms of obsessive–compulsive disorder; but even here the gap between animal model and human counterpart is considerable (it includes, for example, the whole question of the meaning of the phenomena for the individual concerned; and when it comes to symptoms like thought insertion, which require the capacity for second-order thinking, animal models are simply not available.

The principle of necessity is also important as between different groups of patients. For example, in dementia research it is important to work where possible with subjects who still have capacity for consent; or, in general, to work with patients who are not being treated under the Mental Health Act or are in prison. The Jonsen Centre proposals illustrate that, notwithstanding the principle of necessity, it is often important in psychiatry actually to involve the most vulnerable groups (i.e. those with serious mental illness) to ensure that their voice is heard.

(c) Benefit: The calculation of the balance of benefits to risk is complicated in psychiatry by both empirical and evaluative factors. Empirical factors include the lack of an agreed 'corpus' of knowledge noted above. Perhaps even more significant, though, is the diversity of values by which, as we have several times emphasized, psychiatry is characterized. This is important for both sides of the equation: what is an unacceptable risk to one person, may be entirely acceptable to another; what is a clear benefit to one person may be a disbenefit to another.

The Jonsen Centre proposals, in so far as they are confined to gathering information, may appear to present little in the way of risk. This is one reason why audit is often considered not to require ethical review. We will see in a moment that this is over-simplified. But it is important to be aware just how risk-laden non-invasive techniques like interviewing may be. The standard paradigms of high risk in research are patients being given a new drug or subjected to an 'experimental' operation. Far less calculable though are the effects of being asked a series of probing questions, or, merely, of being 'recruited' into a trial in the first place. Randomization, too, the basis of modern research methods, may be a highly adverse experience where subjects feel that they or their relatives have been denied standard treatments.

(d) Consent: Both limbs of the consent formula – freedom of choice and information – may be problematic in psychiatric research. We will look at these briefly before applying them to the Jonsen proposals.

Constraints on freedom of choice may be external or internal. External constraints arise from the unequal power relationship between doctors and patients. Pressure to take part in research is rarely overt: but concerns for one's treatment, or inducements, may amount to strong covert pressures. Patients who are being treated on an involuntary basis, and mentally abnormal offenders in prisons or other institutions, are particularly vulnerable in this respect.

Internal constraints on freedom of choice are generated in a number of ways by different kinds of psychopathology: people who are depressed, or suffering from long-term schizophrenia, are sometimes unduly compliant; obsessive–compulsive disorders may involve a pathological inability to make up one's mind; and patients suffering from psychotic disorders may have aberrant (and often concealed) motivations. A psychotically depressed man, for example, agreed to take part in a research project which involved having some blood taken. He appeared to understand what was being asked of him and to be fully capable of consenting to this procedure. Subsequently, however, it was discovered that his interpretation of the situation had been that he was to be executed. He welcomed this because his profound delusions of guilt led him to believe that he deserved to die and that everyone around him would be better off if he were dead.

Psychopathology may also generate problems for the information limb of the consent formula. Thus, patients with dementia may be unable to retain or recall even quite limited amounts of new information. Depression slows information processing. Anxiety may block it altogether. Hypomania involves marked distractibility.

> **ACTIVITY:** These are striking examples that can arise in relation to consent. To what extent do you think that this is a problem for psychiatry alone? Later in this chapter we shall be going on to explore the concept of consent in more detail.

Problems of this kind, furthermore, complicate the general problem in research ethics of how much information is required for consent to be valid. In clinical work, in the UK, a 'prudent doctor' standard (set by the 'Bolam' test) still prevails. Even in clinical work, though, law and practice are moving towards a 'prudent patient' test. In research, this is already the norm (reflecting the more exacting standards arising from the difference of intent between research and clinical work). Thus the Royal College of Physicians suggests that 'any benefits and hazards' must be explained to research subjects (RCP, 1990). The standard set by the Royal College of Psychiatrists' Guidelines is 'important' risks, what is 'important' being a matter for a research ethics committee, which should 'apply common-sense to decide what level of risk would be likely to affect a reasonable person's decision'. (Psychiatric Bulletin, 1990). This is helpful advice, then.

We can now apply these general principles to the Jonsen proposals. Taking Stage 2 first, which involves interviewing key informants, consent is clearly an issue. Among the key informants will be those suffering from severe mental illness whose capacity to consent may be in question. We return later to the general problem of research with patients unable to consent. But in this case, the general approach recommended by The Royal College of Psychiatrists' Guidelines seems apposite. The research subjects concerned are living in the community and hence are unlikely to be wholly without the capacity for consent to an interview. Moreover, the aim of the interview, to elicit their opinions on the success or otherwise of the local mental health services, is very much in their best interests. To be excluded from the research would indeed be clearly against their interests. On the other hand, there is clearly an issue of power relations (patients may feel the answers they give could prejudice their future care); and it is important that the process of consent is carefully geared to the capacities of those concerned. On these issues, the Committee felt they needed further information. In particular, they wanted to see the patient information sheet and consent form.

Stage 1 of the proposals, however, which

Christine Ready had somewhat discounted in her original letter to the Chair of the Research Ethics Committee, in fact appeared more problematic. The difficulty the Committee identified was that Stage 1 appeared to involve the release of confidential, and potentially sensitive, information to a third party (the Centre researcher) without consent. This would amount to a clear and potentially serious breach of confidentiality.

ACTIVITY: How did you get on with your attempt to use these principles to analyse the Jonsen case? We began this section by investigating the nature of medical research and have ended it by elaborating some principles of research ethics. As we come to the end of this first section of the chapter, we would like you to stop for a few moments and take a look at the checklist you have been constructing as you read the case. Is there anything you feel ought to be added to the list at this stage? Remember that the checklist is to be framed as a set of questions one would ask oneself when assessing the ethical implications of a piece of research.

Below is a list of some of the questions we came up with.

- Is the proposed research going to offer some benefit? Is it going to answer the proposed question? Is this an important question?
- Is it necessary for this research to be carried out on human subjects? Could the answers be gained in the laboratory, or by animal studies?
- What is the balance of harms and risks likely to occur as a result of the research?
- Is there a Patient Information Sheet? Is this clear and accessible to the research subjects who will be asked to participate in the study?
- Are the subjects going to be asked to give their consent? Will this consent be valid? Is there a consent form? Is it clear (as above)? Who will be asking the potential subjects for their consent?
- Is it clear to the subjects that they can withdraw from the study at any time and that this will not affect the quality of their treatment?
- Does it make it clear that the subject can refuse to participate and that this too will not affect the treatment received?

Section 2: Valid consent

ACTIVITY: On the basis of what you have learned from this chapter thus far we would like you now to consider the research proposal described below. What do you think are the central ethical questions it raises? Bearing in mind all the issues, would you let them proceed? If not, what suggestions would you make?

A CASE OF GENETIC RESEARCH

The research ethics committee of a major teaching hospital receives a proposal from researchers associated with a major migraine clinic asking for permission to do gene tests on their clinic patients and their families. The researchers are particularly interested to discover whether one variant of a gene called ApoE is associated with migraine.

Most of the patients at the clinic are young. The clinic has an excellent reputation and good loyalty from its patients. Indeed, the research ethics committee knows that the researchers concerned are one of the teams in the hospital with an international reputation for excellent research.

A problem arises, however, because the team mentions in its application that, in addition to its suspected association with migraine, variants of the ApoE gene they wish to study may also be associated with an early age onset of Alzheimer's disease. Because of this they suggest that they should keep the genetic information they get to themselves and not advise the patients and families.

They say, rightly, that the implications of having the ApoE allele are not completely clear, and in any case they have neither the time nor the money to organize counselling. They also say that their study is very much related to migraine, and that if there is a risk of Alzheimer's disease, the onset will be many years in the future, and telling people would only create unnecessary worry.

ACTIVITY: What are the arguments for and against allowing the research to proceed as proposed?

When we read the case, we thought that the main ethical concern with this case outline is the question of the extent to which subjects are adequately informed about the research.

In a nutshell, a proper consent is a clear, open, intentional – and, we might usefully add, true – statement by the subject that he understands what he is about to do and that he freely chooses to do it. This is possible only where two conditions have been met: first: his choice must be based on his possessing and understanding all the information which is relevant to making the choice; and second the choice must have been made freely, without pressure. There are, of course, difficulties in knowing quite how much is 'all that is relevant' and in knowing quite what is to count as pressure [. . .] But unless it can reasonably be said that the two conditions have been met, then a proper consent has not been given (Evans and Evans, 1996: 78–79).

ACTIVITY: The question of just how much information is reasonably required for the subject to have given his or her valid consent is an important question. For the requirement for consent to be voluntary, competent and informed may appear on a strict definition to rule out virtually all research. How should we go about deciding whether a research subject is going to be giving a valid informed consent? What is it to be 'reasonably informed'?

As Evans and Evans point out above, one of the most fundamental principles in the ethics of medical research is that no one should be enrolled onto a research study without their explicit consent. This clearly means a great deal more than that they have simply said 'I agree' or have signed the bottom of a consent form. In this section we shall be exploring the ethical issues which arise in relation to the question of consent in medical research. Start by reading an extended extract from a paper by Richard Ashcroft in which he addresses the role of informed consent in medical research. He investigates the extent to which the concept of 'explicit informed consent' can act alone as a criterion of ethical research on human subjects and looks at the types of situations in which the criterion may have to be modified, for example in situations where potential research subjects are incapable of providing explicit consent and yet research on them seems to be ethical under certain circumstances.

Autonomy and informed consent in the ethics of the randomized controlled trial: philosophical perspectives

Richard Ashcroft
(In Ashcroft et al., 1997)

Introduction

There are two central principles in human experimentation ethics. The first is that the experiment should be scientifically sound and present a fair proportionality of risk to benefit to the subject. This is uncontroversial, although it can be difficult to spell out this principle in detail in practical situations. The second principle is that no one should be enrolled into an experiment without their express, informed consent. In what follows I examine the arguments used to defend this second principle, and the arguments used to defend departures from it (including the ways departures are sometimes tacitly brought about sans argument). I do not discuss the legal context of the consent doctrine, which is not specific to clinical experimentation, and which is in any case well known. Nor do I discuss in depth the arguments about consent by minors or the mentally ill.

The randomized controlled clinical trial is a type of experiment on human subjects. As such, it falls within the domain of the 'Nuremberg Code', and the 'World Medical Association Declaration of Helsinki'.[1,2] Both of these codes were framed with the Nuremberg War Crimes trials in mind, and sought to specify minimal conditions on human experimentation, such that basic human rights should be protected and respected in all experiments which use human beings as subjects. The aim of these codes is essentially protective; and the philosophical premise of the rights which are

described – or perhaps stipulated or constituted – by these declarations is individualist.[3,4] In other words, each individual's well-being and integrity takes precedence over the interests of the social body, especially the fraction of the social body which is the state.[5,6] This is, of course, directly targeted against totalitarian doctrines which hold that on certain occasions, or for certain groups of subjects, the interests of the state (or the remainder of the social body) are taken to be rights, and to take precedence over those of the individual subject.

I will concentrate discussion on the Nuremberg codes provisions, because it is the simplest, clearest and oldest relevant code on ethics of experimentation. The later Helsinki codes preserve substantially the same position, but devote much more attention to explaining the notions of risk and benefit, which clarifies some considerations about fair risks for incompetent subjects. Arguably, the Helsinki codes weaken the force of the Nuremberg principles, however, and for clarity about the stakes in the debates on consent I concentrate on their original expression in the Nuremberg code.

ACTIVITY: It is clear that the Nazi experiments involved a gross violation of individual human rights, but to what extent do you think it is true to say that individual rights should always take precedence over the public interest or benefit?

One factor which seems to creep in at this stage is the question of the balance between the need for informed consent and public benefit to be gained from the research. Taking the case above, for example, it might be the case that informing the research subjects about the link with Alzheimer's would mean that no one would be willing to take part in the research. Are there situations or types of research in which you consider the informed consent of research subjects to be less important or to be outweighed by the public interest in the research? What, for example, about research involving linking a great many patient records? How would you go about deciding whether and to what extent informed consent was required in such research? What are the dangers associated with justifying research solely on the basis of public interest? What are the dangers of justifying research solely on the basis of informed consent?

Voluntary consent

The first principle of the Nuremberg code states that for research to be ethical, 'the voluntary consent of the human subject is absolutely essential'. In other words, each and every subject in the experiment must give their voluntary consent to be part of the experiment. As this stands it is very unclear what is required; is it enough to say to a subject 'would you like to take part in an experiment?' without saying any more? And would an affirmative reply constitute consent in the required sense? Not yet, because the test of voluntariness may not be passed. And as this test of voluntariness is the nub of the matter, we cannot leave it with the investigating physician's own satisfaction that the patient (or healthy volunteer) has consented voluntarily. Indeed, remembering that the Nuremberg Code has a legal dimension as well as an ethical one, some criterion assessable by a third party is required.[7]

Not only is the principle much more vague than its simplicity seems to imply, it has also some medically puzzling features. It seems to rule out any experimental procedures where the normal condition of the subject is such as to rule out voluntary, or even involuntary consent. Under this test, no experiments seem possible in emergency medicine, in perinatology, in psychiatry or clinical psychology, and probably in most paediatric medicine. Arguably, it disallows any research on pregnant women, not because the women cannot give consent, but because the foetuses cannot.[8] The principle is quite explicit: and so-called proxy consent is no consent at all.[9,10]

ACTIVITY: How would you deal with the question of consent in cases where explicit consent is not possible? Ashcroft goes on next to look at how the principle of voluntary consent might be modified in order that it both provide adequate protection and also allow ethical research to proceed.

Premises of the consent requirement

Let us examine now the premises of the argument for voluntary consent. In the first place, we took it that the principle of voluntary consent is a moral rule. Next, the principle takes as read the principle of individualism as mentioned at the outset. Thirdly, there is a clear distinction between experimental and other sorts of medical care.[11,12,13] Fourthly, there is the presumption that human subjects need protecting.[14]

If we want to avoid the conclusion that much medical research will become impossible if we grant the principle of voluntary consent, then we will need to weaken or discard one or more of these premises. Before we do this, let us reflect on what this principle does not say.

Nothing philosophical is asserted about voluntariness or autonomy or personhood: but it is clear that each human subject – whatever we take that to mean – must voluntarily consent to taking part in the experiment, whatever voluntary consent is.[15,16,17] The words here have – at least – their common-sense meaning. So an unconscious patient has not consented, for example.[18,19,20,21] Nor has a member of a football club consented to participate, simply because his club chairman has indicated that his club as a corporate body will participate in the experiment. Only human subjects are mentioned in the principle, and whatever a collective is, it is not a human subject.

The principle makes no claim to sufficiency. We can easily imagine 'experiments' where a number of human subjects voluntarily consent to take part, but we would not (as outsiders) regard these experiments as ethical. The authors of the Nuremberg Code reflect this point, by following the principle of voluntary consent with a series of nine other principles. The bulk of these concern experimental risks and scientific utility and competence. The final two principles state the right of the subject to leave the experiment at any time (subject to a condition which I will discuss later) and the obligation of the researcher to terminate the experiment if the experiment becomes, in its process, dangerous to the subject. This last principle, stating the investigator's duty to terminate an experiment early under certain conditions, will prove troublesome when we look at randomised controlled trials.

ACTIVITY: Can you think of experiments in which we might consider it to be the case that even if someone gave their informed consent, the research would be unethical? If so, it seems Ashcroft is right to suggest that voluntary consent is by itself insufficient to cover all the ethical issues.

The final element about which the Nuremberg Code is silent is the element which the Helsinki Declaration faces directly: the nature of specifically medical obligations to patient subjects in biomedical research. Nothing in the Nuremberg Code is intended to have specific relevance to this issue. This is slightly puzzling because the Nuremberg Code is addressed to the medical profession and speaks of 'Permissible Medical Experiments'. But nothing is said concerning the experimenter's obligations vis a vis the Hippocratic code of medical ethics (or indeed any other vademecum of medical obligations, responsibilities and purposes). The authors of the Code state that most experiments, to the best of their belief, do 'conform to the ethics of the medical profession generally'.

Note at this point that medical ethics is conceived not on an individual basis but a collective one: the duties of the doctor are framed as elements of a professional ethic, not as duties analytically derivable from the concept of medicine. There is something of a tension in later developments of medical ethics between perspectives which emphasise the collective and traditional, or socio-legal, foundations of medical right, and those which emphasise supposedly self-evident principles of medical good practice (substantively or procedurally justified).

The question of the relationship between the principle of voluntary consent and the ethics of routine medical practice is open, so far as the Nuremberg Code indicates. It may be that the principle of voluntary consent is an additional and independent principle which supplements those of medical ethics in experimental contexts. Or, it could be that the principle of voluntary consent is logically independent of the ordinary principles of medical ethics, and the possibility exists that the two sets of principles will conflict in some situation. Or, it could be that the principle of voluntary consent applies in all experimental situations involving human subjects, and the principles of medical ethics amplify and supplement this principle in just those cases where the experiment has some medical significance; for instance where the human subject has been enrolled into the experiment qua patient.

Most of the experiments (or pseudo-experiments) which the authors of the Code had in mind were experiments of no direct medical merit for the subjects (not all of the experiments were medically uninformative, although many were, and there has been some debate about whether the use of the results of these experiments was legitimate, given the way in which the results were obtained). And many were of no direct medical relevance at all, being natural-historical or physiological in character. As such, these experiments could not be considered part of normal or innovative medical care. The point of the principle of voluntary consent was to ensure that experiments of this kind were legitimate, subject to consent. Naturally, in many cases the conduct of these experiments would require medical help to be on hand, or indeed that the investigator be a medical professional. Whether all such experiments had to be carried out under the scrutiny and professional ethics of the medical profession is probably an issue in disciplinary politics rather than law or ethics. So, as far as ethics is concerned, we can rule out the first possibility that human experimentation is a specialized branch of medicine, and should be governed by medical ethics as supplemented by the principle of voluntary consent. On the other hand, we can accept without further comment the argument that the principle applies to all human subject experiments, but needs supplementing with the ethics of medical care when the experiment is carried out using subjects who are patients (even if their patienthood has nothing to do directly with the topic of the experiment). Or can we?

ACTIVITY: Ashcroft raises an interesting question here about the relationship between the ethics of medical research and the ethics of medicine more broadly. To what extent does the principle of respect for voluntary consent conflict with other ethical demands in medicine and in such situations what ought to be done?

Is consent consistent with beneficence?

The second possibility (having dismissed the first and accepted the third) is that the principle of voluntary consent conflicts – either always or on occasion – with sound medical ethics. We saw that the raw principle seems to conflict with medicine in some common cases (children, the mentally incompetent, etc.). Many writers have argued that medical experiments – especially the randomized controlled trial – involve a conflict of principles, or, on many accounts, of roles.[22,23,24] The role conflict they have in mind is the conflict between the investigator as doctor and the investigator as scientist; and to complicate matters further we could balance that with a conflict of roles between the individual as patient and the individual as subject.

ACTIVITY: Make a list of situations in which steadfast adherence to the principle of voluntary consent might go against the duty to benefit the patient. What ought to be done in such situations? What other kinds of ethical arguments are there which would demand that we override the subject's consent, and when?

Does duty override consent?

Given the protection-oriented nature of the Nuremberg Code, it is natural to emphasize the duties of the investigating physician and the rights of the patient-subject. Also, in context, it is natural to suppose that arguments about the rights of the physician and the duties of the patient-subject are

to be resisted. The sort of duty which could be conceived and which the authors of the Code want to resist is a duty on the part of the patient to society at large.[25,26,27,28] What the authors presumably want to resist here is not the idea that I may regard myself as owing a duty to my fellow citizens, or to my species, but that society may impose such a duty upon me, with attendant sanctions. A natural analogy might be drawn between the duties a soldier owes to his state and the duties a patient might be taken to owe; and, in particular, the duties a citizen owes to the state in the sense of an obligation to undergo military conscription. The core of the obligation to undergo conscription is the so-called 'free-rider' problem, where individuals enjoy the use of some social good (for instance civil liberty) without contributing to the social (and economic) costs necessary for the maintenance of that good. Conscription aims, among other things, to distribute fairly the chances of paying with injury or death the military costs of a state's liberty, in such a way as to avoid the free-rider problems that may be judged to arise if a war is fought with only voluntary enlistment. A similar argument concerns the development of new drugs. Drug development always involves testing for safety and efficacy on human beings. Since some people will be needed to be subjects for any given innovative treatment, is someone who persistently refuses to take part in drug testing as a subject, but who benefits from the outcomes of such testing, to be regarded as immoral? And if they are, what social sanctions might be merited? Related to this is the argument that convicted criminals might be regarded as owing some measure of participation in human experimentation as part of their 'debt to society', either because they have partially forfeited their right to refuse consent, or as a full or partial substitute for their penal servitude.[29,30,31,32]

ACTIVITY: To what extent is it reasonable to say that we have a social duty to participate in medical research? If this is the case what are the limits of such a duty? Ashcroft goes on in the next part of his paper to provide an argument about social and civic responsibility to deal with conflict between public interest and informed consent. As you read it consider how we decide the balance ethically? Do you think we might have an obligation to participate in some sort of medical research? What kind? What are the limits?

The relevance of these arguments, which have an alarming sound to the liberal ear, is that many of them were tacitly or explicitly accepted in many states at the time the Nuremberg Code was being framed. And furthermore, the statist character of these arguments may be regarded as tendentious, but the moral arguments from analogy to what most liberal democracies (and perhaps all states) are prepared to accept are not trivial to refute. It is better to understand the refusal to press the analogy as founded not on self-vindicating moral principles, but on a stipulation that this is the set of moral standards in this limited area which the global community will now adopt and commit ourselves to abide by. The problem with this is that the principles of the Nuremberg Code were in part intended to be self-evident moral principles, against which the activities of figures such as Dr Josef Mengele could be judged. Later revelations about experiments carried out by Allied states following (tacitly or explicitly) the analogy between conscription and a 'duty' to participate in experimentation only underline the ironies of the Nuremberg stipulations; they do not, for all that, detract from the rightness of those stipulations.[33,34,35,36]

Duty and voluntary action

The gap that must be kept open is the gap between recognition that one may morally be under some partial obligation to take part in human experiments in the medical field and a statist position where this duty can be imposed upon citizens. One argument which may assist us is the argument that where military and fiscal obligations are citizenship duties, rather than social duties; and the putative duty to participate in

medical experiments is if anything, social, and not connected with citizenship. The analogy here that could be stressed is between the need for suitable subjects for medical experiments and the need for volunteer blood-donors. Another analogy may be with duties to charitable giving and to voluntary work in the community. Duties of this kind admit of a variety of interpretations, although most people will admit them, whatever their rationale for doing so. It might be that the religious tenets one adheres to stress charitable giving, for instance. A key feature of duties of this kind is that typically they are only regarded as meaningfully satisfied when the duty is voluntarily performed. There is a complication here: many states partially replace this duty with another kind of duty, the duty to pay progressive taxes as a redistributive measure, or as part of a welfare programme. This sort of enforceable duty is sometimes argued to be destructive of charitable virtues, and many resent doing under obligation what they would happily do out of charity. This type of argument is often made by communitarians.

So once again we return to voluntariness, as referred to in the Nuremberg Code, where we first met it as a barrier to coerced participation, and now we meet it as what makes participation morally significant. This consideration was not in the minds of the authors of the code, however. At this point I should underline the claim that the statist argument about obligations to participate, and the state's right to demand participation rests on an elision of citizen and social duties. It is the defining characteristic of totalitarianism that it conflates the political and social spheres; and so the refusal to accept human experimentation without voluntary consent is all of a piece with the authors of the Code's rejection of National Socialist ideology. We should recall in this connection two of the statist's arguments. The first is the argument from the economic free-rider problem; and the second is the construction a statist may put on consent by analogy with consent to be governed.

Free-riding

The relevance of the first of these arguments will become plain if we consider that the free-rider problem is drawn from economic theory, rather than pure political theory; and this draws our attention to the point that the free-rider problem is a problem for any collective organisation, not only the state. It is also relevant to systems of healthcare considered as partially or fully autonomous of the state apparatus. Typically insurance-funded healthcare systems handle free-ridership *vis à vis* medical experimentation not by penalising non-participants, but by rewarding participants with partial or total waiver of treatment fees. In fact, this oversimplifies: hospitals do not charge patients in trials for the costs of the drug being trialled, recovering the cost either from some research agency, or in kind from the drug companies. And many insurance companies will not pay for experimental treatments, but only for accepted treatments. And, the costs of the experiment are borne not by the subjects, but by future patients and present and future taxpayers. This raises the issue of whether this waiver of payment should be understood as an inducement to participate, and more of that in a moment. Healthcare systems, such as the British National Health Service, which impose no costs on patients, have no financial mechanism for encouraging patients not to be free-riders, and rely instead on a mixture of desperation, altruism, and (perhaps) paternalism to encourage participation. And, the social risk which accompanies this method is that the parallel membership of the British state and the British NHS which is enjoyed by all citizens of the United Kingdom might encourage an investigator to treat this not as parallel membership of two institutions, but as membership of a single institution, thus eliding the citizen and social duties. This, arguably, took place in the United States in the notorious Tuskegee experiments, and this interpretation might be put on the cases reported by Beecher and Pappworth in their famous 'human guinea pig' exposés of the 1960s.[37,38,39] And these works were of great importance in establishing the 'informed consent' test in research ethics, as relevant not only in court judgements about totalitarian regimes, but also in liberal democratic states.

> **ACTIVITY:** Ashcroft argues that it is reasonable and possible to talk about a duty and responsibility to the public interest and at the same time to resist the 'statist' approach. This is because in the one case the responsibility is founded in a voluntary choice whereas in the other it is founded in an erosion of citizenship and of 'social duty'. Do you agree with the argument? If not, why not? If so, why?

'Inferring' consent

The relevance of the second argument is as follows. Is there an analogy between political consent and consent to participation in a medical experiment? In political theory only some minority positions hold that the consent of the people to be governed is irrelevant to the legitimacy of the state (a minority nowadays, that is!). However, with the exception of anarchists and some theorists of direct democracy (as exemplified, perhaps, by the Swiss), almost all democratic theorists regard consent as a variable which only needs to be measured relatively infrequently, and can be assumed to behave smoothly between measurements. Consent to any particular political decision or piece of legislation is taken to be consequent on the so-called electoral mandate: and this is an assumption with bite. It is never normally regarded as a sufficient argument in court that I cannot be regarded as guilty under some law unless I accept that law as binding upon me.

One might make an analogy between this and the medical case as follows. We have separated out the medical and the state spheres, let us assume, but surely once a patient presents himself he can be taken to have consented to be treated, whatever that may involve. And if the treatment administered is experimental, but consistent with what some reasonable doctor might do in the circumstances (and this is – very roughly – the 'Bolam' test applied in English law), then the spirit of the consent can be said to have been respected.

'Medically indicated' treatment

Various elements of medical phraseology reflect this theory of what role consent plays, in particular the concept of 'medically indicated treatment'. Where there is a choice of treatments, with differing effects, but which are probably indifferent with respect to their efficacy with respect to the patient's primary condition, only then may the doctor ask the patient's opinion about which course of treatment they would prefer. While the doctor may discuss the treatment preferences with the patient well before this point is reached, there is no expectation that this is morally or legally required. This perspective on the role of consent and the doctor's expertise is frequently known as paternalist, because it is founded upon the notion that 'doctor knows best'.[40,41] But while it has a paternalist flavour, if it is problematic that is because the notion of consent is notoriously difficult to pin down, particularly in the medical context.[42,43,44] Even the paradigm of competent consent – informed, voluntary and autonomous consent by an educated and reflective adult – has an inferential component, for instance in surgery, especially under general anaesthetic (or even prior to its administration, where something like an advance directive is implied).

We need to distinguish inference to consent which is based on a counterfactual reconstruction of what this subject would say – if they were conscious or mentally competent, from inferred consent of the cognitive type; and both of these kinds of consent need to be distinguished from inferred consent based on what we can call role-expectation.

Cognitive inferred consent

This is my consent for you to do a certain procedure under an accurate description for laymen, from which it can be inferred that whatever is technically necessary to fill in the detail in carrying out that procedure is consented to as well, even though I cannot explicitly be said to consent to it. This sort of consent involves an element of trust in the competence and expertise of the doctor,

which involves in its turn a standard of 'what reasonable medical opinion would accept'. There is a continuum here with my acceptance that the doctor has correctly diagnosed my condition, without my need to verify this myself. I have a right to expect that the doctor knows what he is doing, and why he is doing it.

Counterfactual reconstruction of consent

This also builds on inference from what the patient explicitly consents to prior to operating, or prior to temporary incompetence. It is involved in situations where some course of action has been consented to, and some additional course of action may become indicated, or perhaps convenient, in the course of treatment, when the patient is unable to be consulted. A typical example might be appendectomy in the course of some operation on the digestive tract unconnected with appendix problems; this is sometimes done as a preventive measure, and for convenience, although this is less commonly done without prior consent than it used to be. In any case, it is risky to extend consent in this way because the extension is so unreliable, as the recent case shows of a surgeon carrying out a 'medically indicated' abortion in the course of some surgery, without prior consent. In many cases this inference will be straightforwardly illegal, under criminal law, because it involves an illicit 'touch', that is, a common assault (or worse). This extension quickly shades into what I claim is illegitimate inference to consent, viz. consent inferred from role-expectation.

Paternalism

In this case, rather than building in a limited way on consent to some specific course of action, a doctor may judge that simply because a patient has put himself into his hands, the patient may be taken to have certain expectations of what a doctor is, and infers the patient's consent to whatever the doctor deems necessary without further consultation. This is the essence of medical paternalism. In fact, it has only been agreed that medical paternalism is ethically unsatisfactory in relatively recent times. Less than 20 years ago, articles in the Journal of Medical Ethics (the leading journal in the subject in the UK, frequently read and contributed to by the medical professions as well as the bioethics community) were published making the defence of paternalism (not in so many words!) on the grounds that 'informed consent' was prima facie impossible, and so consent could be obtained by the investigating doctor referring himself to the patient's appointed medical representative.[41] And occasional defences of paternalism are still published, usually based on some argument about information and comprehension.

Arguments of this kind have an important truth, as consultation of empirical articles about actual patient comprehension indicate. Patients, for a variety of reasons, linguistic, educational, psychological and social, frequently do not fully comprehend what they are being asked to consent to, or why, or in what their consent consists, or how far it extends.[45,46] And this is so on most tests – the most telling being the test of recollection: can they, after a decent short interval recall what they have consented to?[47,48] Whether one is entitled to conclude from this that the consent process is a waste of time, or dispensable at any rate, is a moot point, and one that has occupied much space in the medical and ethical journals. My opinion is that there is something suspicious about drawing absolute conclusions concerning the utility of patient consent from facts about the difficulty of achieving it. This is especially to be resisted when much of that difficulty may be regarded as founded upon imperfections in communication.

ACTIVITY: Ashcroft argues that the claim that subjects often or even sometimes find procedures difficult to understand cannot count as a justification for over-riding their consent. Particularly when this is because of difficulties of communication. List the kinds of factors that might make informed consent difficult in this way.

These imperfections may be regarded as being of three kinds. The first kind, the linguistic barrier, is contingent, where some individual or group of patients is unable to understand the information given, either because the information is insufficiently informative, or because the language used is obscure, or because, simply, the patient or doctor is not fully at home in the language being used (perhaps, as in a case reported in the *British Medical Journal* recently, they are first generation immigrants from Vietnam who have learnt English late in life).[49] Here all that is required is that efforts be made to ensure that these contingent imperfections in communication are removed.

The second kind of imperfection, cognitive barriers, might be regarded as necessary: simply, no non-medical professional can reasonably be expected to understand the details of the medical procedure, and so basing the requirement for consent upon a requirement that the patient understand those details would make consent almost impossible to obtain. Consequent upon that would be the necessity of abandoning the experiment. However, the number of experiments where the patient cannot be given a balanced and comprehensible description of the experiment, such that he understands and can make a decision about consent must be vanishingly small.

The third kind of imperfection, social distortions, may be regarded as contingent but 'structural'; that is the contingency relates not to any facts about the individual patient, doctor or treatment, but to social facts. The sort of social facts which are relevant are facts connected with social structure and what Habermas calls 'systematic distortions in communication', which are founded in power relations.[50] Examples of this include: patients not understanding that they are entitled not to give consent; patients not understanding the scientific purpose of the trial and supposing that the novel innovation is (a) more effective and (b) will be administered to them (when they may be randomized to the alternative arm); patients interest in consent to being treated not being equivalent to the doctor's interest in consent to advance medical knowledge; differential attitudes in particular socio-cultural groups to the need for consensual decision-making and appropriate processes for making decisions; differential capacities and opportunities to exercise patients' rights.[51]

All of these 'distortions' to the process of giving voluntary consent can be related in part to social structural factors, and as such are properly the domain of social research rather than philosophy or medicine. But there are three main points to be noted here. The first is that the social context of the consent process (both the micro-context of the sick patient in the interview room in the surgery or hospital, and the wider social, political, cultural and economic contexts of the patient) is relevant to the quality and significance of consent. The second is that consent is obtained in a situation where power is involved in quite complex ways. And the third is that consent is a sort of action (technically, a speech act of a certain kind), such that there are conditions under which verbal consent fails to be consent in the relevant way.

The Nuremberg Code gives an explicit gloss to the meaning of 'voluntary consent' which indicates that the authors recognized that consent was an action involving understanding. The paragraph reads:

This [sc., voluntary consent] means that the person involved should have legal capacity to give consent; should be so situated as to be able to exercise free power of choice, without the intervention of any element of force, fraud, deceit, duress, overreaching, or ulterior form of constraint or coercion; and should have sufficient knowledge and comprehension of the elements of the subject matter involved as to enable him to make an understanding and enlightened decision. The latter element requires that before the acceptance of an affirmative decision by the experimental subject there should be made known to him the nature, duration, and purpose of the experiment; the method and means by which it is to be conducted; all inconveniences and hazards reasonably to be expected; and the effects upon his health or person which may possibly come from his participation in the experiment. (The Nuremberg Code is reproduced in full later in this chapter.)

This statement tells us quite a lot about the meaning of voluntariness. It tells us that consent is

genuine only when free from intentional duress, and only when the giver is in a position to understand the significance and extent of what he is assenting to. In some ways this makes the consent requirement even more restrictive than the naked formulation, because it adds additional tests: notably the core of what later is known as 'informed consent'. Most of the literature on informed consent – and it is very extensive – concentrates on this question of what informed consent should be said to consist in. But it is also interesting that some tests we might set for assent to be consent are not mentioned, here or in any of the subsequent Codes. For instance, we might regard consent given under conditions of desperation as no more genuine than consent given under conditions of duress. And the ways in which desperation can be socially generated are numerous – not only the gravity and severity of an illness, but also economic need, for instance. And consent under desperation usually contains an intention that the novel treatment be received, and so (in the randomised controlled trial) does not intend randomised assignment.[52]

That this is so is illustrated by the subversion of randomisation by AIDS sufferers in certain treatment trials in the late 1980s. This is a fine point. Arguably, these patients acted unethically in giving apparent consent to enrol under the treatment protocol, thus rendering the data in these trials almost useless (although usable to some extent under some interpretations), and perhaps necessitating further trials to retest the hypothesis. But on their part the argument that to be offered a choice between getting the drug, probability 0.5, and getting nothing was not a fair set of alternatives under the circumstances. That this is so has been recognized increasingly in AIDS trials, although multi-armed trials are considerably more expensive, require greater quantities of the probably rare, possibly dangerous experimental drug, and need the enrolment of proportionately more patients.[53]

Conclusion

That the tests an experimental procedure should pass are more restrictive than those we place upon 'ordinary' treatment is not surprising. But what are these tests designed to achieve? As noted above, the tests on consent are meant to distinguish valid consent from invalid pseudo-consents, specifying relevant features of each; and consent itself is meant to ensure that patients are protected from undergoing risks and harms without their knowledge and agreement. Their force, in the Nuremberg Code at least, is to force doctors to seek consent, a matter which the code is quite explicit about, making it a duty upon doctors in the third paragraph of the first section of the Code:

The duty and responsibility for ascertaining the quality of the consent rests upon each individual who initiates, directs or engages in the experiment. It is a personal duty and responsibility which may not be delegated to another with impunity.

A slightly curious feature of this formulation is that it makes of each doctor – in the first instance – his own gatekeeper. Later, both in Britain and in the United States, an additional institution was created, the Local Research Ethics Committee or Institutional Review Board, to oversee the implementation of this requirement and to assess all research for their ethical status (at least *prima facie*).[54,55,56] However, as yet no mechanism exists for ensuring that the researcher will actually do what he says he will in his proposal, and the 'with impunity' sentence in the Code is the weaker for this omission.[57,58] Certain mechanisms exist for enforcing this protective rule, notably the public sanction of the medical journals, which may refuse to publish studies conducted without valid consent processes, and the possibility of medical negligence torts in the case of experimental procedures carried out *sans* consent.[59,60,61] Out and out fraud with respect to consent is uncommon, so far as we know, and two doctors who forged signatures on consent forms were recently struck off by the General Medical Council's professional conduct committee.[62,63]

ACTIVITY: Thus far in this section we have investigated the concept of informed consent by means of a reading exercise using Richard Ashcroft's paper. It seems clear, taking into account the limitations described by Ashcroft, that being informed constitutes at least part of what it means for consent to be valid. He has also pointed out some other requirements, notably that such consent should be competent and uncoerced. In the second part of this section we go on to investigate these requirements by means of a reading exercise on a paper by the Finnish medical lawyer, Salla Lötjönen. Before you start reading the paper, we would like you to take a few minutes to consider the various ways in which obtaining valid consent might prove difficult in practice. If you were a member of a research ethics committee, what questions would you want to ask the researchers in order to ensure that the consent they would obtain would be valid? Then begin your reading of the paper.

Ethical and legal issues concerning the involvement of vulnerable groups in medical research

Salla Lötjönen

In the aftermath of the Second World War and during the trial of the doctors who took part in the inhuman experiments carried out during the Nazi era, the Nuremberg Code was drafted, in 1947. The first and foremost criterion of the Code was the voluntary consent of the human subject which is also recognized in the United Nations Covenant on Civil and Political Rights (1966). Since then, the scope of the requirement for a free and uncoerced consent to experimentation has raised a considerable amount of discussion and it has been the basis for many additional international documents. Mostly, the discussion has concerned the voluntariness or the capacity of experimental subjects.

Voluntariness

The voluntariness of the experimental subject comes into question most of all with regard to institutionalised persons, i.e. prisoners, soldiers, patients subject to involuntary treatment, and patients staying permanently in nursing homes, etc. There are some views which regard institutionalisation as such as excluding voluntariness (e.g. Kaimowitz v Michigan Department of Mental Health). The fear has been that the institution's management or staff could unduly influence the self-determination of the subjects towards participation, or that potential research subjects in an institution would at least regard their choice restricted even if that was not actually the case. It has also been proposed that subjects might participate in a research project in the hope of benefits such as early release, more attention, or simply a change in the daily routine, which have been thought to be inappropriate incentives for participation.

It is questionable whether such incentives really differ significantly from the incentives used at present outside of such settings, which include financial benefit, free or sometimes even better access to treatment or access to a better monitored treatment. Additionally, the groups that are often involved in participating research projects are medical students and hospital staff. Until recently, only few guidelines or conventions have taken these groups to deserve special protection. For example, the Declaration of Helsinki or the Council of Europe Convention on Human Rights and Biomedicine (referred hereafter as the Biomedicine Convention) in their present form do not include provisions protecting these groups, even though the chance for at least indirect pressure from their superiors or colleagues can be obvious. Moreover, these groups often take part in research that is not likely to have any direct health benefit to them which makes their use as experimental subjects even more problematic.

ACTIVITY: Stop here for a moment and consider the following case. In the light of the previous few paragraphs and using your checklist we would like you to analyse the case and to list the arguments in favour of the research being allowed to proceed and

those against. In the end, after having considered both sets of arguments, what would you decide, and why?

A case of payment for research

A research project focusing on specific CSF enzyme levels in neurological disease requires control measures. For this purpose, healthy volunteers are required who are willing to undergo lumbar puncture. Recruitment is slow. The researchers have funding and propose to pay each volunteer £800 in order to increase the recruitment rate. The volunteers are properly informed about the procedure and its risks and give valid consent to take part in the research. However, most would not have given consent were it not for the £800.

Now continue with your reading of the paper.

Competence

Recently, the hottest debate in Europe has not been on the voluntariness but on the competence of research subjects. The two concerns can overlap, as in the case of a patient who receives involuntary psychiatric care for his or her mental illness. In the 1960s, a physician called Henry Beecher identified several research projects which had used children, often suffering from mental disability, as research subjects. Probably the best known of them, the Willowbrook study (Krugman et al., 1965), concerned mentally retarded children in an institution who were deliberately infected with hepatitis in order to examine the efficacy of the vaccine in preparation.

In the light of Willowbrook and several other studies, it is understandable that there are voices that would prefer to ban research on incompetent subjects. However, there is another side to the coin. If medical research on minors and other incompetents were to be banned altogether, gathering scientifically valid information on their development and diagnostics or finding suitable medication for childhood diseases or, e.g. Alzheimer's disease, would be seriously hindered. What is needed is a compromise that aims to protect the incompetent as well as to give science some space to explore.

Self-determination

What makes minors and incompetent adults special is, of course, their impaired ability to decide for themselves. Although in most countries the capacity to decide over one's own body does not strictly follow the age of majority, setting a clear line on whether a person is competent to make a health-related decision has proven to be very problematic. In some countries, strict age limits or tests of capacity have been imposed, in some others more flexible formulations on the sufficient level of understanding have been set. The level of involvement of persons with impaired decision-making ability in research can be categorized in the following way: (a) independent consent (full capacity), (b) assent (both the consent of the subject and his or her proxy are required), (c) refusal (objection is valid despite incompetence and proxy consent).

One very interesting factor is the emphasis that is placed on the right of self-determination of the incompetent in medical research compared to medical treatment. Children can be taken as an example here. Whereas competence for deciding over minor, purely therapeutic measures can be achieved in quite an early age, competence for deciding independently on research procedures is considerably harder to achieve. A link can be made to the comparison of levels of competence required in consenting and refusing treatment. As the latter may bring some negative consequences to the incompetent person, his or her right to self-determination does not seem to stand on its own, but on a more consequentialist ground, on the outcome of the procedure (see, e.g. Re W).

The same may be said of the incompetent adult. In contrast to minors, adults enjoy a presumption of competence which seems to alter the situation in favour of the adult in terms of stronger involvement in decision-making. Additionally, adults who have been competent earlier, may have had the opportunity to state their opinion before becoming incompetent. In that case, their previous wishes should be given the same weight as advance directives. One could, however, think of a situation of an adult incompetent who has previously (e.g. at the early stages of dementia) stated his willingness to participate in research, but along with deteriorating mental capacity has become afraid of physicians and medical procedures. Should the previously stated will of the patient still be respected? That question will remain unanswered here. A lot will always stay within the discretion of the medical profession and depend on the circumstances of the individual case.

Nevertheless, as the outcome of the research procedure seems to weigh more than the autonomy of the patient in medical research, it leads to a situation where the refusal of the subject is his or her strongest means of self-determination. This right is very strongly protected, and the required level of competence is taken to be very low. When the Medical Research Act (No. 488 of Statutes, 9 April 1999) was drafted in Finland for example, a child as young as 5 was proposed to be given the right to refuse a research procedure. In the present Act, no definite age limits have remained, but the relevance of objection has been left to be determined by the age and maturity of the minor. In comparison, the refusal of an adult incompetent is always considered sufficient.

Proxy decision-making

If the subject is incompetent to decide for him or herself and he or she does not object, who can then decide on their behalf? In the case of a minor, the parents or the local authority have the power to make decisions over the child as his or her legal guardians. However, in the case of an adult, there are usually no provisions that make someone automatically his or her legal representative as in the case of a minor.

The legal representation of adult incompetents has been settled differently in various jurisdictions. In England and Wales, nobody, not even the courts, has strictly speaking the authority to decide on behalf of the adult incompetent at present. In the case of Re F, the House of Lords decided that a doctor, acting in the patient's 'best interests' and on the basis of the general principle of necessity, could decide for the incompetent patient. Although the courts did not have the power to act as proxies on the basis of their inherent jurisdiction, they could, however, give a declaration on whether the proposed procedure was in the patient's 'best interests'.

It was expected that the forthcoming legislation in England and Wales on proxy decision-making on behalf of mentally incapacitated adults would address also the issue of medical research, but according to the Government policy statement 'Making Decisions', medical research will not be specifically touched upon at this point. According to the statement, however, the Continuing Powers of Attorney (CPA) delegated by the patient in case of incompetence may also entail healthcare decisions and therefore apply to medical research as well. The other alternative for proxy decision-making, the court appointed manager, would only have the powers that the court, after taking all relevant factors into account, considers necessary to vest the manager. The statement leaves it open whether they may include also a power to consent to research.

In the Finnish Medical Research Act, Section 7 of the Act states that incompetent adults may be research subjects in cases where written consent has been given by 'their close relative or other relative or legal representative'. The selection of people is thereby made quite extensive and may result in problems in a case of disagreement in the family. However, as the right to refuse is interpreted widely in medical research, it could follow that in the case of disagreement amongst the patient's relatives, one relative refusing to give consent would be sufficient to prevent the subject's participation.

ACTIVITY: Stop here for a moment and consider the question: should it ever be possible for someone other than the potential research subject to consent to their involvement in a research project? Try to think of two arguments for and two against.

Scope of proxy decision-making

What then is the scope of proxy decision-making in medical research? Taking part in medical research is by definition not solely concerned with the patient's best interests. Here, a distinction between therapeutic and non-therapeutic research must be made. After all, with therapeutic research, the treatment given is at least connected to the patient's condition and may be of significant benefit to him or her. In fortunate cases, the experimental treatment may prove to be more beneficial to the patient than the standard treatment. Leaving aside the debate on so-called 'placebo-controlled' trials, very few objections towards incompetents taking part in therapeutic research have been made and proxy decision-making has been considered acceptable in therapeutic research at least in principle.

The problem then becomes clearly visible in non-therapeutic research. When the sole legal criterion in almost all of the European countries for proxy decision-making has followed the general rule of best interests of the incompetent person, how can an infringement of the incompetent person's bodily integrity be justified if there is no potential health benefit to be expected?

In England, the already mentioned case of Re F followed the general principle of 'best interests' leaving it for the courts to decide whether the proposed procedure was in the best interests of the incompetent patient. Later, in the case of Re Y, the High Court of Justice gave more flesh to the interpretation of the 'best interests' criteria. It ruled that harvesting bone marrow from a severely mentally and physically disabled person to be used as a bone marrow transplant for her sister would be lawful. The court based its ruling on the grounds that preventing the death of Miss Y's sister would be for her 'emotional, psychological and social benefit' as the family was a particularly close one. It has been suggested that neither of the cases can be applied to solve the problem of proxy decision-making for medical research on adult incompetents because even a wide interpretation of the 'best interests' criteria hardly ever would be met in non-therapeutic medical research.

There seems to be a conflict here that cannot be solved using the traditional criteria. One suggestion to resolve the conflict is formulated in the Biomedicine Convention which has been adopted, e.g. into Finnish legislation. It provides a compromise that is needed to bridge the aim of protection and fear of exploitation into a constructive solution. It makes a distinction (as does the Helsinki Declaration) between whether the procedure has an expected therapeutic benefit to the patient or not. According to the Convention, in exceptional circumstances and under the protective provisions of national law, also non-therapeutic research on the incompetent is allowed. The provisions on non-therapeutic medical research on the incompetent in the Convention are based on two criteria: societal necessity and the principle of minimal risk. Both of them have to be simultaneously fulfilled.

> **ACTIVITY: Stop here for a moment and consider the distinction between therapeutic and non-therapeutic research. This is a distinction which, despite appearing very prominently, as Lötjönen points out, in the Declaration of Helsinki, has been the subject of a great deal of disagreement recently. To what extent do you think it is possible and important to make such a distinction?**

Societal necessity

Societal necessity stems from the claim that if research on incapacitated persons was not permitted this might in fact work against the interests of the group such a ban was designed to protect. If non-therapeutic research on the incompetent were prohibited altogether, existing medicines could not be tested on children before they reach

the market and the physicians treating these patients would have to base their decision-making on estimating the right dosage using their own discretion instead of scientifically valid data. Mental illnesses could not be researched on effectively, and certain illnesses of the ageing population would also be left without due regard.

The use of the term 'societal necessity' may be misleading in the sense that it may not be the society at large whose interests are at stake, but merely the group that the incompetent person belongs to. In order to ensure that the best interests of the subject are not interfered with for a purpose other than the original aim, provisions have been drafted so that if the prospect of benefit in taking part in the research is not directed to the subject him or herself, it should be directed 'to other persons in the same age category or afflicted with the same disease or disorder or having the same condition' (Article 17, para 2). Another illustration of the necessity argument is visible in the provision which states that if the research of comparable effectiveness can be carried out on individuals capable of giving consent, research on incompetent subjects may not be undertaken even in the case of therapeutic research (Article 17, para 1).

A third aspect to the notion of 'societal necessity' does not apply only to vulnerable groups but addresses research ethics in general. It touches the general aims and the quality of the project. For example, if the design of the project is flawed, if it is merely duplicating what has already been scientifically proven or if the results are more directed to advance commercial rather than medical interests, the reason for conducting the project is medically speaking futile and therefore cannot fulfil the 'societal necessity' criteria.

Minimal risk

The other condition for conducting non-therapeutic research on incompetents is the criteria of minimal risk. The research must not entail more than a 'minimal risk and a minimal burden' to the subject (Article 17, para 2). This requirement resembles closely one of the interpretations given to the 'best interests' criteria, namely the criteria according to which the parental powers extend to cover also procedures which are not considered to be 'against the best interests' of the patient, e.g. taking a blood sample (S v S, W v Official Solicitor). In the explanatory report of the Biomedicine Convention some examples have been given as to what the term 'minimal risk' might mean. With regard to children, it lists 'ultrasonic scanning when replacing X-ray examinations or invasive diagnostic measures, incidental blood samples from newborns without respiratory problems in order to establish the necessary oxygen content for premature infants and discovering the causes and improving treatment of leukaemia in children for example by taking a blood sample'. The list is by no means complete. However, as can be seen from the list, a procedure is not considered acceptable or unacceptable merely on the basis of a consideration of the risk it poses, but the risk is also evaluated in comparison to the aim of the research project.

Role of ethics committees

Ethical research on incompetent persons involves a lot of weighing and balancing of different aspects. Very often there is no legislation (as in, e.g. England and Wales, see, however, Kennedy and Grubb (1998)) or clear guidelines to be given on deciding on competence or making the risk–benefit calculations which are of central importance in deciding over the ethics and legality of the research concerned. Fortunately, such decisions are not left solely for the researchers to decide, but they can and shall get an approval of the proposed research project from the relevant ethics committees that are equipped to give a more objective opinion on the project. On the condition that the research ethics committees are provided with adequate resources and training to be able to efficiently supervise medical research involving vulnerable groups, some of the restrictions of medical research could be loosened according to the example given by the

Biomedicine Convention. As already said, this leaves a heavy responsibility for the ethics committees and the need for ascertaining the public confidence is apparent. As most of the documents processed by the committees are confidential, the general trust shall be maintained by paying special attention to the composition of the committees in order to ensure the objectivity of its decision-making.

ACTIVITY: At this point stop for a moment and, taking into account what you have read in the section so far, make a list of all the elements you consider to be required for consent to be valid. Next make a list of the various ways and circumstances in which these criteria are unlikely to have been met. Add these points to your checklist.

At the end of this section our checklist has added the following questions:

- Are the research subjects giving their informed consent?
- Are the research subjects competent to participate in the research?
- Are the research subjects subject to any form of coercion?
- Are the research subjects in a dependent relationship with the researcher?
- Is participation in the research in the subject's best interests?
- How big are the risks associated with the research?
- What are the likely benefits of the research?

Section 3: Ethical implications of research methods

In the previous two sections we have looked at the question of what counts as medical research and we have also looked at some of the criteria by which we might judge whether or not a project is ethical. In the previous section we looked at the importance of valid consent. In this section we shall be going on to explore the ethical implications of scientific methodology. We will explore these questions in relation to a case of some research which was carried out on HIV infection and transmission in developing countries and caused an international debate about whether or not it was ethical. In fact, the research caused so much dispute within the bioethics community that it led to demands for a revision of the Helsinki Declaration itself, the international declaration against which the ethical acceptability of research is usually compared. Such was the controversy. Now read through the outline of the case: As you read it through, think about the ethical questions it raises and put these on your checklist.

A question to bear in mind as you read through the following case is this. How do we balance the potential benefits of medical research against the risks to individual research subjects (or even to communities)?

ACTIVITY: Can research that is beneficial and to which valid consent has been given, still be unethical? In this section we will be going on to explore whether it is ever possible to answer yes to this question. Some of the situations to be considered are:

- When the risk posed by the research is so great that even if subjects consented the research would still be unethical.
- When the research question is not worth investigating, perhaps because it has already been answered before.
- If the research methodology does not offer the likelihood of achieving the proposed aims.
- If the research method has an injustice built into it.
- Consent to participate in placebo-controlled trials.

THE CASE OF HIV DRUG TRIALS IN DEVELOPING COUNTRIES

It is estimated by the National Institutes of Health that there are, or soon will be, 6 million pregnant women in the developing world infected with HIV. Maternal–infant transmission of HIV occurs in approximately 15 per cent of cases. At present, approximately 1000 HIV+ babies are born each day, a high proportion in the developing world.

A particular regimen of the antiretroviral drug zidovudine has been shown by research in the United States and in France to reduce the risk of such transmission by up to 66 per cent. The 'triple combination' regimen, as it is known, which involves three stages (oral doses whilst pregnant, intravenous doses during labour and further oral doses, for the child, up until six weeks after birth), is claimed to be too expensive for widespread use in the developing world [$800 per mother and infant according to Varmus and Satcher (1997). This is 600 times the annual per capita allocation for healthcare in Malawi]. Were it possible to develop an effective regimen of the drug which was less expensive than triple combination therapy and cheap enough for widespread use in the developing world, it would clearly have the potential to avoid the infection of a very large number of babies. In order to investigate the success of a lower dosage of the drug, researchers considered two alternative study designs. The first approach considered was to run a trial comparing a new cheaper regimen with placebo. The second approach considered was to compare the new regimen with triple combination therapy.

The approach adopted was the first. Between 1995 and 1997, a programme of 15 trials, co-ordinated by UNAIDS, was carried out on 12 000 women in various parts of the developing world (Ethiopia, Ivory Coast, Uganda, Zimbabwe, Tanzania, South Africa, Malawi, Kenya and Burkina Faso). The research was carried out by researchers funded by the United States, France, Belgium, Denmark and South Africa.

The use of a placebo-controlled trial meant that only half of the women who were all HIV-positive actually received the drug. The other half of the women involved in the trial received a placebo. The research took place in countries where pregnant women with HIV would not normally receive such treatment.

Had the trials been carried out in the 'developed world', they would have been considered unethical. The Declaration of Helsinki [revised in 1989, Hong Kong] states that,

The potential benefits, hazards and discomfort of a new method should be weighed against the advantages of the best current diagnostic and therapeutic methods.

However, given the absence of any such treatment locally, the researchers felt that the trials were justified because, without them, the women who received the reduced dose therapy and those who received the placebo would both have received nothing. The trial it was claimed would leave no one worse off than they would otherwise have been: some women would receive treatment they would not otherwise have had and those who received placebos would be no worse off than they would otherwise have been.

It was also felt by the researchers that a placebo-controlled trial would produce results more quickly than a treatment-controlled approach.

> **ACTIVITY: Before you go on, stop here for a moment and consider whether this research project is an ethical one. If not why not? If so, why? Imagine that you are a member of the ethics committee that had to decide whether or not to approve this project. Make a list of arguments for and another of arguments against allowing the project to proceed. We will be asking you to return to this list at the end of this section.**

Many critics have argued that the trials were unethical and that the ethical way to have conducted such trials would have been to test the new regimen of the drug against the triple combination therapy. They argue that not to do so was inevitably to allow research subjects to receive treatment (or absence thereof), which fell below that which is currently considered 'best practice' and contravenes the Declaration of Helsinki.

In order to assess the arguments for and against the trials, we would now like you to read two papers. The first is by Udo Schüklenk, the Head of the Centre for Bioethics and Human Rights at Johannesburg's University of the Witwatersrand Faculty of Health Sciences in South Africa and argues that the trials were unethical. As you do so,

note down the arguments used and add them to the list you have begun. We will then ask you to read a paper that argues in favour of the trials.

In his paper Udo Schüklenk addresses the issue of the HIV trials and of what constitutes an ethical approach to research in the developing world in the light of current attempts to change the Declaration of Helsinki and other research ethics guidelines.

Clinical research in developing countries: trials and tribulations

Udo Schüklenk

Two pivotal international research ethics documents are currently undergoing substantial revisions. These documents are The World Medical Association's (WMA) Declaration of Helsinki, and the Council for International Organisations of Medical Sciences' (CIOMS) International Ethical Guidelines for Biomedical Research Involving Human Subjects. Both documents are of fundamental importance with regard to the conduct of international collaborative research. The United Nations AIDS organisation's Ethical Review Committee demands 'assurance that the Principal Investigator has confirmed in writing that the research will be conducted in conformity with the Declaration of Helsinki.'[65]

There is nothing unusual, of course, about research ethics guidelines evolving over time to adjust to changing societal perceptions about what is and what is not ethical. However, opponents of many of the proposed changes argue that this time we are faced with changes that constitute a major threat to the few research ethics protections that are currently afforded to research subjects in developing countries.

Proposed changes to the Declaration of Helsinki[66]

The most contentious of the proposed changes is the one proposing different standards of care, depending on where a given trial takes place. The current text of the Declaration requires that in any research clinical trial 'every patient should be assured of the best proven diagnostic and therapeutic method'. The proposed change adds to this sentence '. . . that would otherwise be available to him or her'. The implications of this seemingly innocuous change are wide ranging. Should this proposed change succeed in becoming the new wording of the Declaration of Helsinki, we would find ourselves with two sets of research ethics standards – one for people in rich countries, and one for subjects living in poor countries.

Suppose you are German and you participate in a preventive HIV vaccine trial. If something unfortunately goes wrong during the trial, and you get infected with HIV, or you get sick after the trial, you fortunately live in a society with functioning public healthcare, hence you will be taken care of by German medical doctors. Triple combination therapy will not only keep you alive, it will even allow you to go back to work one day, or else you'll be furnished with a disability pension that allows you to live a decent life.

Imagine now that you are a participant in a preventive AIDS vaccine trial that takes place in Uganda or Ivory Coast. The resources of the healthcare system are stretched far beyond its limits. Combination therapy is unaffordable, and it is certainly not the local standard of care. If you are one of the 30 per cent or so of volunteers of any such trial who has a serious misconception of the nature of the trial, and as a consequence of that misconception you get HIV infected and sick, under the proposed watered-down version of the Declaration of Helsinki, you will only receive whatever the local standard of care is. In economic terms, clearly, that is an excellent deal for any pharmaceutical multinational on the look-out for cheap research subjects. In any developed country, such an organization would have to foot the substantial bill to provide their research subjects with the best local standards of care, while in many developing countries the outlay would be negligible to non-existent.

Furthermore, the idea that there is such a thing as a local standard of care is problematic. The reality is that it is a standard of care dictated by prices Western pharmaceutical multinationals set regardless of the consequences for millions of people in developing countries. It allows the introduction of placebo controls in clinical trials that would be considered unethical in Western countries. A case in point is the now infamous mother–child HIV transmission prevention trials. This has been discussed widely in the medical and bioethical literature. What was offered as an ethical reason for the introduction of a placebo control in this trial was not a medical reason. It proposed that none of the women in the trial was worse off. The reason for this claim is that the local standard of care in Thailand, Uganda and any of the other developing countries participating in this trial was no intervention and those who got AZT, a proven intervention and the standard of care for developed nations were better off than they would otherwise have been. Those who got a placebo were not worse off, because if they had not participated they would not have received AZT either.

Quite obviously, what we have in these trials is the proposed change to the Declaration of Helsinki in action; exploiting the vulnerability of poor research subjects in countries where AZT is made unaffordable by the price its manufacturer sets. Even the pseudo-justification, that these trials had to be done, in order to produce affordable drugs for people living in developing countries, proves to be a smokescreen. The lower-dosage regimen that was the result of these trials is so expensively priced by its manufacturer that even the health minister of South Africa which is a middle income country announced that she would not fund this intervention because it doesn't constitute, in the local environment, a cost-effective means of HIV prevention. I proposed some time ago that, for this reason alone, these trials should have never taken place.[66] The bottom line of this proposal is that it is acceptable to withhold a proven intervention for purely economic reasons. Without going too much into the details of the economical aspects of this problem, it should be mentioned here that the international trade regime allows for compulsory licensing of drugs in developing countries if lives are at risk. The US Government threatened the South African Government with trade sanctions if it made use of this provision. The South African Government planned to compulsorily license a whole range of AIDS drugs in order to manufacture them locally at affordable prices in order to save the lives of millions of infected citizens of that country. The US intervention made that impossible. Ethical justifications of the trials in question, and of the local-standards-of-care concept tend to ignore these vital facts.[67]

Despite ample evidence of seriously deficient informed consent procedures in developing countries[68] the proposed changes permit waivers of informed consent when the research involves only a 'slight risk'. Clearly, what constitutes a 'slight risk' depends very much on the interpretation of individuals, in this case the principal investigators. In societies where most research subjects could not afford the costly litigation that is possible in Western countries, reducing the informed consent-based requirements is deeply disconcerting.

> ACTIVITY: What arguments did you manage to identify in the paper?

We listed the following:
(a) To allow the trials to go ahead is to condone the existence of two sets of research ethics standards: one for the rich and another for the poor. This is a literal case of 'double-standards' and is unjust.
(b) Those who participate in the research in the developing world are, in any case, more at risk and more vulnerable by virtue of the fact that they live in countries with lower standards of care. This ought to be a reason for providing them with more protection rather than less.
(c) The idea of a 'local standard of care' is problematic because any such standard is inevitably determined both by international relations between the developed and developing world and by the pricing policies of pharmaceutical companies and this ought not to form the

basis of an assessment of the ethics of a research trial.
(d) Even the cheaper regimen is unlikely to be cheap enough for the developing world.
(e) Placebo-controlled trials are not necessarily quicker than other forms of trial if the number of participants is high enough.

> We would now like you go on to read the next section in which we outline the case for such trials as presented in a joint statement by two of the organizations funding the research, 'The Conduct of Clinical Trials of Maternal–Infant Transmission of HIV Supported by the United States Department of Health and Human Services in Developing Countries'.

A defence of HIV trials in the developing world

(based on NIH, CDC Statement)

In a joint statement [NIH and CDC, 1997] the Directors of the two organizations funding the research trials, the National Institutes for Health and the Centres for Disease Control and Prevention in the US [http: //www.nih.gov/news/mathiv/mathiv.htm, 1997], made the case for the research trials. The statement begins by reiterating the desperate need for the development of less expensive treatments for the developing world.

One regimen of antiretroviral therapy has been shown to reduce substantially the likelihood of maternal–infant transmission of HIV. The identification of this successful regimen was the result of the National Institutes of Health's AIDS Clinical Trials Group protocol 076 (ACTG 076 or 076) in 1994. In spite of this knowledge, approximately 1000 HIV-infected infants are born each day, the vast majority of them in developing countries. This occurs, in part, because the regimen proven to be effective is simply not feasible as a standard of prevention in much of the developing world.

There are two reasons for this lack of feasibility. Firstly, to follow the regimen that has proven efficacy requires that the women be reached early in prenatal care; be tested for and counseled concerning their HIV status; comply with a lengthy oral treatment regimen; receive intravenous administration of the antiretroviral zidovudine (ZDV or AZT) during labor and delivery; and refrain from breastfeeding. Additionally, the newborns must receive 6 weeks of oral AZT therapy. During and after the time the mother and infant are treated with AZT, both must be carefully monitored for adverse effects of exposure to this drug. In the developing world countries that are the sites of these studies, these requirements could seldom be achieved, even under the infrequent circumstance when women present early enough for the screening and care requirements of the 076 therapeutic regimen to be implemented. Secondly, the wholesale drug costs for the AZT in the 076 regimen are estimated to be in excess of $800, an amount far greater than these developing countries could afford as standard care. [. . .] Less complex and expensive alternatives are urgently needed to address the staggering impact of maternal–infant transmission of HIV in developing countries.

The authors go on to point out that this type of research trial was specifically called for by the World Health Organization's 'Recommendations from the Meeting on Prevention of Mother-to-Infant Transmission of HIV by Use of Antiretrovirals, Geneva 23–25 June 1994', on the grounds that it offered the best chance to get results quickly. The World Health Organization document argues that,

Since the ZDV regimen studied in ACTG 076 is not applicable in those parts of the world where most MTI transmission of HIV occurs, placebo-controlled trials offer the best option for obtaining rapid and scientifically valid results.

In addition to their argument that placebo controlled trials would get results quicker than treatment-controlled trials the WHO also argued that,

[Triple combination therapy] is not applicable [in the developing world] because of its cost and operational requirements. In those parts of the world, the choice of a

placebo for the control group of a randomized trial would be appropriate as there is currently no effective alternative for HIV-infected pregnant women.

The WHO guidelines are taken by the NIH and CDC to:

. . . clearly indicate that the in-country healthcare capabilities of each country in which maternal–infant HIV transmission research is to be conducted must be used to define the type of research which is ethical and therefore permissible in that country.
. . . [Many of the] arguments against the NIH and CDC supported studies appear to rest on the proposition that it is unethical to conduct a clinical trial unless it offers all participants a chance to receive an effective intervention if such is available anywhere in the world, even if it is not available at the site of the clinical trial. Ideally, this would be so for all clinical trials for all therapies. But the reality is that often it is not possible. The very purpose of the NIH and CDC supported studies of maternal–infant transmission of HIV in developing countries is to identify interventions other than those of 076 [triple combination] and we agree with the WHO Geneva panel's recommendation 2 that:

. . . it should be emphasized that the results of ACTG 076 are only directly applicable to a specific population. Moreover, the ZDV regimen employed in the ACTG 076 study has a number of features (cost, logistical issues, among others) which limit its general applicability. Therefore, no global recommendations regarding use of ZDV to prevent MTI transmission of HIV can be made.

The joint NIH and CDC statement argues that the 'primary consideration' when making decisions about what constitutes an ethical research project in the developing world ought to be the extent to which, once the research has been completed, will the population represented by the study participants benefit from the results of the project? They go on to argue on the basis of this claim that to carry out research on the triple combination treatment would in fact actually itself have been unethical because it would have been testing a treatment which stands no chance of becoming standard treatment locally.

The International Ethical Guidelines for Biomedical Research Involving Human Subjects that were prepared by the Council for International Organisations of Medical Sciences (CIOMS) in collaboration with WHO are:

. . . intended to indicate how the ethical principles embodied in the Declaration [of Helsinki] could be effectively applied in developing countries.

To evaluate interventions that they could not implement realistically would be exploitative of those in the participant country since there would be no likelihood of meeting requirement 15 of the Guidelines that obliges:

. . . any product developed [through] such research will be made reasonably available to the inhabitants of the host community or country at the completion of successful testing . . .

Therefore, we have determined that the more compelling ethical argument is against using a regimen that if found to be superior in the study could not possibly be used in the prevention of maternal–infant transmission of HIV in the host country. Turning once again to Malawi for example, health officials there refused to permit the conduct of a study involving a full course regimen of AZT (such as that used in ACTG 076) because they believed it would be unethical to undertake such a study in Malawi given that its very limited resources and poor health infrastructure make the introduction of AZT as standard treatment for HIV-infected pregnant women unfeasible. Instead, the health officials wanted research on alternative treatment approaches that might reduce maternal–infant transmission of HIV. The justification and ethical foundation for the NIH- and CDC-supported studies incorporate the reality that the clinical trials are examining other alternatives that could actually be used for the majority of HIV-infected pregnant women and mothers in the countries in which the clinical trials are being carried out.

ACTIVITY: We would now like you to reread this defence of the trials and, as you do so, attempt to identify the various arguments used. Compare them with your own list.

We came up with the following:
(a) Without the trial none of the women who took part in the trial would have been receiving treatment. No one is worse off as a result and at least some women and infants are better off. This is not to mention the knowledge and information gained as a result of the trial going ahead.
(b) There is a desperate need for the drugs. Placebo-controlled trials will get results more quickly than treatment-controlled trials. This means the developing world will benefit more quickly from the research and lives will be saved.
(c) The primary ethical question is 'would the local community benefit from the research?' They would not benefit from triple combination because it will never become standard treatment. Therefore such research would itself have been unethical. Placebo-controlled trials offer a real comparison between the proposed treatment and conditions at the sites as they are now and offer the prospect of real benefit to the local community.
(d) Expert bodies such as the WHO and some local governments had called for the research.

ACTIVITY: Now, having read these two sets of arguments and having listed your own, return to the activity with which you began this section. Imagine you were the member of an ethics committee which had been asked to approve these trials. Compare the arguments. Which do you find the most persuasive? What are your reasons? Write 250 words justifying your decision.

Key points: At the end of this section we had added the following questions to our research ethics checklist:
• Are the risks posed by the research so great that even if subjects consented the research would still be unethical.

- Is the research question worth investigating?
- Does the research methodology offer the likelihood of achieving the proposed aims?
- Does the research method have an injustice built into it?
- What is the broader social setting?
- Consent to participate in placebo-controlled trials.
- Are there risks to others than those who are being asked for their consent?

Section 4: The benefits and harms of medical research

We introduced this chapter on research ethics by raising the ethical implications of the tension between the harms and benefits of medical research. As we have seen through the sections preceding this one, the ethical review of medical research projects will always involve to some extent a consideration of both the question of how to protect the rights, interests and health of research subjects, and the question of how best to ensure that such research advances medical knowledge and contributes to the wellbeing of real people. We have seen in the case of the Nazi Doctors however, that to talk about 'balancing individual rights against benefits for the larger community' can begin to look like the first step on a very dangerous slippery slope unless certain protections are built into such 'balancing'. This was recognized by the creators of the Nuremberg Code, who felt that, whilst it may be true to say that in some cases our participation as research subjects may well advance the well-being of our fellow human beings through development of medicine, the choice of whether or not to engage in a particular piece of research ought always to be one for the research subjects themselves (unless very strict other criteria have been met, e.g., in the case of research on children and incompetent adults or in the use of patient records). We have already explored some of the ethical issues related to questions of valid consent. In the final section of this chapter, we shall be considering the benefits and harms of medical research.

ACTIVITY: We would like you to begin by reading the Nuremberg Code. As you read through the code make a note of any ways it suggests your checklist might be extended. The Nuremberg Code was written shortly after the Second World War. Are there any developments in modern medicine or society which have occurred since then about which you feel the Nuremberg Code would not be able to provide us with ethical guidance? To what extent do you think research ethics ought to change with changing social circumstances and medical advances? If you could rewrite the code how would you change it?

The Nuremberg Code

From 'Trials of War Criminals Before the Nuremberg Military Tribunals Under Control Council Law No. 10', Volume 2, Nuremberg, October 1946 – April 1949 (Washington DC: US Government Printing Office, 1949), pp. 181–182.

The great weight of the evidence before us is to the effect that certain types of medical experiments on human beings, when kept within reasonably well-defined bounds, conform to the ethics of the medical profession generally. The protagonists of the practice of human experimentation justify their views on the basis that such experiments yield results for the good of society that are unprocurable by other methods or means of study. All agree, however, that certain basic principles must be observed in order to satisfy moral, ethical and legal concepts.

(a) The voluntary consent of the human subject is absolutely essential. This means that the person involved should have legal capacity to give consent ; should be so situated as to be able to exercise free power of choice, without the intervention of any element of force, fraud, deceit, duress, overreaching, or other ulterior form of constraint or coercion; and should have sufficient knowledge and comprehension of the elements of the subject matter involved as to enable him to make an understanding and enlightened decision. This later element requires that before the acceptance of an affirmative decision by the experimental subject there should be made known to him the nature, duration and purpose of the experiment; the method and means by which it is to be conducted; all inconveniences and hazards reasonably to be expected; and the effects upon his health or person which may possibly come from his participation in the experiment. The duty and responsibility for ascertaining the quality of the consent rests upon each individual who initiates, directs or engages in the experiment. It is a personal duty and responsibility which may not be delegated to another with impunity.

(b) The experiment should be such as to yield fruitful results for the good of society, unprocurable by other methods or means of study, and not random and unnecessary in nature.

(c) The experiment should be so designed and based on the results of animal experimentation and a knowledge of the natural history of the disease or other problems under study that the anticipated results will justify the performance of the experiment.

(d) The experiment should be so conducted as to avoid all unnecessary physical and mental suffering and injury.

(e) No experiment should be conducted where there is an a priori reason to believe that death or disabling injury will occur; except perhaps, in those experiments where the experimental physicians also serve as subjects.

(f) The degree of risk to be taken should never exceed that determined by the humanitarian importance of the problem to be solved by the experiment.

(g) Proper preparation should be made and adequate facilities provided to protect the experimental subject against even remote possibilities of injury, disability or death.

(h) The experiment should be conducted only by scientifically qualified persons. The highest degree of skill and care should be required through all stages of the experiment of those who conduct or engage in the experiment.

(i) During the course of the experiment the human subject should be at liberty to bring the experiment to an end if he has reached the physical or mental state where continuation of the experiment seems to him to be impossible.

(j) During the course of the experiment, the scientist in charge must be prepared to terminate the experiment at any stage, if he has probable cause to believe in the exercise of good faith, superior skill and careful judgement required of him that a continuation of the experiment is likely to result in injury, disability, or death to the experimental subject.

ACTIVITY: Stop here for a moment and reread the fifth principle of the code. What are the ethical implications of the proposal that under certain circumstances researchers might ethically use themselves as research subjects in potentially fatal experiments? Should a person, even a medical researcher, ever be able to consent (even if freely and in full understanding) to participate in research which puts their own life at risk? If not, why not? Can you think of any counter examples?

As the penultimate key points activity in this section we would now like you to return to the research ethics checklist you have been constructing as you have worked your way through this chapter. Below is a summary of some of the questions we noted as we worked through the various activities. Have a look at it in the light of your own and critically assess it. Remember that the list is meant to take the form of a series of questions one might ask a researcher or ask oneself about a research project.

AN INCOMPLETE RESEARCH ETHICS CHECKLIST

- What is the balance of harms and risks likely to occur as a result of the research? Is the proposed research going to offer some benefit?
- Is the study going to answer the proposed question?
- Is it necessary for this research to be carried out on human subjects? Could the answers be gained in the laboratory, or by animal studies?
- Are the subjects going to be asked to give their consent?

- Is there a consent form? Is it clear and understandable?
- Who will be asking the potential subjects for their consent?
- Are the research subjects giving their informed consent? Will subjects have sufficient information to be able to consent?
- Is there a Patient Information Sheet?
- Is this information presented clearly and in a way subjects will be able to understand?
- Are the research subjects competent to participate in the research?
- Are the research subjects subject to any form of coercion?
- Are the research subjects in a dependent relationship with the researcher?
- Is participation in the research in the subject's best interests?
- Is it clear to the subjects that they can withdraw from the study at any time and that this will not affect the quality of their treatment?
- Is it made clear that the subject can refuse to participate and that this too will not affect the treatment received?
- How big are the risks associated with the research? Does the study put subjects at unacceptable risk?
- Might the validity of the research subjects' consent be questioned as a result of their distress or vulnerability.
- Why is the research to be carried out on incompetent and vulnerable patients? Could such groups lose out as a result of not being researched?
- Does the research involve deceit or covert methods?
- Is the research question worth investigating? Has it been done before?
- Does the methodology offer the likelihood of achieving aims?
- Is the confidentiality of the research subjects protected?
- Are the risks posed by the research so great that even if subjects consented the research would still be unethical.
- Does the research method have an injustice built into it?

- What is the broader social setting?
- Are there risks to others than those who are being asked for their consent?

> ACTIVITY: As we come to the end of this chapter we would like to finish our consideration of the ethics of medical research by considering another case. Using your checklist consider the following research proposal and list the arguments in favour and against the research being allowed to proceed. Make a decision and provide a justification for it.

A CASE OF RESEARCH INTO THE USE OF RIGHT HEART CATHETERS

Following concern expressed by members of staff at the Hospital about the perceived risks involved in the use of right heart catheters in proposed research with healthy volunteers into the physiology of heart failure, the Research Ethics Committee decided to carry out an ethical review of this issue. The committee was aware that a number of studies involving right heart catheters had already been conducted in Switzerland, Italy, Sweden, Canada, USA (Connors et al., 1996). These studies, however, were on critically ill patients and combined with existing therapy, mostly in heart transplant patients. However, the proposed research was to be carried out on healthy volunteers in order to better understand the physiology of heart function. The procedure to be followed was as follows:

The procedure

A small sheath is passed into a vein near the elbow joint under local anesthesia. Under radiographic control, the tube is directed through the heart into the veins draining blood from the heart, brain and kidneys.

The whole procedure lasts about 6 hours and some back pain might be experienced through lying horizontally during this period.

The ethical review

In addition to the usual members of the committee, a number of staff members familiar with the use of right heart catheters, and those with known expertise in the procedure, were invited to contribute to the discussion.

The following issues were raised with relation to the use of right heart catheters in research.

- What are the risks?

The risks of pulmonary artery catheters have yet to be formally evaluated, with randomized studies yet to be conducted. The procedures are done by experienced staff only. 674 procedures of this kind have been carried out at the Hospital since 1981 and have all been free from adverse events.

The risks to normal volunteers are no greater than those encountered in daily life. The risk of death or serious disability is said to be no greater than that of being struck by lightning. There is a small risk of injury to a blood vessel associated with the organ being investigated by placement of the catheters. The advancement of the catheter to the right side of the heart may cause the development of an abnormal heart rhythm. This can be alleviated by removal of the catheter or by giving appropriate therapy. There is a small risk of bleeding once the catheters are removed and an extremely low risk of blockage of the artery at the puncture site.

- If fluoroscopic guidance was used, is there an associated radiation risk?

The radioisotope used is equivalent to the amount of radiation one would expect to be exposed to in everyday life every 12 hours. The dose of radiation required for placement of the catheters is less than 30 per cent of the accepted annual limit for members of the public, but numerous exposures should be avoided.

- What other risks are there?

There is some risk of pulmonary arterial rupture. If, however, 'Float to wedge' techniques are used to determine wedge pressure, this avoids the risk of pulmonary arterial rupture.

There can be some risk associated with the puncture site, i.e. neck or arm. If entry is through the arm, this is much lower.

- Can volunteers to non-therapeutic research of this kind really be said to be making a voluntary decision to participate? Are volunteers who feel that they may benefit from the research in the future really making a voluntary decision to participate in research? (Declaration of Helsinki, III, 2.)

Conclusions/ guidance

In the light of their discussion, the members of the committee came to the following conclusions.

It was felt that the use of right heart catheters *may* be justified in some cases if it conforms to the following minimum requirements but that the actual evaluation and ethical review of applications should be carried out on a case-by-case basis.

- Only experienced operators are to do the procedures.
- To be used for right heart studies only
- 'Float to wedge' only to avoid pulmonary artery rupture.
- Entry through arm.
- Thought to be given to alternative, non-invasive methods of obtaining readings.
- Thought to be given to conducting a randomized trial to ascertain the risks.
- To ensure volunteer autonomy, the Explanatory Statement is to:

clearly outline the risk of death and serious injury;

include a comparison of risks (e.g. to daily life);

indicate the level of operator experience;

indicate the non-therapeutic nature of the research.

Suggestions for further reading

Evans, D. and Evans, M. (1996). *A Decent Proposal: Ethical Review of Clinical Research*, Chichester: Wiley.

Grodin, M. and Glantz, L. (Eds.) (1994). *Children and Research Subjects: Science, Ethics and Law*. New York: Oxford University Press.

Kennedy I, and Grubb, A. (1998). Research and experimentation. In *Principles of Medical Law*, ed. I. Kennedy and I. Grubb, pp. 714–746. Oxford: Oxford University Press.

McNeil, P. (1992). *The Ethics and Politics of Human Experimentation*. Cambridge: Cambridge University Press.

Smith, T. (1999). *Ethics in Medical Research: A Handbook of Good Practice*. Cambridge: Cambridge University Press.

Vanderpool, H. Y. (ed.) (1996). *The Ethics of Research involving Human Subjects: Facing the 21st Century*. Frederick, MD: University Publishing Group.

References and Notes for this chapter

1 Annas, G.J. and Grodin, M.A. (eds.) (1992). *The Nazi Doctors and the Nuremberg Code: Human Rights in Human Experimentation*. Oxford: Oxford University Press.

2 Advisory Commission on Human Radiation Experiments Research Ethics and the Medical Profession. (1996). *Journal of the American Medical Association*, **276**, 403–9.

3 Caplan, A.L. (1992). Is there a duty to serve as a subject in biomedical research? In *If I were a Rich Man Could I Buy a Pancreas? And Other Essays on the Ethics of Healthcare*, ed. A.L. Caplan, Bloomington: Indiana University Press. Chap. 6.

4 Emson, H.E. (1992). Rights, duties and responsibilities in healthcare, *Journal of Applied Philosophy*, **9**, 3–11.

5 Rothman, D.J. (1987). Ethics and human experimentation: Henry Beecher revisited. *New England Journal of Medicine*, **317**, 1195–9.

6 Jones, J.H. (1993). *Bad Blood: The Tuskegee Syphilis Experiment*. Gelncoe: Free Press.

7 Annas, G.J. (1992). The Nuremberg Code in US courts: ethics versus expediency. In *The Nazi Doctors and the Nuremberg Code: Human Rights in Human Experimentation*, ed. G.J. Annas and M.A. Grodin, Oxford: Oxford University Press.

8 Bush, J.K. (1994). The industry perspective on the inclusion of women in clinical trials. *Academic Medicine*, **69**, 708–15; Dresser, R. (1992). Wanted: single, white male for medical research. *Hastings Center report* **22** (**Jan/Feb**); 24–9; McCarthy, C.R. (1994). Historical background of clinical trials involving women and minorities. *Academic Medicine*, **69**, 695–8; Mastroianni, A.C., Faden, R. and Federman, D. (1994). Women and health research: a report from the Institute of Medicine. *Kennedy Institute of Ethics Journal*, 1994: **4**, 55–61; Merton, V. (1993). The exclusion of the pregnant, pregnable and once-pregnable people (a.k.a. women) from biomedical research. *American Journal of Law and Medicine*, **XIX**, 369–451; Merkatz, R.B. and Junod, S.W. (1994). Historical background of changes in FDA policy on the study and evaluation of drugs in women. *Academic Medicine*, **69**, 703–7.

9 Warren, C.A.B. and Karner, T.X. (1990). Permissions and the social context. *American Sociologist*, Summer, 116–35.

10 Lesser, H. (1989). Obligation and consent. *Journal of Medical Ethics*, **15**, 195–6.

11 Freedman, B., Fuks, A. and Weijer, C. (1992). Demarcating research and treatment: a systematic approach for the analysis of the ethics of clinical research. *Clinical Research*, **40**, 653–60.

12 Reiser, S.J. (1978). Human experimentation and the convergence of medical research and patient care. *Annals of the AAPSS*, **437**, 8–18.

13 Reiser, S.J. (1994). Criteria for standard versus experimental therapy. *Health Affairs*, **13**, 127–36

14 *Op. cit.* Note 3.

15 Allmark, P. (1994). An argument against the use of the concept of 'persons' in health care ethics. *Journal of Advanced Nursing*, **19**, 29–35.

16 Gillon, R. (1993). Autonomy, respect for autonomy and weakness of the will. *Journal of Medical Ethics*, **19**, 195–6.

17 Pellegrino, E.D. (1990). The relationship of autonomy and integrity in medical ethics. *Bulletin of the Pan-American Health Organization*, **24**; 361–71.

18 Karlawish, J.H.T. and Hall, J.B. (1996). The controversy over emergency research: a review of the issues and suggestions for a resolution. *American Journal of Respiratory Critical Care Medicine*, **153**, 499–506.

19 Sheldon, T. (1995). Consent is not always essential, say Dutch experts. *British Medical Journal*, **310**, 1355–6

20 Jonas, C. and Soutoul, J.H. (1993). Biomedical research in incapacitated people according to French law. *Medical Law*, **12**, 567–72

21 Hodgkinson, D.W., Gray, A.J., Dala, B., Wilson, P., Szawarski, Z., Sensky, T., Gillet, G. and Yates, D.W. (1995). Doctor's legal position in treating temporarily incompetent patients, *British Medical Journal*, **311**, 115–18.

22 Gifford, F. (1986). The conflict between randomized clinical trials and the therapeutic obligation. *Journal of Medicine and Philosophy*, **11**, 347–66.

23 Shumm, D.S. and Speece, R.G. (1993). Ethical issues and clinical trials. *Drugs*, **46**, 579–84.

24 Perry, C.B. (1994). Conflicts of interest and the physician's duty to inform. *American Journal of Medicine*, **96**, 375–80.

25 *Op. cit.* Note 3.

26 Emson, H.E. (1992). Rights, duties and responsibilities in healthcare. *Journal of Applied Philosophy*, **9**, 3–11.

27 Jonas, H. (1969). Philosophical reflections on experimenting with human subjects. *Daedalus*, **98**, 219–47.

28 Fethe, C. (1993). Beyond voluntary consent: Hans Jonas on the moral requirements of human experimentation. *Journal of Medical Ethics*, 19–103.

29 Rothman, D.J. (1987). Ethics and human experimentation: Henry Beecher revisited. *New England Journal of Medicine*, **317**, 1195–9.

30 Beecher, H.K. (1970). *Research and the Individual*. London: J. and A. Churchill.

31 Beecher, H.K. (1966). Ethics and clinical research. *New England Journal of Medicine*, **274**, 1354–60.

32 Popper, S.E. and McCloskey, K. (1995). Ethics in human experimentation: historical perspectives. *Military Medicine*, **160**, 7–11.

33 Buchanan, A. (1996). Judging the past: the case of the human radiation experiments. *Hastings Center Report*, **26** (May/June); 25–30.

34 Burchell, H.B. (1992). Vicissitudes in clinical trial research: subjects, participants, patients. *Controlled Clinical Trials*, **13**, 185–9.

35 Evered, D.C. and Halnan, K.E. (1995). Deadly experiments. *British Medical Journal*, **311**, 192.

36 Pappworth, M.H. (1990). 'Human guinea pigs' – a history. *British Medical Journal*, **301**, 1456–60.

37 *Op. cit.* Note 30.

38 *Op. cit.* Note 31.

39 *Op. cit.* Note 36.

40 Tobias, J.S. and Souhami, R.L. (1993). Fully informed consent can be needlessly cruel. *British Medical Journal*, **307**, 1199–201.

41 Garnham, J.C. (1975). Some observations on informed consent in non-therapeutic research. *Journal of Medical Ethics*, **1**, 138–45.

42 Byrne, P. (1988). Medical research and the human subject: problems of consent and control in the UK experience. *Annals of the NY Academy of Sciences*, **530**, 144–53.

43 Reiser, S.J. and Knudsen, P. (1993). Protecting research subjects after consent: the case for the 'research intermediary' *IRB* **15**, 10–11.

44 Silverman, W.A. (1989). The myth of informed consent: in daily practice and in clinical trials. *Journal of Medical Ethics*, **15**, 6–11.

45 Silverman, W.A. and Altman, D.G. (1996). Patients' preferences and randomized trials. *Lancet*, **347**, 171–4.

46 Rosenzweig, S. (1933). The experimental situation as a psychological problem. *Psychological Review*, **40**, 337–54.

47 Daugherty, C., Ratain, M.J., Grochowski, E., Stocking, C., Kodish, E., Mick, R. and Siegler, M. (1995). Perceptions of cancer patients and their physicians involved in Phase trials. *Journal of Clinical Oncology*, **13**, 1062–72.

48 Susman, E.J., Dorn. L.D. and Fletcher J.C. (1992). Participation in biomedical research: the consent process as viewed by children, adolescents, young adults and physicians. *Journal of Pediatrics*, **121**, 547–52.

49 Nguyen-Van-Tam, J.S. and Madeley, R.J. (1996). Vietnamese people in study may have had language difficulties. *British Medical Journal*, **313**, 48.

50 Habermas, J. (1979). *Communication and the Evolution of Society*. London: Heinemann Educational.

51 Alderson, P. (1995). Consent, and the social context. *Nursing Ethics*, **2**, 347–50; Alderson, P. (1988). Trust in informed consent. *IME Bulletin* (July) 17–19; Andreasson, S., Parmander, M. and Allebeck, P. A. (1990). A trial that failed, and the reasons why: comparing the Minnesota model with outpatient treatment and non-treatment for alcohol disorders. *Scandinavian Journal of Social Medicine*, **18**, 221–4; Angell, M. (1984). Patients' preferences in randomised clinical trials. *New England Journal of Medicine*, **310**, 1385–7; Beech, C.L. (1995). Compliance in clinical trials. *AIDS*, **9**, 1–10; Brownlea, A. (1987). Participation: myths, realities and prognosis. *Social Science and Medicine*, **25**, 605–14; Daugherty, C.K., Ratain, M.J. and Siegler, M. (1995). Pushing the envelope: informed consent in Phase I trials. *Annals of Oncology*, **6**, 321–3; DeLuca, S.A., Korcuska, L.A., Oberstar, B.H. Rosenthal, M.L., Welsh, P.A. and Topol, E.J. (1995). Are we providing true informed consent in cardiovascular clinical trials? *Journal of Cardiovascular Nursing*, **9**(3), 54–61; Fox, R. (1996). What do patients want from medical research. *Journal of the Royal Society of Medicine*, **89**, 301–2; Gostin, L.O. (1995). Informed consent, cultural sensitivity and respect for persons. *Journal of the American Medical Association* **274**, 844–5; Grimshaw, J.M. (1990). Clinical trials: patient perspectives. *AIDS*, **4**, Suppl. 1, S207–8; Joseph, R.R. (1994). Viewpoints and concerns of a clinical trial participant. *Cancer*, **74**, 2692–3; Kotwall, C.A., Mahoneym L.J., Myers, R.E. and Decoste, L. (1992). Reasons for non-entry in randomised clinical trials for breast cancer: a single institutional study. *Journal of Surgical Oncology*, **50**, 125–9; Lilleyman, J.S. (1995). Informed consent: how informed and consent to what? *Pediatric Hematology and Oncology*, **12**(6); xiii–xvi; Llewellyn-Thomas, H.A., McGreal, M.J., Thiel, E.C., Fine, S., and Erlichman, C. (1991). Patients' willingness to enter clinical trials: measuring the association with perceived benefit and preference for decision participation. *Social Science and Medicine*, **32**, 35–42; McGrath, P. (1995). It's OK to say no! A discussion of ethical issues arising from informed consent to chemotherapy. *Cancer Nursing*, **18**, 97–103; Winn, R.J. (1994). Obstacles to the accrual of patients to clinical trials in the community setting. *Seminars in Oncology*, **21**(4, Suppl. 7), 112–17.

52 Logue, G. and Wear, S. (1995). A desperate solution: individual autonomy and the double-blind controlled experiment. *Journal of Medicine and Philosophy*, **20**, 57–64.

53 Epstein, S. (1991). Democratic science? AIDS activism and the contested construction of knowledge. *Socialist Review,* **21**, 35–64.

54 Benson, P.R. (1989). The social control of human biomedical research: an overview and review of the literature. *Social Science and Medicine,* **29**, 1–12.

55 McKay, C.R. (1995). The evolution of the institutional review board: a brief overview of its history. *Clinical Research and Regulatory Affairs,* **12**, 65–94.

56 McNeill, P.M. (1993). *The Ethics and Politics of Human Experimentation.* Cambridge: Cambridge University Press.

57 Byrne, P. (1988). Medical research and the human subject: problems of consent and control in the UK experience. *Annals of the New York Academy of Sciences,* **530**, 144–53.

58 Reiser, S.J. and Knudsen, P. (1993). Protecting research subjects after consent: the case for the 'Research Intermediary' *IRB,* **15**, 10–11.

59 DeBakey, L. (1974). Ethically questionable data: publish or reject? *Clinical Research,* **22**, 113–21.

60 Rosner, F., Bennet, A.J., Cassell, E.J. et al. (1991). The ethics of using scientific data obtained by immoral means. *New York State Journal of Medicine,* **91**, 54–9.

61 Smith, R. (1996). Commentary: the importance of patients' consent for publication. *British Medical Journal,* 313; 6.

62 Carnall, D. (1996). Doctor struck off for scientific fraud. *British Medical Journal,* **312**, 44

63 Dyer, O. (1996). GP struck off for fraud in drug trials. *British Medical Journal,* **312**, 798.

64 UNAIDS Ethical Review Committee (1998). Provisional Terms of Reference and Procedures. *Journal International de Bioethique,* **9**(4), 125–28, 126.

65 This paragraph relies heavily on information provided to me by Dr Peter Lurie of *Public Citizen,* Dr Bebe Loff, Monash University Faculty of Medicine, and Dr Richard Nicholson, Editor of the *Bulletin of Medical Ethics.*

66 Schüklenk, U. (1998). Unethical perinatal HIV transmission trials establish bad precedent. *Bioethics,* **12**, 312–19.

67 See, e.g. Crouch, R.A. and Arras, J.D. (1998). AZT trials and tribulations. *Hastings Center Report,* **28**(6), 26–34.

68 Queiroz de Fonsecoa, F.O. and Lie, R.K. (1995). Informed consent to preventive AIDS vaccine trials in Brazil. *AIDS and Public Policy Journal,* **10**, 22–6. Karim, Q.A. Karim, S.S.A. et al. (1998). Informed consent for HIV testing in a South African Hospital: is it truly informed and truly voluntary? *American Journal of Public Health,* **88**: 637–40.

Part II

Vulnerability, truth-telling, competence and confidentiality

Long-term care

Introduction

Open any book on medical ethics and look at the contents page. Look at the front page of any national newspaper. In nearly all cases the focus will be on dramatic cases, crisis situations or situations in which clinicians and families are faced with what are often called 'ethical dilemmas'. The fact is though that the day-to-day practice of medicine and healthcare more generally is not like this. The danger of this concentration on crises is that it creates the impression that medicine and healthcare is otherwise ethically unproblematic. Nurses and doctors and other healthcare professionals know that this is not the case. Many of the most difficult and, indeed the most interesting, ethical aspects of healthcare are those that arise in daily and long-term care. In this chapter we investigate ethical issues relating to long-term care, such as truth-telling and deception, confidentiality, the ethics of mealtimes and feeding, of mobility, the ethical difficulties raised by work with patients suffering from dementia, dealing with intimate relationships between patients, and so on.

Section 1: Truth-telling

THE CASE OF MR D

Sixty-eight-year-old Mr D, who has moderate dementia of the Alzheimer's type, lives at home with his wife. He is active and fit, which makes him quite demanding for Mrs D to nurse, given that he is also prone to wander and to forget where he lives. She welcomes the respite given by his attendance at a day-care centre, which he enjoys: he is very sociable.

Lately, however, Mr D has become worried about going to the day-care centre because he thinks he is losing time off work. He has never really stopped believing that he is still employed, although his increasing dementia forced him to retire 6 years ago. Now he insists that he cannot afford time to 'relax' because his deadlines at work are too pressing. There have been unseemly tussles with the staff of the day-care centre van when it comes to collect Mr D, and Mrs D is embarrassed by the scenes in front of the house. She is also increasingly exhausted because she is no longer getting the respite she needs.

Missing the company of the day-care centre has made Mr D morose and irritable, increasing the tensions at home. He has also become increasingly obsessive, muttering that 'he never has any time any more' and complaining that his work burdens seem to grow and grow. He desperately needs more time at the office, he says angrily, and blames his wife for being unable to drive, so that she cannot take him to work.

The ambulance staff have suggested to Mrs D that she could tell her husband that the van is a taxi, calling to take him to work. They are sure that the staff at the centre will go along with the fiction that this is Mr D's new office. These little deceptions happen all the time with patients like Mr D, they reassure her: sometimes patients are given medications in secret at the day-care centre, for example. Somehow Mrs D doesn't actually find this terribly reassuring *(based on a case in Hope and Oppenheimer, 1996).*

> **ACTIVITY: Stop here for a moment and ask yourself what should be done in the case of Mr D. What ethical issues are involved? Make a list of the arguments for and against telling him that the day-care centre van is his taxi to work.**

What arguments for and against the deception did you come up with? Here are some of the arguments we came up with.

Arguments for:
- The burden on Mrs D will be greatly reduced if she is spared the scenes and given time to recuperate from her heavy burdens in providing long-term care for Mr D.
- It is unlikely that Mr D will find out the truth; the day-care centre staff can be trusted to keep up the fiction.
- Long-term care arrangements for Mr D are otherwise satisfactory, and he can be maintained at home, with respite care, for a longer period. Alternative nursing home arrangements may be difficult to set up, and costly.
- No one is harmed and everyone benefits: Mr D benefits from, and enjoys, his day-care centre; his obsession will be reduced; Mrs D will get the rest she needs.

Arguments against:
- Mrs D is not happy about the deception.
- Mr D may be very angry if he finds out he has

been lied to, and may refuse to attend the centre ever again.
- This 'little' lie may lead to others; already the staff suggest that deception is routine, extending even to administration of medicines in secret which would be taboo on a psychiatric ward, in such countries as the UK (Hope, 1996) and Germany (Wolf, 1996). A climate of deception is easily created but not so easily undone.
- There is a shift from 'reality orientation' towards the 'validation' of Mr D's delusions if we accept that he should be lied to rather than being confronted with them as delusions. Arguably, this breaches the clinical duty of care (Widdershoven, 1996).

You may have noticed that virtually all of these arguments are concerned with the likely consequences (harmful or beneficial) of deception of this kind. Perhaps the strongest arguments against deception, however, are those which are sometimes called deontological or 'duty-based'. From a deontological perspective we might say that we have a duty to tell the truth and that:
- Deceiving Mr D in this way is simply dishonest. Lying is morally wrong. It diminishes the status of the person being lied to, denying him or her the opportunity to act as a free agent on the basis of correct information. It manipulates and uses people in an unacceptable way. This is inconsistent with respect for Mr D's dignity and integrity.

But is this last argument necessarily true? Many practitioners would find it very moralistic. Some might argue that ethical absolutes like this have no place in clinical practice, that pragmatic considerations should win the day (and probably that Mr D should be deceived for his own good). But if you look at some of the arguments for the deception, you'll find that they, too, have an ethical component. Look, for example, at the argument that 'no one is harmed and everyone benefits'. This eminently pragmatic argument actually rests on moral principles.

> **ACTIVITY: Stop here for a moment and consider what the underlying principles are.**

The answer may seem so obvious as not to be worth stating: that we have an obligation to maximize benefit and minimize harm. If the first principle of clinical practice is 'first do no harm' (*primum non nocere)*, we would have to be certain that no clinical harm will come to Mr D from the deception. We might want to distinguish clinical harm from social harm, such as marital stress, which seems less obviously the concern of the practitioner. However, if staying at home all the time increases the risk that Mr D will become more anxious or that his dementia will worsen, we might argue that avoiding the deception does in fact impose a risk of clinical harm. Conversely, if Mr D discovers that he has been lied to and then refuses to co-operate with his caregivers, clinical harm could also result.

Similarly, the argument that everyone benefits rests on a slightly different conception of the practitioner's duties: to benefit patients positively, not just to avoid harming them. Conceivably that might extend to a view that their long-term benefit outweighs any short-term harm, so that 'first do no harm' could be overridden. For example, even if it is admitted that there is a risk of short-term harm in deceiving Mr D, one might argue that the chance of successful long-term care management is increased if we take the small risks entailed in lying to him. On the other hand, someone who was committed to benefiting patients first and foremost might equally well argue that the benefits of lying to Mr D are by no means clear. Perhaps there is some other, less obvious treatment strategy which might achieve comparable benefit and avoid the wrong of lying?

So the principles of doing no harm (sometimes called *non-maleficence)* or maximizing benefit (sometimes called *beneficence)* don't actually tell us which way to jump in the case of Mr D. At this early stage of the chapter, it's not as crucial to find a solution as to suggest that the comparatively 'ordinary' and 'everyday' kind of case which Mr D represents does raise ethical dilemmas which need careful analysis. Very often, practical arguments actually rest on ethical disputes.

ACTIVITY: Your final activity in this section forms a bridge to later parts of the chapter. We would like you to begin reading an article by the Dutch philosopher and medical ethicist Guy Widdershoven, 'Truth and truth-telling'. The first section of the article appears here, but your reading of it will be resumed later in the chapter. As you read this first part of Widdershoven's article, ask yourself what the implications are (a) for the case of Mr D, and (b) for long-term care of the elderly more generally.

Truth and truth-telling

Guy Widdershoven

Truth is an important value in our lives. We do not want to be deceived, and we usually find it difficult to deceive others. Yet truth-telling is not a simple matter. Often we are not sure whether we should tell somebody else what we know, or how we ought to tell it. In every long-term relationship, a lot goes on which could be told, but actually is not. One might decide not to say what one actually thinks because it would take too much trouble to explain. One might refrain from correcting another person's views, because doing so would not be productive. In such cases it seems better to remain silent than to tell the truth. But how exactly can we justify such actions (or maybe better: omissions)?

In healthcare, several approaches to the issue of truth-telling can be found. The first is developed by defenders of principlism in biomedical ethics. They hold that the decision whether or not to tell the truth can be made by applying various principles, especially the principle of respect for autonomy and the principle of beneficence, to the case at hand. The second set of approaches are based upon a therapeutic perspective. This approach can be applied in various ways. Within the therapeutic perspective, some, the proponents of Reality Orientation Therapy (ROT), claim that truth-telling is crucial because it helps the patient (especially the demented patient) to orient himself in the world. Telling the truth is helpful because it keeps patients in touch with reality. Others, whilst also starting from a therapeutic perspective, deny that truth-telling is of itself therapeutically helpful and argue for a process of validation, claiming that one should not confront patients with reality, but attune to their way of meaning-making.

> ACTIVITY: Stop reading here for a moment and think about what these different approaches might say about Mr D. Has our discussion so far left any of these perspectives out?

We would say that so far we have discussed Mr D's case mainly in terms of principlism and Reality Orientation Therapy. We looked at the force of doing no harm and the hope of benefit, drawing on the principles of non-maleficence and beneficence. We also mentioned an argument against lying to Mr D which turns out to be derived from Reality Orientation Therapy: that there is a shift from confronting Mr D with reality to validating his delusions if we tell him the ambulance is a taxi to work. But we have not looked explicitly at the rightness or wrongness of validation: we merely assumed that it was a bad thing.

Now continue with your reading of Widdershoven's article.

THE CASE OF THE FORGETFUL MOURNER

In 1995, the *Hastings Center Report* published a case study, titled 'The forgetful mourner'. In it an 86-year-old woman has been admitted to a nursing home following the heart attack of her son, with whom she lived. After 2 years, her son dies. She attends the funeral. Yet afterwards she continues to ask for her son, as though he were still alive. When she is told that he is dead, she shows much distress. Each time the staff try to explain the situation to her, she reacts as though she is hearing the news for the first time.

The staff do not know what to do. Should they keep trying to tell her the truth, or should they remain silent about her son's death? In the latter

case, she might become convinced that her son is neglecting her, which might cause her a great deal of emotional pain. The doctors think that it is necessary to try and convince her that her son is dead. After 15 attempts without success a nurse proposes to dress her in the clothes which she wore at the funeral. The dress seems to remind her of her son. She speaks gently of him. After the ritual, she no longer asks for him. Yet she continues to mention his name every now and then.

In medical ethics, the issue of truth-telling is seen as an instance of medical ethical problems in general. Medical ethical problems are characterised by a conflict of principles (Beauchamp and Childress, 1994). The principles which are relevant to medical ethics are: respect for autonomy, beneficence, non-maleficence and justice. Ethical problems arise when these principles call for different kinds of actions. Respect for autonomy might mean that one executes the conscious wishes of a patient even if these are not in his own interest. In such a case, respect for autonomy conflicts with beneficence. According to principlism, the doctor should weigh the principles, and follow the principle which is the most important in the case at hand.

The issue of truth-telling can easily be integrated into this approach. On the one hand, the principle of respect for autonomy urges us to tell the truth to a patient. In hiding the truth, we do not take him seriously. On the other hand, the principle of beneficence might entail that we care for the patient's well-being by not telling him what we know. He might become upset by the news, and his condition may get worse. The caregiver has to become aware of such conflicts, and judge what is best in the concrete situation. By balancing the principles, the caregiver can decide what to do in a justified way.

Applying the principlist approach to the case described above (the 'forgetful mourner'), the first significant thing is the evident tension between respect for the patient and acting in the patient's best interest. Respecting the patient would mean continuing to tell her the truth. But since this results in distress, the patient's well-being is seriously harmed by this procedure. Therefore, one should consider ending the attempt to make her see the truth. In this case, one might argue that the policy of the doctors should have been ended long before they actually stopped. The harm done seems to be much larger than any possible gain. After ending the attempts to tell her the truth, one might try and look for means to make her more at ease. The intervention of the nurse can be regarded as aimed to comfort the patient. This intervention is not inspired by respect for autonomy, it is motivated by the wish to enhance the patient's well-being. Both in theory and in practice, beneficence appears to be stronger than respect for autonomy. The principlist approach to the problem of truth-telling emphasizes tensions experienced by the caregiver. The caregiver feels the need to respect the patient, or to enhance his well-being. Within the dominant principlist approach, it might be said that the patient's feelings are not relevant to medical ethics.

In therapeutic approaches to care for the elderly, in contrast to those which are principlist, especially in relation to care for people with dementia, the perspective is radically different. The emphasis is not on the moral considerations of the caregiver, but on the experiences of the carereceiver. Reality Orientation Therapy (ROT) and validation are two, mutually conflicting, approaches in this field; yet they have in common the claim that interventions should focus upon the condition of the carereceiver.

ACTIVITY: Take a moment to think about Widdershoven's use of the term 'therapeutic' here. Does it sound unfamiliar? How does his use of the term differ from its more everyday usage? Bear this in mind as you continue with your reading of Widdershoven's paper and try to get a clear picture of what he means by a therapeutic approach to healthcare.

According to ROT one should stimulate and actively help elderly people to keep in contact with reality, or to regain contact with it. The idea is that, by giving the right information about the environment and about the things that are going on around the patient, one can help him to orient himself better. Caregivers applying ROT constantly comment upon their actions ('now we are going to wash, and next you will get dressed; would you like to put on your red dress? Here it is . . .', etc.). They ask the patient about his life, using aids such as photographs to help the patient remember important people, such as parents or children. They will correct the patient if he is mistaken, and help him if he is not able to use the right words or perform the right actions all by himself.

Telling the truth is a fundamental aspect of ROT. One should not keep silent about what is happening, even if the patient has trouble in understanding it. One should not refrain from correcting the patient's mistakes, albeit in a gentle way. The aim of ROT is not to confront people with their mistakes, but to help to correct them. Applying principles of ROT to the case described above, one should not focus upon feelings of obligation or guilt on the part of the caregiver, but on the experience of the patient. One should try to make the patient aware of the fact that her son is dead, in such a way that she can accept it. One might use a photograph of the son, or another memory of him, to explain about his death. Actually, the intervention of the nurse functioned in this way: it somehow reminded the woman of the funeral, and thus made her son's death real for her. From a therapeutic perspective, it is important that the patient feels safe and comfortable. In this respect, the attempts of the staff to tell her the truth right away were not adequate. They did not help her accept the facts, but made her afraid. Telling the truth is not a virtue in itself, it has to be told in a way that is conducive to helping the patient to orient herself better, and to regain access to reality. The nurse's ritual appears to be a good way to convey the truth to the woman. It brings her in contact with reality in a productive way.

A second therapeutic intervention which focuses upon the patient's experiences is validation. Instead of telling the patient what is actually the case, as in ROT, one focuses upon the patient's feelings. The idea is not to enhance the patient's view of reality, but to show interest, and to accept the patient as he is. Strange or objectively wrong utterances may have a meaning for the patient. It is important to grasp this meaning, and help the patient to formulate it. The crux of validation is to make contact with the patient. A good way of doing this is to respond in a bodily way, by hugging for example.

Truth-telling plays hardly any role in validation. The objective situation is not important; the emphasis is on the patient's feelings. Telling the truth might easily lead to frustration. Focusing upon truth or falseness might also obscure why a person or event is meaningful for the patient. Instead of correcting the patient's views, one should find out what his utterances mean.

Applying the technique of validation to the case of the forgetful mourner, one would try to understand the patient's feelings about her son. From this perspective one should not try to tell her that he is dead, but focus on the fact that he obviously is important to her, and elaborate upon this. If the patient mentions her son, one might react by commenting that she obviously misses him very much. In this way, the patient is invited to express her feelings about her son. In this process, a mixture of feelings, both positive and negative, may come up. Thereby, the patient may be induced to rework her past, and to develop a new sense of self. From this perspective, the attempts of the staff to 'break the news to her' are clearly incompetent. She becomes so upset that she is not able to experience any feelings about her son. The intervention of the nurse is much more helpful; it evidently enables the woman to give her son a new place in her life. The nurse's intervention is not a matter of truth-telling at all; afterwards the woman still does not really know that her son is dead, but she has developed a new relationship towards him.

ACTIVITY: What do you think about this sugges-tion? Does it resonate with your own experience?

We will end our reading of Widdershoven there for now, but we shall be returning to the article in Section 3. Let's now end this section by relating what you have just read back to the case of Mr D with which we began the chapter.

In long-term care, where relationships with patients can be established and where patients' values and preferences may come to be known more deeply than in acute care, the question of truth-telling is linked to how the patient construes reality. Although Mr D is moderately demented, his construction of reality is still important. (This relates back to whether carers should validate or challenge how the patient sees the world.)

A principlist approach to the case of Mr D might analyse it in terms of the concepts of autonomy, beneficence and non-maleficence and in terms of the conflicts between them. For example, Mr D's autonomous right to be told the truth might be seen to be in conflict with the view that 'everyone benefits and no one is harmed' by telling him a little white lie.

A therapeutic perspective might focus instead on how Mr D construes reality. Telling him that the ambulance is his taxi to work risks confirming his delusional construction of reality. Telling him the truth, according to Reality Orientation Therapy, might arguably keep him in better touch with reality. But so far that strategy does not appear to be working; it only results in painful scenes – just as staff attempts to tell 'the forgetful mourner' that her son was dead only succeeded in upsetting her.

Perhaps an alternative validation-based approach which respects Mr D's view of the world might be to ask what work represents to Mr D. Why is it so important? – or more accurately, why is the loss of it so important? Is there any way in which he could be made to recognize the truth – that he is no longer working – in a similarly inventive manner to that which the nurse devised for bringing the reality of the son's death home to the 'forgetful mourner?'

We will leave you with this question for now. Truth-telling, as illustrated by the everyday cases of Mr D and of the 'forgetful mourner', raises

issues about how we approach practical and
ethical dilemmas in long-term care, but it does
not exhaust the list of those dilemmas: far from it.
In Sections 2 and 3 we will discuss a range of other
common ethical quandaries in long-term care,
analysing them in some of the terms to which
Section 1 has introduced you but extending our
analysis into new areas as well.

In each of those sections, we will follow the plan
of Section 1, beginning with an everyday case in
long-term care and drawing out the implications.
This may seem odd: medical ethics is more often
conceived of in terms of 'big' issues such as euthanasia. But as the Swedish nursing lecturers Anne-
Cathrine Matthiasson and Maja Hemberg have
perceptively written,

Ethics is concerned with how we ought to act toward
one another. What is good and bad, what is right and
wrong when acting toward another individual? Within
the study of medical ethics, these questions are often
equated with dramatic decisions about life and death, or
consequences of the latest advances within medical
technology and research. Ethics, however, is not only
concerned with the spectacular or with questions of life
and death. In general wards of hospitals or in nursing
homes, particularly in the daily care of the elderly, lies a
type of everyday ethics with countless small down-to-
earth decisions concerning the various aspects of care.
These actions are not subject to analysis every time they
are performed. Rather, they reflect consciously or
unconsciously the fundamental attitudes which carers
express in their everyday actions. In seeking assistance
in concrete situations, it is therefore imperative that we
are aware of the values upon which we base our
reflection (Mattiasson and Hemberg, 1997, p. 1).

**ACTIVITY: Stop here for a moment and make a list
of the key points raised by this section.**

Section 2: Autonomy, competence and confidentiality

Restraint, wandering and mobility

We begin this section with another everyday sort
of case in long-term care of the elderly, provided
by Tony Hope, an English medical ethicist and
old-age psychiatrist.

THE CASE OF MRS B

Mrs B, who suffers from moderate to severe
Alzheimer's disease, frequently wanders from the
nursing home where she is living. She has poor
traffic sense. Not long ago, she wandered out into
the road. A car swerved to avoid her and crashed
into a tree. The driver suffered mild bruising and
was very shaken, but was not seriously hurt.

**ACTIVITY: Consider how you would act in this case
if you were responsible for Mrs B's care? Jot down
some possible options and the arguments for and
against them.**

You probably found yourself balancing Mrs B's
'right' to wander freely, without restraint, against
the risk of harm to herself and the public. The
usual analysis of Mrs B's case would pit her 'right
to wander', based on a claim that her autonomy
should be protected for as long as possible,
against the harm to others and to herself which
might result from her wandering. In her own best
interests, should she be prevented from wandering? There are also the interests of others to consider. Whether or not the motorist was seriously
hurt this time, a fatal accident could occur next
time. So perhaps you found yourself considering
whether she should be restrained from wandering; alternatively, you might have considered
tracking or tagging, depending on the legitimacy
of those strategies in the legal and professional
codes of your country.

Compared to Mr D, Mrs B seems much less able
to decide for herself, although walking around

freely still seems important to her view of the world. She may well be incompetent to judge the risk to both herself and to others from her wandering; whereas Mr D's understanding of his situation has fluctuated. Competence is a crucial concept in law, dictating different treatment strategies for competent and incompetent patients. As Hope summarizes the distinction,

A competent adult has a right to refuse any, even life-saving, treatment. To impose a treatment without consent would amount to battery. The only grounds for restraining a competent adult without consent (against their will) is for the protection of others (in which case the restraint would normally be more a matter for the police than for health professionals). An incompetent adult should normally be treated on the basis of their best interests (Hope, 1997).

Truth-telling, the issue in the case of Mr D, is premised on the assumption that the patient is to some degree competent to understand the truth and act on it. In the case of Mr D, what the carers actually hoped was that he would act on a lie – that the day-care centre ambulance was a taxi to his office – but they still treated him as able to act on information that was given to him, as competent in that sense. In English law, the test of competence is threefold: understanding the information given, believing the information, and being able to weigh it up in deciding whether to accept or refuse a proposed intervention (Re C, 1994).

But although truth-telling and negotiation are not so much the issue here as in the previous example, autonomy is still relevant. Barring Mrs B from walking around the grounds is likely to feel like imprisoning her to her carers, whether it is done by means of a locked door, sedation, or tracking devices. It feels like a significant invasion of her rights, even though she is almost certainly not competent. There are risks of elder abuse if such strategies are followed too frequently, and most professionals are sensitive to this – although, as Tony Hope's analysis below demonstrates, they may not feel they can let their sensitivity be the only consideration.

In balancing best interests, the degrees of risk and harm need to be weighed against the distress caused by restraint and the loss of pleasure due to the loss of freedom. In my view, arguments against the use of restraints either on the grounds of loss of dignity or on the grounds that it is important for people with dementia to be given the same freedom as normal people should not be given much weight. It could be argued that restraining Mrs B constitutes an abuse. Alternatively, it could be argued that allowing her to wander, risking grave harm, is also a form of abuse – an example of neglect (Hope, 1997).

But what about cases in which the patient is less obviously incompetent, although the risks of harm are just as serious? Take the case of Mr A, summarized below.

THE CASE OF MR A

Mr A is a 72-year-old retired railway conductor who lives with his wife in the house of their 43-year-old daughter and her family. Still active on the family smallholding, he is increasingly frustrated by difficulties in operating machinery and in finding his way about the house. Accompanied by his wife and daughter, he visited Dr B's clinic for memory disturbance, where he was diagnosed with hypertension, arteriosclerotic occlusive disease, and multiple subcortical perivascular lesions on a computer scan of his brain. The overall diagnosis was subcortical vascular dementia with a moderate degree of impairment. It emerged that Mr A also had considerable impairment of his short-term memory (e.g. telephone numbers) and long-term recall (e.g. names of old friends). However, he denied strenuously that his mental powers were in any way impaired.

In the course of the consultation, Dr B asked Mr A whether he drove a car. Mr A replied that he did, and Dr B warned him that he should stop, from a medical point of view – because of his memory impairment. Mr A absolutely refused to consider stopping: he was in perfectly good health, he insisted, and still very fit. 'I'm a lot better driver than all those young lunatics!' Mr A's daughter broke in at this point to describe two small car accidents which her father had recently caused. Mr A then announced, out of the blue, that he had just decided to buy a new car. If there was any problem, it lay in the old car, not in his driving. And there the matter rested, at least in the doctor's consultation.

Privately, Mr A's wife and daughter agreed between themselves that the only possible solution was to hide the car keys. But Mr A managed to locate them, and drove off to a reunion of his railway colleagues without any incident. When he returned, it was with a new copy of the car keys, and a bad mood that lasted for days at home. Mr A's wife has now lost any will to prevent her husband from driving: she can't bear his anger, she says, and in any case he was perfectly all right last time he drove. Perhaps he doesn't have dementia after all, she remarked to the doctor on her own next visit to his surgery.

> ACTIVITY: How would you analyse this case? Think in terms of (a) the possible decisions which Dr B could take and (b) the reasoning behind those decisions.

Dr B's options range from doing nothing to full-scale psychiatric interventions. In-between lies the option of reporting Mr B to the driver licensing authorities, on the grounds that he is a danger to others. However, that would raise issues about confidentiality in the doctor–patient relationship. This is one element in the reasoning which might enter into Dr B's decision: that information obtained in the course of doctor–patient consultation is normally private, and that it would be wrong to reveal it to the licensing authorities.

In most countries, however, the obligation of confidentiality is not absolute. Where public interest in disclosure outweighs the public interest in ensuring confidentiality, health professionals are permitted – though normally not obliged – to breach confidentiality (Montgomery, 1997, p. 257). 'Most countries have legislation which gives to the doctor the right to be freed from the obligation of confidentiality, when there is a danger to the health or life of other people' (Dalla Vorgia,

1997). The exact scope of the obligation varies from country to country, as do guidelines issued to practitioners by their professional bodies. In the UK, General Medical Council guidelines allow disclosure to prevent a risk of death or serious harm to others, and do require doctors to inform the Driver and Vehicle Licensing Authority of any patient who is unfit to drive but cannot be persuaded to stop. In Italy, the 1995 code of medical ethics suggests that public interest in disclosure extends to a duty to inform partners or family of a patient's HIV-positive status, even without the patient's consent (Fineschi et al., 1997, p. 242).

Other limitations on absolute confidentiality may occur in cases of child abuse or of dangerous psychiatric patients being discharged into the community: here again, disclosure of confidential information may be permitted. (See, for example, an English case involving a patient in a secure hospital who challenged disclosure of a confidential psychiatric report on his dangerousness to the medical director of the hospital and to the Home Office: *W* v. *Egdell*, 1990.) UK case law holds that professionals may disclose confidences in order to protect the public, provided three conditions are satisfied:

- There must be a real and serious danger to the public
- Disclosure must be to a person or body with a legitimate interest in receiving the information
- Disclosure must be strictly limited to the information about risk, not all the patient's details (Montgomery, 1997, pp. 259–60).

What lies behind the general duty of confidentiality? (Even if Dr B can breach that duty – after further attempts to persuade Mr A to stop driving voluntarily – it is not a duty lightly to be broken.) We might seem to be back with the principles of autonomy versus beneficence again, as we were in one possible interpretation of the case of Mr D in the previous section. That is, Mr A's autonomy, his right to judge his own competence to drive and the freedom which driving brings, would have to be balanced against enhancing public safety by reporting him. This is certainly one set of considerations that Dr B might be considering. But we saw in the previous section that there are alternative ways of analysis, too: in that case, involving truth-telling, in terms of validation vs. Reality Orientation Therapy. Whereas in the principlist approach tensions experienced by the caregiver were to the fore, both validation and ROT focus on the condition of the care receiver, according to Widdershoven. For example, in the case of Mr A, trying to understand his condition on a personal level might involve asking why mobility is so important to him. Does he miss the daily travel which his job as a railway conductor used to give him, for example?

> **ACTIVITY:** Now read the following analysis of the case of Mr A by Tony Hope. As you read, ask yourself whether Hope is offering an alternative to a principlist analysis, or a more sophisticated version of it. How does he construe autonomy?

A commentary on the Case of Mr A

Tony Hope

At first sight this case may appear to be a conflict between respecting Mr A's autonomous desire to drive, and the risk he poses to others. However, it is not as straightforward as that. Consider first autonomy. What would it be to respect his autonomy, to allow him to do what he now wants (i.e. to drive); or to do what he might have said about this situation prior to his dementia?

It is normally only considered possible to 'respect someone's autonomy' if that person is competent with regard to the decision to be made. Is this man competent to make a decision about whether he should drive? Two important considerations in making a decision are the risk to others and the risk to oneself. Since Mr A is not aware that he is suffering from dementia and does not appear to understand these two risks, I do not think that he is competent to make a decision about his driving.

In these circumstances, respecting autonomy is more a question of respecting the view he would have had before the onset of dementia than respecting his current desire to drive. Therefore, from the point of view of autonomy, the key issue is what he might have said about the situation had he been asked about it prior to the dementia. I suspect that most people would say that they would prefer to be prevented from driving in these circumstances rather than risk seriously harming another person. However, I have no good evidence for this belief, and in any case the issue here is what would Mr A have wanted.

Thus, I see the conflict in this vignette as being between the value and pleasure which Mr A gets from continuing driving (this might include the value of retaining some independence, over and above simply the pleasure from driving) against the risks he poses to other people and himself. Most countries have laws to prevent some people from driving, principally because of the risk which they pose to other people. Such laws typically prevent people with certain illnesses such as epilepsy from driving (under certain conditions) as well as preventing those who have been found guilty of certain criminal offences from driving. Society deems it right to prevent people from driving if they pose an excessive risk to others, even if this overrides their own autonomous views.

Of course, all driving poses a risk to others, so that as a society we clearly have judged that some risk can be taken in the interests of individuals and society from allowing most adults to drive. Thus the issue seems to be that at some point the risk to others outweighs the benefit to the individual. In England, at any rate, an assessment of how much a person wants to drive, or even how valuable it is to a person to drive, is not considered relevant. For example, the criteria as to what frequency of epileptic fits should prevent a person from driving do not differ depending on how much pleasure a person gets from driving, or whether driving is a necessary part of his job. In the UK the criterion for epilepsy is that you can only drive if you have been free from fits for 2 years (or have only had fits whilst asleep for the last 3 years).

Thus it would seem that the issue of whether a person ought to be prevented from driving should essentially be a question of whether the risk that person poses to others is greater than some threshold. What risk does Mr A pose? Presumably he poses a greater risk than he did before the dementia. But that by itself would not justify stopping him driving on the grounds of risk to other people. Does he pose a greater risk than many normal 18-year-old men? Let us suppose that the figures suggest that people with the degree of dementia of Mr A actually pose less risk of harm than do young adult males, who have a relatively high accident rate. Is there any justification for allowing the 18-year-old to drive, but not Mr A? Here are some possible justifications:

(a) The fact that Mr A poses a greater risk than previously. However, this does not justify banning Mr A whilst allowing the 18-year-old to drive.

(b) The combination of increased risk plus the fact that he is no longer fully competent. Suppose an 18-year-old man drives dangerously and causes an accident. He would be held fully responsible for what he had done. However, were Mr A to cause an accident, he is likely not to be considered responsible. Although the question of whether or not the driver could be held responsible does not help the victim of the accident, it does provide the victim with the potential for some kind of redress, either civil or criminal. But this argument does not seem to me a convincing reason for treating Mr A differently from the young man.

(c) If Mr A were to cause an accident, his insurance company might well not pay compensation to the victim, on the grounds that the company was not aware that Mr A suffered from dementia. Thus, unlike the victim of the 18-year-old driver, whose age is a known risk factor to the insurance company (and who pays a higher premium accordingly), Mr A's victim would receive no compensation. This seems to me to provide a powerful reason why either the doctor or Mr A's family should inform the insurance company of Mr A's condition. However, if the company were still willing to insure Mr A (perhaps at higher cost), it does not seem to me to provide a reason to prevent Mr A from driving.

(d) The most powerful argument for preventing Mr A from driving is that this is what Mr A would have wanted had he been asked when competent. My view is based on an empirical belief (which might be false) that most people would be concerned not to cause an accident through having dementia but no insight into it.

At the end of his analysis Tony Hope returns to the interesting re-interpretation of autonomy which he offered at the beginning. In this view, autonomy is not simply doing what you please, but acting in a responsible, competent manner. Really respecting Mr A's autonomy doesn't mean giving in to his current desires, lacking in insight into his condition or concern for the risks he imposes on others. It means treating him as a rational moral agent, and holding him to the standards of responsibility that a rational agent would accept. Respect for persons in this view means treating others as 'citizens of the kingdom of ends' (in the words of the eighteenth-century philosopher Immanuel Kant): as moral agents, not objects of care. It has been argued by other modern medical ethicists that autonomy in this sense means honouring the patient's ability to behave unselfishly, rather than giving him everything he wants (Lindemann Nelson and Lindemann Nelson, 1995).

To return to the question which we asked you to consider while you were doing this activity, Hope can thus be seen as using both a principlist and a non-principlist approach to analysing the case of Mr A. Whilst he concentrates first on the principles of autonomy and beneficence, he notes immediately that they are too simplistic as usually presented. His elaboration of autonomy turns out to be rather more like the approach suggested by Widdershoven, in fact. Rather than simply accepting Mr A's desire to drive at face value, as an expression of his autonomy, Hope asks whether it is a competent and responsible wish. If not, it needs questioning in much the same way that Reality Orientation Therapy suggested in the previous case examples.

Autonomy and its critics

In this section we move from case examples to two extended critiques of the conventional approach to autonomy, relating these more theoretical analyses back to the cases so far introduced and to management of long-term care in general.

ACTIVITY: We would like you to begin with a reading exercise on an article by Ruud ter Meulen, a psychologist and medical ethicist at the Institute for Bioethics in the Netherlands: 'Care for dependent elderly persons and respect for autonomy.' As you read, ask yourself what the implications are for practice of the broader view of autonomy which Ter Meulen suggests. How would it affect the case of Mr A? or a case from your own experience?

Care for dependent elderly persons and respect for autonomy

Ruud ter Meulen

The safeguarding of autonomy is an important principle in care for the chronically ill. This is particularly true in the care of the dependent elderly. Policies in most European countries are aimed at allowing elderly dependent people live in their own homes for as long as possible. Even once they have left their own homes, autonomy continues to be an important consideration in care management. In many nursing homes, elderly patients are given maximum opportunity for independent living and for shared decision-making. As an example, I refer to a 1993 policy paper of the Dutch Association of Nursing Home Care (NVVZ), which states that nursing home care should be about more than mere physical management. Instead, it should be aimed at making itself

superfluous: at reducing, stabilizing or even removing the requirement for care. In communication with the client, caregivers should respect individuals' choices as much as possible, in order to enable clients to live their lives according to their own values.

In this context, autonomy is defined as participation and the right to self-determination. Autonomy is commonly defined in various ways: as 'self-rule', 'making your own choices,' or 'being able to live independently'. The right to self-determination is a necessary condition for realising one's autonomy. However, the question is whether it is a sufficient condition for autonomy. If we are given the opportunity to determine our own lives, do we need more than a mere formal right to self-determination?

In this paper I will argue for a broad concept of autonomy in which aspects of identity and identification play an important role. This broadening of the concept of autonomy will be preceded by a philosophical and sociological critique of the way autonomy is usually conceived in healthcare ethics. This broad concept of autonomy will be illustrated in long-term care management for chronically ill and dependent elderly persons.

In healthcare and healthcare ethics, the concept of autonomy is for the most part exclusively described as the freedom to make choices and to follow one's own preferences. 'Freedom' is often defined negatively, that is 'not hindered by others'. According to the American philosopher George Agich in his book *Autonomy in Long-term Care* (1993), this negative idea of freedom comes from the political sphere, where it is meant to safeguard individuals from interventions by the state in their own personal affairs. In respect to the relations between individuals, particularly in the care of dependent elderly, this liberal ideology is inadequate. Liberalism has achieved the important right of individuals not to be harmed in their own physical and mental integrity. The right to information, the principle of free and informed consent and the safeguarding of privacy are important and enduring moral principles in our healthcare system, and they apply to the care of dependent elderly persons as well. Nevertheless, the relations between individuals would be impoverished if they were exclusively defined in these terms. Such relationships will have a predominantly formal and procedural character, but would lack sufficient moral, psychological or emotional content.

Agich directs our attention to discussions in American psychiatry, where, in his view, the right to self-determination has degenerated into 'a right to rot'. In that context, the ideal of freedom is radically explained as the right of individuals 'to be left alone'. Legal procedures have increasingly disrupted the relationship between physicians and other care professionals on the one hand, and patients on the other. However, in European healthcare systems, one can observe the same tendencies. In the Netherlands, for example, physicians are increasingly afraid of a lawsuit for 'malpractice'. As a consequence, they tend to adopt a defensive attitude and limit their services to necessary care, on the condition that patients have given their explicit consent.

The relationship between individuals, particularly that between patients and healthcare professionals, will turn then into a predominantly contractual relationship. This is a relationship which is defined in terms of rights and allows no room for personal virtues like solidarity and personal involvement. The change into a contract-like healthcare system can be illustrated by the transition from nursing home care to home care, which in many European countries is an important policy in elderly care: care 'in the community'. Although this policy may appear to increase the autonomy of the elderly, in the negative sense of being free from intervention, they may as a result fall into a 'black hole' of loneliness and neglect.

In healthcare ethics, the concept of autonomy is based on the philosophical concept of the person, particularly the concept of the person as advocated by Immanuel Kant. According to Kant the person is a rational and free being who can determine his own actions, independent of both his natural circumstances or the desires and inclinations of his own body. Freedom, Kant says, is the following of duty. This means that man should act

according to duties which are unconditionally and at all times binding for every person (according to one formulation of Kant's 'categorical imperative'). When there is no respect for the freedom of the person, *one loses the possibility of acting morally.*

In healthcare ethics, we are often encouraged to follow Kant in considering the person as an individual and rational being, whose autonomous decisions should be respected. However, there is an important difference between Kant and contemporary health ethics. While Kant sees the freedom of the person as embodied in acting from duty, in healthcare ethics freedom is merely seen as a freedom to decide on one's own body and mind, without any reference to a universal duty. Thus, the difference is between autonomy as self-legislation (Kant) and autonomy as 'self-determination' (healthcare ethics).

> **ACTIVITY: Stop for a moment and consider this important distinction, which reaches out beyond healthcare ethics into our entire popular conception of freedom and autonomy. What implications does it have?**

Ter Meulen is making a similar point to that raised by Tony Hope in his discussion of Mr A's 'freedom' to drive. Mr A interprets his autonomy as freedom to continue driving, regardless of the consequences for others. In ter Meulen's interpretation of Kant, this is not justifiable. The autonomous decisions which deserve respect are those which coincide with the categorical imperative, which is also formulated as 'Act according to that principle which you could will to become a universal law.' But if everyone behaved as Mr A wants to, there would be utter carnage on the roads. Autonomy means choosing one's wishes to conform with reason, not simply giving in to every passing whim – like Mr A's abrupt decision to buy a new car just to prove that he can do what he likes. Whereas Hope, however, had to rely on empirical evidence that most people recognize responsibilities to others – which might or might not have been true of Mr A before his dementia – ter Meulen is relying on a philosophical rather than an empirical argument. Now continue with your reading of ter Meulen's paper.

In healthcare ethics, the only limit to freedom is the autonomy or freedom of another person. That is, the choices which one makes may not result in an unacceptable or unreasonable limitation of another person's freedom to choose. In fact, this view on autonomy is more close to the liberal social ethics of John Stuart Mill than to the philosophy of Immanuel Kant. In healthcare ethics, autonomy is usually defined as the freedom to make choices, particularly the freedom to decide on one's own body and mind. The only limit to this freedom is the autonomy or freedom of another person. That is, the choices which one makes may not result in an unacceptable limitation of the freedom to choose of another person. In case of conflicts, one should reasonably argue or negotiate to reach a mutual agreement.

> ACTIVITY: Think about how this view of autonomy as limited only by harm to others is illustrated by the case of Mrs B's wandering. Bear this in mind as you continue now with your reading of the rest of the paper.

Basing itself on this liberal social ethic, mainstream healthcare ethics reflects the self-image of the individual in modern bourgeois culture, in which freedom, individuality and rationality are central values. This self-image, however, is an ideological construct: it is partly both an adequate and an inadequate reflection of the social reality.

The concept of autonomy in healthcare ethics is adequate insofar as individuals are expected to behave rationally and self-consciously and to treat other persons with due respect. Violence or authoritarian commands are not accepted: disagreements between persons ought to be resolved by negotiation and deliberation. This culture of negotiation has replaced the culture of commands which disappeared in our society in the past century. As a consequence, the content of the relationships between individuals has been liberalized. However, the way people get along

with each other is subject to strict rules: there is an increased tolerance for various kinds of relationships between individuals, but only on the condition of mutual agreement and free consent.

The rise of the culture of negotiation can be considered the sociological background for the strong emphasis in healthcare ethics on the principle of free and informed consent: physicians should respect the wishes and preferences of their patients and should try to reach agreement concerning their medical treatment by way of negotiation. The patient should know what he wants and should express his preferences clearly to the physician. The traditional authority of the physician has been removed and replaced with a democratic relationship based on negotiation and mutual respect. In the phrase of the American medical ethicist Tristram Engelhardt, 'To be a person is to be a possible negotiator' (Engelhardt, 1988).

> ACTIVITY: What are the advantages and disadvantages of the 'culture of negotiation' in relation to elderly patients? You might consider it to be an advantage, for example, that routine is less likely to dominate these days, and that patients are involved in negotiating about their own care, even in small matters such as choosing what clothes to put on (to use the example from Widdershoven). One disadvantage of the 'culture of negotiation' is that it forces elderly people to conform to a model of the 'consumerist' individual which probably did not obtain when they were growing up: they may be more accustomed to obeying authority for its own sake. If patients don't actually want a democratic relationship with their doctor, is it right to force one on them?

The individualistic and rationalistic concept of autonomy is inadequate because it ignores the social processes which underpin the appeal to negotiation and mutual respect. According to the German sociologist Norbert Elias, this concept of the person as an independent actor is a fiction, or as he himself puts it, 'an artefact of human thinking that is characteristic of a certain level in the development of human self-experience' (Elias, 1971). Elias conceives of the individual as someone 'who in his relationship with other human persons possesses a higher or lower degree of autonomy, but who will never reach total or absolute autonomy, who during his life is fundamentally thrown into a world with others and indeed is necessarily dependent on these others'.

The individualistic concept of autonomy is also criticized by other sociologists and philosophers, who point to increased alienation in modern culture: the sense of community and of solidarity has been replaced by individualism and egoism. According to this view, public morality has fallen apart: every individual has his own goals and his own standards of right and wrong. The narcissistic concentration on one's own individuality has resulted in a decrease of unity with the group. According to Cushman (1990), in the second half of the twentieth century individuals have been confronted with an absence of community ties and shared systems of meaning. This has resulted in feelings of emptiness or an 'empty self'. Another consequence of this process is a fragmentation of public morality, in which every individual has his own moral standards based on his own feelings and intuitions. The problem of moral pluralism in contemporary society and the difficulty of reaching a moral consensus is closely linked to the impossibility of the modern narcissistic personality to find a moral standard outside himself.

The concept of autonomy in mainstream healthcare ethics does not acknowledge these social determinations. It presupposes rationality, individuality and self-determination, ignoring the social structures in which these characteristics play a role. The concept of autonomy then, needs to be corrected: the emphasis on autonomous individuality should be adjusted towards a social and relational concept of the person, which pays attention to the social context in which the person realizes him or herself. I want to mention three aspects of autonomy which are not recognized in contemporary health ethics, but which can be part of this broader concept: 'identification', 'identity' and 'sense of meaning'. Each of these aspects of autonomy requires a social context for its develop-

ment. In his study on autonomy in long-term care George Agich also makes a strong plea for a social concept of autonomy. According to Agich the view of man as a rational and free individual is an abstraction of reality. In reality, individuals are not so much directed by rational decisions as they are by the image of themselves. Acting autonomously means that you identify yourself with your own actions and practice. This kind of approach does not see autonomy as a quality of an abstract rational self, but as the way individuals experience themselves in reality. In this view of autonomy, psychological processes like 'identification' play an important role. When I can identify myself with my behaviour or with the results of this behaviour, I feel autonomous. When I write an article such as this, and I can identify myself with its creation, I experience a certain degree of autonomy. This experience can also accompany the writing itself: the more I can lose myself in an activity, the more I experience myself as an autonomous being. Autonomy is in this view never finished or 'ready': it is a process, by which the person develops himself and realises himself. Being autonomous means to develop oneself, not in the direction of an abstract ideal, but by way of a continuous identification with changing circumstances.

This means that care for dependent elderly people should be organized in such a way, that the elderly person can identify herself with her own behaviour and with her changing environment. Respect for autonomy should not be limited to dramatic medical treatments, for example nontreatment decisions at the end of life, but should be a continuous process in daily care. It means, for example, that elderly persons in a nursing home are given the opportunity to make meaningful choices, particularly regarding daily care and daily activities. Rosalie Kane and Arthur Caplan (1990) talk about 'everyday ethics': particularly in normal interactions and daily care, there are many possibilities and obstacles for the realisation of autonomy. This can mean that people may make their own choices regarding 'sleeping and feeding' times or the clothes they want to wear. In every nursing home one needs a regime, but not at the expense of a social sphere in which individuals can express their own individuality.

ACTIVITY: What would it mean in practice to organize the care of the elderly in the way described?

One may wonder whether autonomy and dependency can co-exist. A chronic disease has in many cases a profound impact on the life of those who are afflicted by it. Life-plans are disrupted, while social relationships and everyday activities are often seriously hindered. These dramatic changes often have a serious consequences for the experience of one's own 'identity'. Kathy Charmaz (1987) talks about a 'constant struggle': people who are suffering from a chronic or enduring disease have to fight continually for their own identity, adjusting themselves to their handicaps, pain and loneliness. The promotion of autonomy is not in contradiction with the dependency caused by chronic disease: in view of his chronic diseases, a person who finds him or herself to be dependent and vulnerable needs support by his environment to find a new identity or to adjust the previous one. Particularly in those circumstances, he or she needs to recognize himself or herself in the choices he or she makes. Opportunities should be offered then to make these choices a reality. In this process of identification and of regaining or restoring autonomy, the relationship with caregivers is extremely important. Autonomy, conceived as development of one's identity, is a relational process. It requires the solidarity and commitment of the caregiver.

However, to safeguard or restore autonomy, one needs not only the commitment of the caregiver, but also a sense of 'meaning' of what it is to be old, particularly of being dependent. Individuals do have some sense of meaning, but it may be fragmented and not articulated. The articulation of this individual sense of meaning of life and old age is hindered by the fact that, as a society, we have great difficulty giving meaning to old age and dependency. While in former times ageing was considered a normal process of existence, in modern times it seems a practical problem which

can be solved by scientific research and technology. We live in a society in which being young seems to be the absolute norm.

Of course, it is important to stay healthy and active as long as possible during the course of our life. However, we must realize that our lives do come to an end, in spite of all attempts at rejuvenation. We also have to realize that this end is often preceded by a period of debilitating diseases and handicaps. Because we value youth and activity in such a strong way, we are not able to give meaning to our dependencies. Yet the acceptance and integration of dependency is an important condition for realizing autonomy.

The lack of a shared system of meaning is closely linked to the emergence of the negotiating culture. In a society based on negotiation, there is no fixed norm or criterion. There are only rules for mutual relationships (freely consent to), not for the content of these relationships. The only certainty lies in one's own self, in one's own feelings. This narcissistic quest for the self, this absolute triumph of the 'me', is breaking down old fences and old traditions, like 'age' and 'generation'. Traditions cannot offer any guidance any more; in fact they hinder the development of the self.

Here I want to refer to what the Canadian philosopher Charles Taylor has called the 'horizon of meaning' (Taylor, 1991). According to Taylor, we can realize our identity only when we experience ourselves as part of a whole, that is within a spiritual or cultural tradition. The influence of liberal ideology on our culture has resulted in greater political rights. However, it has also resulted in the disappearance of a horizon of meaning, a cultural framework of values which gives meaning to individual and societal experience. The price to be paid for this freedom is a sense of meaninglessness and triviality.

What we need, Taylor says, is an 'art of retrieval'. That is, an attempt to regain senses of meaning that have been lost during the past, particularly the meaning of old age. Such a horizon of meaning is a necessary condition for realising our identity. By regaining a commonly shared horizon of meaning, there will be growth of mutual ties and a decrease of the fragmentation of society into separate individuals. A shared interpretation of ageing and dependency may prevent the relationships between carers and elderly care recipients from becoming impoverished as a result of the individualization process. Horizons of meaning are in this respect an important and necessary supplement to the one-sided and narrow political–liberal interpretation of the concept of autonomy.

Ter Meulen stresses identification with one's actions, support from caregivers in adjusting to the new dependent identity, and realization by caregivers that our society loads unattractive and burdensome meanings onto old age. Above all, he sees autonomy as created in relationship – in contrast to the usual notion of 'finding oneself'. In practical terms – for example, the case of Mr A – ter Meulen's 'broad' concept of autonomy would suggest helping the patient to recover self-respect despite dependency, perhaps employing 'lateral thinking' like that demonstrated by the nurse in the case of the forgetful mourner. Clearly Mr A's sense of himself is intimately linked to mobility and to being in control: both, not so incidentally, characteristics of his old job. Although Dr B would not be betraying confidentiality if he reported Mr A to the licensing authorities – and indeed, in many countries his professional code would require him to do so – there also needs to be some consideration of how Mr A can adjust to the loss of mobility without the loss of autonomy in the sense of relational identity. Hiding the car keys – understandable response though it is – doesn't address this problem, and only makes Mr A angrier. Instead, it would seem that Dr B has to assist Mr A's wife and daughter more overtly in their consultations, in challenging Mr A's limited, egoistic view of autonomy and in negotiating other ways in which he can remain mobile without posing a threat to others.

The emphasis on the self as constructed through relationship, which emerged so strongly in ter Meulen's article, is shared with many feminist approaches to moral philosophy and medical ethics. Like ter Meulen's analysis, such feminist approaches emerge originally from psychology and psychiatry, particularly the work of the American psychologist Carol Gilligan (1982). Like ter Meulen's 'broad' model, the approaches suggest that autonomy is too often narrowly construed, with unfavourable consequences for those who do not fit the 'rational consumer of health services' mould. In the final reading for this section, Gwen Adshead, a psychotherapist, forensic psychiatrist and medical ethicist, discusses autonomy from this perspective. Her focus, too, is on constructing a richer model of identity, but she adds an another new dimension to this chapter in that she does not construe long-term care solely in terms of the elderly: rather, psychiatric patients are her principal interest, of all ages (Adshead and Dickenson, 1993).

Autonomy, feminism and psychiatric patients

Gwen Adshead

Within the individualistic tradition of Western philosophy and political thought, autonomy is an essential feature of both personhood and citizenship. But this central position of autonomy hides an enduring tension between the identity of the person as an individual and their connection to groups of others, either small scale (e.g. the family) or larger scale (e.g. the political domain). In this article I am going to explore the connections between identities: the individual identity and the group identity. I am going to suggest that feminist perspectives may enrich the debate about the nature of psychological identities, their relationship with each other, and with concepts of autonomy. I will also attempt to link the feminist perspective with a psychological perspective, drawing on ideas about psychological development, based on attachment theory.

Traditional views of autonomy involve a vision of individual personhood which is both separate from others and hierarchical. Full autonomy is linked with rationality, 'untainted by desire', in Kant's phrase – reflecting a view of reason which excludes affects and feelings and links those aspects of mental life with irrationality. Another traditional view appears to draw on Darwinian notions of the survival of the fittest, so that decisions which do not further one's own interests are perceived as being suspect, and only self-interest is natural. The link between the two lies in the understanding of emotions as being both irrational in themselves (and therefore tending to diminish autonomy) and causing us to take decisions which are biased and therefore irrational.

ACTIVITY: Stop here for a moment and think about Mr A's emotions: his anger, for example. Do you view that as diminishing his autonomy? Arguably Mr A uses his anger in order to get what he wants, in quite a rational manner. Does that undermine Adshead's argument that emotion is generally perceived as irrational and as tending to diminish autonomy?

However, it appears that there are some limitations to the scope of exercising autonomy: a notion of 'good enough autonomy'. For example, recently in the UK the press reported a case where a woman would not donate bone marrow to her dying sister because she was afraid of needles. Initial press reports were critical of her, as not being free to refuse. The newspaper view seemed to be that she could not claim that the domain in which she exercised her personal autonomy was both discrete and private. Rather, she had a duty to help her sister regardless of her own preferences, presumably because of the connection between them. (Of course it might be argued that it is only women whose autonomy is conceived as limited, because they should be caring towards others.)

When autonomy is exercised in an extreme way, without any consideration of connection to others, this is sometimes called a lack of empathy, classically said to be a defining criterion for psychopathic states. Persons in psychopathic states frequently do describe a profound sense of disconnection from others. In both clinical and non-clinical settings, a lack of connection with others is a significant contributor to the capacity to harm others. Descriptions of training of Nazi soldiers demonstrate the importance of the deconstruction of empathy in Nazi Germany: freedom from undue influence indeed.

If extremes of autonomy are pathological, and there is a strong intuition that we ought sometimes to consider other interests than our own, then clearly both the exercise of autonomy and the state of being autonomous involve connections and relationships with others in a more complex way than is suggested by traditional views. Contemporary writings from different theoretical perspectives suggest an interest in concepts such as altruism (Wilson, 1993), intuition (Vogel, 1997) or the origins of virtue (Ridley, 1996). Within moral philosophy there has been some acknowledgement that the emotions are part of the capacity to be rational (Oakley, 1992) and that concepts of autonomy have to account for those many states in life when we are less able to exercise autonomy, and when we are both vulnerable to others' coercion and dependent on their assistance. The standard of independence traditionally conceptualised as being essential to autonomy will be too high for some, as the Canadian feminist theorist and medical ethicist Susan Sherwin has illustrated (Sherwin, 1993).

ACTIVITY: Think of examples from long-term care which illustrate this combination of being 'both vulnerable to others' coercion and dependent on their assistance.

Indeed, it is recent feminist theory which has mounted the most consistent and sustained attack on traditional notions of autonomy. Can feminist theory offer a better account of autonomy? – one which preserves the aspect of protection from interference and oppression by more powerful others, but acknowledges the need for connection to others, especially those with whom we are in relationship. There are two areas of social relationship which are relevant to the concept of autonomy, and which have been subject to feminist analysis: power relations and caring relations.

A complete explication of power relations cannot be offered here. Most significantly, feminist theory questions unequal distributions of power (especially between the sexes) and the devaluation of those who are deemed to be 'different' from the status quo, as defined by status quo setters. In addition, feminist writers have questioned the devaluing of those who are deemed to be powerless. Where there is a strict hierarchy of power, those who have none are devalued: first because they have no power in the sense of agency, and second because they are perceived to be lower in the hierarchy, and thus vulnerable.

> **ACTIVITY: How might these points be particularly relevant to long-term care? Clearly, elderly people receiving long-term care are one of the most vulnerable groups in society, and are one with little power. It is also true that a high proportion are women. Furthermore, given the earlier demise of men and the typical pattern whereby women marry men older rather than younger than themselves, women are less likely to be cared for by a spouse than men are.**

Women, of course, are not essentially vulnerable, unless both difference from status quo holders (male) and biological difference are taken to define vulnerability and indicate reduced agency at any number of levels. But feminist questioning of traditional power structures has allowed the asking of another question: is vulnerability a problem? Or is it an essential part of human experience, without which we might not be human?

The question of vulnerability raises the area of caring relationships. Traditionally, the feminine gender role is associated with caring (Showalter, 1987), so that being female implies principal responsibility for the care and maintenance of relationships, and the protection of dependency and dependants. Gilligan (1982) has found some evidence that different ethical perspectives may be associated with gender role (not sex): a rights-based perspective in males and a care-based perspective in females. Gilligan presents these two perspectives on ethical reasoning as complementary and not mutually exclusive.

A more connected vision of autonomy, which addresses dependency needs, is not a sexist one, which applies only to women. Men also are dependent, and it is likely that some sexist practice is related to male gender role escapism and intolerance of dependency. For men and women alike, we might argue for a wider conceptual revision of the traditional view of autonomy. We might see autonomy as 'interstitial' (Agich, 1990) in the gaps between people and within their relationships. Accounts of autonomy need to include the concept of dependency and its effect on identity.

To be fully autonomous is to be located in a network, rather than an isolated dot in the universe. This accords with notions of best psychological health, where mutual interdependence is seen as being a goal of mature development, and detached isolation in terms of self is seen as being potentially pathological. Narrative theories of self imply relationships between a narrator and one who listens, dialogue rather than monologue.

If personal identity were understood in this way, then a richer account of autonomy might be possible. Autonomy, and the exercise of autonomy, would include accounts of the self as embedded in relationships. Agency would recognize the connections between persons in relationship, and understand those as relevant to ethical decision-making. *Many people have multiple commitments,* which often conflict: they are all aspects of a person's identity, and in the decision-making process a resolution will have to be achieved which reflects all these aspects of this identity. It simply cannot be a question of work always coming before family (or the reverse), nor of some types of principle always 'trumping' others, because otherwise important aspects of our personal identity and integrity will be lost or devalued. And if we lose our integrity as persons, can we be autonomous? What if we achieved some kind of freedom from interference, but lost our souls in the process? If individual discourse reigns, how will we live together?

ACTIVITY: As your final exercise in this section, ask yourself how Adshead's statement that 'to be fully autonomous is to be located in a network' might apply in the case of Mr A. One point which occurs to us is that although Mr A is exercising his 'individual right' to drive at the expense of his family's mental well-being and the safety of the public, he uses his car to drive to reunions. The car symbolizes connection as much as individual independence. Another point might be that Mr A is so fierce in his 'independence' because at some level he recognizes that he is in fact dependent on his daughter, in whose house he lives.

This concludes Section 2, in which we have moved from two further case studies to conceptually rich and iconoclastic revisions of the key notion of autonomy. In Section 3 we will build on this theoretical and practical reconstruction, with further development of the idea of narrative in ethical issues about long-term care.

ACTIVITY: Before moving on to the next section of the chapter, make a note of the key points raised by this section.

Section 3: Ethics in relationships

THE CASE OF LISA AND MARTIN

Lisa and Martin are elderly residents in a residential home which caters for people who suffer from dementia. In general, both Lisa and Martin seem to be happy and this appears to be largely the result of their relationship with one another. During the day Lisa and Martin are inseparable. They sit holding hands, they flirt with each other and talk or cuddle for most of the time.

However, despite the genuine happiness both

Lisa and Martin experience the staff at the home are concerned about their relationship. It is apparent that Lisa falsely believes that Martin is her husband and that Martin, also falsely, believes that Lisa is his wife.

This poses several problems for the staff. On the one hand, there is the ethical question raised earlier in Section 1 of this chapter of whether they ought to adopt a reality orientation approach or one based on validation. That is, should they encourage the two residents to confront the truth about their relationship or should they respect and validate their feelings and the meaning the relationship has for them? On the other hand, in the case of Lisa and Martin there is a much more pressing ethical dilemma for the staff. For whilst Lisa's husband is in fact deceased, Martin's wife is not and comes to visit him on average once a week. This causes practical as well as ethical problems for the staff.

When Martin's wife visits him, he sometimes recognizes her but sometimes he does not. This naturally upsets his wife and she takes it very hard. Martin's wife does not appear to know about the relationship between Martin and Lisa, however. When she comes to visit, the staff who work in the home try to make sure that Lisa is out or engaged in some activity in another room in order to avoid a confrontation. The problem with this is that Martin and Lisa desperately want to be together and protest and are extremely unhappy when they are separated.

The staff do not know what to do. This is not, they feel, simply a matter of whether or not they should keep Martin's wife in the dark but affects every aspect of managing the home. At bedtime, for example, Martin and Lisa want to sleep together. They have said this when their respective children have been to visit them and when they do so it is apparent to the staff that their children become very upset about this. In fact, the children have told the staff that such behaviour cannot be allowed.

Thus far, the staff who work in the home have respected the wishes of the children and have separated Martin and Lisa at bedtimes despite loud protests. The staff find this very upsetting when they see just how unhappy Lisa and Martin are, but find it very difficult to know what they ought to do.

Commentary on the Case of Lisa and Martin

Tony Hope

This case appears to present a conflict between the interests of Lisa and Martin, on the one hand, and the interests of their families, on the other hand. The interests of nursing home staff, and other residents in the nursing home, should, perhaps, be a further consideration. Before discussing the case of Lisa and Martin directly, I will start by considering a different but related hypothetical situation. That of 'Carla and Stefan'.

Carla and Stefan meet at a conference on bioethics. They form a close sexual relationship. Both are married and have children. They continue their relationship after the conference and separate from their respective spouses. Their spouses and their children are very upset.

In the case of Carla and Stefan we would normally say that no one has the right to prevent their relationship even if we do not approve of what they have done. The understandable distress caused to their families does not provide a justification for others to interfere.

There are two important differences between the situation of Carla and Stefan and that of Lisa and Martin. The first is that Lisa and Martin both suffer from dementia; the second is that the nursing home staff do have a relationship of care towards Lisa and Martin and thus have some special responsibilities towards them. What is the ethical relevance of these two differences?

The issue of the staff's special responsibilities does not seem to me to be critically relevant. Suppose that Carla and Stefan were physically handicapped (say, for example, that they suffered from spinal cord injury resulting in the paralysis of the legs) and required institutional care. If, nevertheless, they were fully competent, I cannot see that the healthcare staff would have the right to interfere in their relationship. They might have the right to restrict their behaviour whilst in the hospital or nursing home for the sake of residents and staff (for example, sexually overt behaviour in the public rooms of the institution): the institution would also be justified in preventing such behaviour between a man and wife. However, the relationship between Stefan and Carla is a matter between them and their respective spouses and not in itself a concern for the healthcare staff. The key difference between the two cases is the impaired mental state in the case of Lisa and Martin.

The concept of 'competence' is generally used to help clarify when it is right for healthcare staff to act against the apparent wishes of patients. In simple terms, a competent patient can refuse any treatment even when such a refusal is clearly against the patient's best interest. However, healthcare staff should generally act in the 'best interests' of incompetent patients. The question of competence is not always straightforward. One important aspect is that competence must be judged with reference to the specific issue. That is, the question should be: is this person competent to refuse this specific treatment – does she understand the aspect relevant to coming to a decision in this case?

Applying this kind of approach to Lisa and Martin raises then two issues: are Lisa and Martin competent to choose to develop this close sexual relationship despite being married to other people; and, what is in their best interests?

It should, at once, be said that an analysis relevant to the question of refusing treatment is rather different from the situation we are currently considering. However, even if the analysis is in theory applicable, it is difficult to apply in practice. Consider first the question of competence. Lisa and Martin appear to be able to recognize each other and to have sufficient memory of the past to sustain their relationship with each other. What exactly does it mean, and what should the criteria be for judging that they are incompetent to sustain this relationship? The key point in doubting their competence would seem to be the fact that Martin only intermittently recognizes his wife, and presumably has no memory of his longstanding relationship with her; and Lisa believes that Martin is her husband. But it is by no means clear that this makes Lisa and Martin incompetent to carry on their relationship.

When we read this we found ourselves asking, why should competence be so important here anyway? One possible response to Hope's analysis of the case thus far would be to point out that engaging in sexual and deeply emotional relationships is never fully a question of competence. We might argue instead that the key question here is the authenticity or otherwise of the emotions felt by Lisa and Martin. But perhaps the two questions are related.

If, as Hope suggests, the dilemma for the staff cannot be resolved through a consideration of 'competence' alone perhaps the concept of 'best interests' might help us to decide what to do. But

as we shall see, Hope goes on to suggest that this approach too, is problematic.

Ronald Dworkin distinguishes between 'critical interests' and 'experiential interests' (Dworkin, 1993). As applied to the situation under consideration, the experiential interests of Lisa and Martin would depend upon their day-to-day experiences. Since Lisa and Martin are, presumably, enjoying their relationship, and not suffering significantly from the distress which they are causing their family, it would seem to be in their experiential best interests for them to be allowed to pursue their relationship uninhibited.

Critical interests refer to those interests we have in the kind of person that we want to be, and our long-term aims, and enduring wishes. Thus a vegetarian might have a 'critical interest' in remaining vegetarian after suffering from dementia, even if, once demented, the person has no memory or understanding of vegetarian principles. If asked to complete an advanced directive, such a vegetarian might state that she wishes to be prevented from eating meat should she, at some stage in the future, become demented and no longer be able to voluntarily restrict her diet.

The strongest argument I believe for restricting the relationship between Lisa and Martin lies in an argument along the following lines. Supposing Martin (or Lisa) had been asked, before the onset of dementia, what he would want to happen if, at some stage in the future, he suffered from dementia and the situation as described in this vignette occurred. Suppose he then said that his relationship with his wife was of great importance to him (a 'critical interest') and that for two reasons he would want those looking after him to prevent his developing and enjoying another relationship. The first is that the mere development of such relationships spoils his conception of his relationship with his wife; and secondly it would distress him greatly to think that he might cause such pain for his wife.

In the present situation, there is no such clear statement. So Hope first considers (again by the use of a thought experiment) what should be done were there good evidence that Martin had made such a statement. Hope starts by asking us to imagine a third case, involving another couple, 'Robert and Catherine'.

Robert is happily married. He is shortly going off to a bioethics conference without his wife. He says to several of his friends that he is worried that he might start to develop a relationship with someone at this conference. He says to his friends that if this were to happen he would want them to do everything in their power to stop such a relationship. Robert subsequently goes to the conference and develops a relationship with Catherine. When his friends learn of this and try to prevent his relationship with Catherine, he tells them to stop interfering.

> **ACTIVITY: The use of thought experiments of this kind in philosophy is designed to throw new light on a philosophical problem (in this case an ethical one) by analogy. What are the similarities and the differences between the case of Robert and Catherine and Lisa and Martin? Now go on to read the rest of this commentary and think about whether or not the use of thought experiments of this kind are useful here and does this particular one work. If so, why?**

Unless there are some extra special circumstances I think that Robert's most recent view has to be respected. Although friends might reasonably try to persuade him, they could not go any further than this.

In the case of Lisa and Martin, there are further circumstances, the critical one being that Martin is now suffering from dementia. It seems to me that this fact of dementia is potentially relevant in two ways. The first comes back to the question of competence. That is, a reason why we should respect his previous and not his current wishes is that his previous wishes were made when competent. This raises problems to do with establishing what exactly competence means in these circumstances. The second difference is to say that he is now ill and his relationship with Lisa is a direct

result of the illness. In order for this to be a reason for countermanding his current desires, it would have to be further argued that the illness has interfered with his 'true self'. On this analysis his views prior to dementia represent his true views which have been obscured by the dementia.

In the present case we do not have this clear evidence of what Martin's and Lisa's views about the current circumstances would have been. We might try to establish what their views would have been, although, clearly the families' accounts are unlikely to be objective on this matter.

So where does this leave us with regard to what the staff should do? I think what it shows is that, in order to justify interference with the relationship between Lisa and Martin all of a number of statements would need to be considered true:

(a) That Lisa and Martin would have wanted their relationship to be broken, had they been asked about this situation before the onset of dementia.

(b) That such 'critical interests' should trump experiential interests.

(c) Either that Lisa and Martin are now incompetent with regard to the understanding of their relationship with each other; or that sense can be made of a distinction between a true self and a false self, and that the true self is represented by their pre-dementia state.

Each of these statements is problematic, and I think therefore, the balance lies on the side of allowing the relationship to continue (whilst trying to minimise the distress to the family).

An issue which I have not considered is what should happen if the analysis leads to a conflict between the interests of Lisa and Martin. That is where on the above analysis we decide that (let's say) Lisa's interests are served by a continuation of the relationship whereas Martin's are not.

> **ACTIVITY: Tony Hope's commentary on the case of Lisa and Martin focuses on the nature of competence and autonomy and on the best interests of the various parties and he comes to the conclusion that Lisa and Martin's relationship ought to be allowed to continue.**

Are you convinced by this argument? If not, why not? In a moment we shall be returning to the article by Guy Widdershoven which you began earlier in this chapter but before we ask you to do this we would like you to read the following commentary by Widdershoven on the case of Lisa and Martin. You will see that it focuses much more on the nature of relationships than Hope's commentary, through an analysis of commitment and meaning in relationship. Whilst you are reading this, we would like you to compare its approach with that taken by Hope and note any crucial differences.

Commentary on the Case of Lisa and Martin

Guy Widdershoven

By engaging in a relationship, people declare a kind of mutual commitment. This is obviously the case in relations of friendship, love or marriage. Yet one never knows what these engagements will actually result in. One does not know what will happen in the future, nor does one know exactly in what way one will act. In deciding to enter into such a commitment, one does not (at least not always) promise to perform specific actions, or to refrain from them, but rather one promises to build up a common life in mutual engagement. Relationships are always to some extent exclusive, in that they imply unique commitments. They are, on the other hand, not entirely exclusive. For, were that to be the case, they would preclude a person from having other (equally unique) commitments. One can never be totally committed to one person, although one may share with this person things which one will not share with any other person.

An important dimension of interpersonal relationships is keeping connected. One has to stay in touch with each other, in order to be able to re-establish the relation of mutual engagement and give it form and substance. One way of keeping connected is building up joint rituals. Keeping connected implies communication, and results in reaching a common perspective.

In the case of Martin and Lisa, several relationships are involved. The first (in order of appearance) is the one between Lisa and Martin. They obviously engage with one another, and are somehow able to build a common future. This relationship clearly has a great experiential richness for both of them. The next relationship is that between Martin and his wife. This relationship is quite problematic. The wife has to face the tragedy of losing her husband. He is no longer the same. As a result she obviously feels ambivalent towards him; she visits him once a week (which is hardly enough to keep connected), and would undoubtedly find it difficult to understand his feelings for Lisa were she to come to know about the relationship. Martin is himself clearly unable to remain 'faithful', since he does not distinguish between his wife and his present lover. In his own way, he keeps in touch with his wife, but clearly loses her by not regarding her as a unique person. The third relationship here is that between Lisa, Martin and their respective children. They do not want to accept any change in the one they have known for so long. But this also precludes them from the very possibility of keeping in touch, and reaching mutuality.

It seems to me that the wife and the children should try to accept the feelings of Martin and Lisa, in order to accept them and to get connected. They will have to re-define their relationship with their demented relative, and acknowledge that the life they had together is no longer possible. This, however, might enable them to build up a new mutuality. Martin's wife might learn to accept his feelings for Lisa, by realizing that he might also want her to build up new relationships (which is not uncommon if the partner is hospitalized). The children might learn to accept the new partner of their parent, as children have to do when parents divorce. This does not mean that the wife and the child have to approve of everything which Lisa and Martin might want to do together. They might try to prevent them from getting married, or to change their wills in order to benefit one another. Such interventions might be justified on the basis of the relationship they have with Lisa and Martin, and the responsibilities which it involves. But in order to act in a engaged way, one should first of all keep connected, and not deny the changes which have evidently taken place.

ACTIVITY: When we were reading this commentary, we felt that the approaches of the two commentators were significantly different and yet in many useful ways, complementary. Interestingly, they both came to the same conclusion, that the relationship ought to be allowed to continue.

Stop for a moment and return to the list you prepared earlier after your first reading of the Lisa and Martin case. Look again at your two lists of arguments, those for allowing the relationship to continue and those against it. In the light of the above commentaries, have you changed your mind? Is it possible to group the types of arguments used into different kinds? When we tried to do this, we found that arguments seemed to fall into two general categories: those which emphasized competence and best interests and, those which were more relationship based and emphasized the meaning of marriage, of commitment and of changes in relationships. At this point you might like to compare the approaches taken here with those adopted earlier in this chapter by Gwen Adshead, Ruud ter Meulen and George Agich.

Traditionally medical ethics has tended to focus on conflicts of interests, questions of autonomy and competence and so on. It seems here that Widdershoven in particular is offering an alternative relationship-based approach which is worth exploring further. In the next section we shall return to Widdershoven's paper on 'Truth and truth-telling' which we began in Section 2. While you read it and complete the activities we ask you to do, we would like you to continue to bear in mind and compare this relationship-based approach with the approaches mentioned elsewhere such as principlism and those used by Tony Hope. Are these approaches in competition with each other? Does adopting one rule out adopting the other or are they complementary?

Four types of practitioner–patient relationship

Now that you have done a number of activities about the ethical issues in long term-care we would like you to read the final section of the paper on truth-telling by Guy Widdershoven which we began earlier. In order to do this properly you'll probably need to go back and refresh your memory about the arguments Widdershoven put forward in the earlier part of his paper to support his claims in this second part.

Truth and truth-telling *(cont.)*

Guy Widdershoven

Thus far in this paper, I have critically examined approaches to truth-telling. I have argued that both the bioethical perspective and the therapeutical perspectives are one-sided in their own way. In the bioethical approach, truth-telling is seen as a moral imperative, which has to be weighed against other values. The focus is upon general principles. In the therapeutic approach, truth-telling is regarded as either functional or dysfunctional to the patient's way of understanding the world he lives in. The emphasis is on the individual patient's way of dealing with his situation. As an alternative to all of these therapeutic approaches, I want now to present a hermeneutic approach to truth-telling. In this approach, truth-telling is not considered as a moral imperative for the care-giver nor as a phenomenon which helps or hinders the patient to orient himself in the world, but as a dialogical endeavour which is part of an ongoing intersubjective relationship.

Beyond principlism and therapy: a hermeneutic perspective

In bioethics, the focus is usually upon general norms and values. Principlism for example, tries to develop methods to make norms and values explicit, and to weigh them in the concrete situation. Truth is an important value, but it can be overruled by other values, especially that of acting in the patient's best interest. A therapeutic approach on the other hand puts the individual patient at the centre. Reality Orientation Therapy and Validation, despite their differences, have in common that they aim to convey a method of listening to the patient and to help him or her to experience the world in a new and richer way. In principlism, universal norms and values decide whether or not the truth should be told; from a therapeutical perspective, the individual patient's experience is decisive.

One might, however, argue that both perspectives, the therapeutic and the principlist, miss the essence of truth-telling. For, in disclosing the truth, we claim that something important is at stake, something which has to be understood and acknowledged by the person whom we tell about it. In telling the truth, we show our engagement with the other. We try to create a mutual endeavour in which the facts we refer to play a crucial role. Truth-telling is not simply a matter of respecting another person by conveying certain important facts to him or her, as the principlist conception seems to imply. It is a means of reaching an understanding about the situation at hand (Habermas, 1980). This implies respect for the other, but it is more than that, since it aims at gaining contact with the other. In truth-telling, we are oriented towards the other as an individual person. Yet this is different from the therapeutical approach, which is not interested in creating mutuality, but only in stimulating the other's experience.

From a hermeneutic perspective, truth-telling aims at creating a joint process of meaning-making. This implies that the truth is not owned by the caregiver, as in the principlist approach. If the care receiver contests the claim to truth, and does not respond appropriately, mutuality is not reached. Thus, the project of the caregiver fails. This does not mean, however, that truth is only rel-

evant in relation to the care receiver's capacity of meaning-making, as in the therapeutic approach. Neither the caregiver, nor the care receiver is in a privileged position. Both are part of a process of mutual engagement, in which truth is not given, but created (Gadamer, 1960).

A hermeneutic reading of the case of the forgetful mourner (which we looked at in Section 1) will emphasize the staff's attempts to reach a shared understanding of the situation. From this perspective, the urge to tell the truth is not primarily the result of a feeling of respect for the patient, but of a need to come to a mutual understanding. The attempts fail, since the woman does not respond. Evidently, the claim to truth, however valid it may seem to the staff, is not accepted by her. She cannot integrate it into her life. At this point, several options are open. One could contend that the woman is just unable to see the truth, because she is incompetent. This would mean that no further communication on this matter would be possible. Or one might conclude that the truth does not matter any more, as long as she is happy. This would imply stopping the attempts to make her aware of her son's death. Again, the possibility of communication would be excluded. A third option would be to try and get into contact with her in such a way that the truth becomes accessible to her in a different way. This is exactly what the nurse's intervention brings about. Crucial to the intervention is the performance of a ritual in which mutuality is created, in that all the participants experience the death of the son together. Thus, the truth is communicated in a non-verbal way. In this process of communication, the partners change. Through the ritual, the incomprehensible death becomes acceptable, and changes into a reality; but this is not specific to the forgetful mourner. For, it is the essence of every human process of mourning (Kübler-Ross, 1982). Thus, the strange reaction of the woman is changed into a common human way of dealing with sorrow. In the end, the ritual changes both the care-receiver's experience of her son's death and the care-giver's experience about her. The

---

result is a communality which did not exist before (Gadamer, 1975).

> **ACTIVITY:** When we were reading this, we began to think about what it might mean in the case of Lisa and Martin. In the case of the forgetful mourner, the patient was dressed in her funeral clothes as a way of helping her to come to terms with the meaning of her situation. What do you think this would mean in the case of Lisa and Martin? Once again this confronts us with the responsibilities of the carer or doctor within the context of the practitioner–patient relationship. What kind of relationship ought one to adopt to those for whom one has a responsibility of care?
>
> Widdershoven argues that each of the ethical approaches and perspectives he described earlier in his paper implies a different answer to the question of what is an ethical relationship between physicians and patients. We would now like you to go on to read this section of Widdershoven's paper and make a note of each of these types of relationship and the perspective with which they are associated.

Four types of professional–patient relationship

The perspectives on truth-telling discussed above imply different views of the professional–patient relationship. In each of the various approaches one may recognize the four models of the physician–patient relationship described by Emanuel and Emanuel (1992). The first is the paternalistic model. In this model the doctor decides, acting in the best interest of the patient. In this model the doctor is the guardian of the patient. The second model is the informative, or consumer model. It is based upon the autonomous choice of the patient, after being informed by the doctor. The values of the patient are considered to be given. In this model the doctor is the technical expert. The third model is the interpretive model. It aims at interpreting the patient's values and implementing the patient's selected intervention. The values of the patient are seen as

inchoate and conflicting, and in need of interpretation. In this model the doctor is a counsellor or adviser. The fourth model is the deliberative model. It is based upon the presupposition that the patient's values are not only in need of interpretation, but also of discussion and deliberation. The doctor is regarded as a friend or teacher. This model is the most radical.

> The conception of patient autonomy is moral self-development; the patient is empowered not simply to follow unexamined preferences or examined values, but to consider, through dialogue, alternative health-related values, their worthiness and their implications for treatment. (p. 2222).

According to the principlist approach, the professional can choose to follow the principle of beneficence, which means that he or she acts in the patient's best interest, or to respect the patient's autonomy, which means that the patient is regarded as a client whose wishes are to be responded to by the professional. In the first case, the professional–patient relationship is paternalistic; in the latter case, it is informative. The therapeutic approach is in line with the inter-

> **ACTIVITY:** Which of the four models do you consider to be closest to Widdershoven's approach?

pretive model of the professional–patient relationship. The professional does not take his or her own views of the situation of the patient for granted (as in the paternalistic model), nor does he or she restrict himself to giving information and executing the patient's wishes (as in the informative model). Rather, he or she acknowledges that the patient's views are not clear, and have to be interpreted. The patient's perspective is central, as in the informative model, but this perspective is not considered to be given. It has rather to be elaborated by the professional. The professional has to listen carefully to the patient's utterances, and help the patient to give meaning to the situation, without imposing his or her own views.

	Informative	Interpretive	Deliberative	Paternalistic
Patient values	Defined, fixed and known to the patient	Inchoate and conflicting requiring elucidation	Open to development and revision through moral discussion	Objective and shared by the physician and patient
Physician's obligation	Providing relevant factual information and implementing patient's selected intervention	Elucidating and interpreting relevant patient values as well as informing the patient and implementing the patient's selected intervention	Articulating and persuading the patient of the most admirable values as well as informing the patient and implementing the patient's selected intervention	Promoting the patient's well-being independent of the patient's current preferences
Conception of patient's autonomy	Choice of, and control over, medical care	Self-understanding relevant to medical care	Moral self-development relevant to medical care	Assenting to objective values
Conception of physician's role	Competent technical expert	Counsellor or adviser	Friend or teacher	Guardian

In the deliberative model of the professional–patient relationship, the professional and the patient both bring in their view of the situation, and engage in a dialogue about what should be done. This model fits to the hermeneutic perspective on truth-telling. Both the caregiver and the care receiver play an active role. In a process of deliberation, the views of the caregiver and the care receiver confronts one another. The aim is to reach a common understanding of the situation, in which the views are no longer opposed to one another, but merge into a shared perspective.

In their paper 'Four models of the physician–patient relationship in the *Journal of the American Medical Association*, **267**, pp. 2221–2226, 1992, the Emanuels use the table above to describe and summarize the four types of relationship and their implications.
They conclude their paper in the following way,

Over the last few decades, the discourse regarding the physician–patient relationship has focused on two extremes: autonomy and paternalism. Many have attacked physicians as paternalistic, urging the empowerment of patients to control their own care. This view, the informative model, has become dominant in bioethics

and legal standards. This model embodies a defective conception of patient autonomy, and it reduces the physician's role to that of a technologist.

The essence of doctoring is a fabric of knowledge, understanding, teaching, and action, in which the caring physician integrates the patient's medical condition and health-related values, makes a recommendation on the appropriate course of action, and tries to persuade the patient of the worthiness of this approach and the values it realises. The physician with a caring attitude is the ideal embodied in the deliberative model, the ideal that should inform laws and policies that regulate the physician–patient interaction.

Finally, it may be worth noting that the four models outlined herein are not limited to the medical realm; they may inform the public conception of other professional interactions as well. We suggest that the ideal relationships between lawyer and client, religious mentor and laity, and educator and student are well described by the deliberative model, at least in some of their essential aspects (p. 2226).

ACTIVITY: Guy Widdershoven and the Emanuels have introduced a different approach to ethics from those based on principles and conflicts of interest. We would like you now to re-read the case of Lisa and

Martin and then to reconsider it in the light of the table and the quote above from the Emanuels. Try to identify what each of the different models would point to as the right way to deal with this case.

Can you think of any weaknesses with the Emanuels' approach? One thing which we wondered about was whether in reality any doctors would fall neatly into any of the models described by the Emanuels, even though their table is based upon sociological research. Is this an accurate description of different actual approaches? Secondly, we wondered whether the deliberative model was always the ethical approach to take. Might there not be at least some circumstances in which paternalism, for example, would be justified? Thirdly we wondered whether there was an ethical hierarchy to these models. If the deliberative model is inappropriate which model ought we to move to next?

Are any of these models more appropriate to long-term care than others? If so, why? Think of a case from your own practice or experience which confronted you with an ethical dilemma. Can you identify which of these models you adopted and why? Should a good doctor be one of these or ought a good doctor to be able to use different types of relationship where appropriate?

In response to this activity one of our critical readers, Mark Wicclair wrote,

In addition to the questions you raise, I would raise the following: There may not be one model to fit all patients. Accordingly, the informative model might be appropriate for patients who have clear preferences and values; the interpretive model may be appropriate for patients who do not have such clearly defined values and preferences; the deliberative model may be appropriate for patients who are conflicted; and the paternalistic model may be appropriate for demented patients or patients who prefer to defer to healthcare professionals. Different models might even be appropriate for different choices by the same patient.

ACTIVITY: Make a list of the key points raised by this section.

Section 4: The meaning and ethical significance of old age

In the final section of this chapter we shall be going on to consider, in the light of our reflections of the importance of relationships, whether there is anything unique about ethics in long-term care. Whilst it is important to remind ourselves that not all long-term care involves the elderly, we shall be using the question of the meaning and ethical significance of old age as the focus of our discussion of ethics in long-term care in this section. As you progress through this section you might like to consider the similarities and differences between long-term care of the elderly and long-term care with other groups.

ACTIVITY: We would now like you to read the following case study and to bear in mind whilst you do so what kinds of relationships are being described and how a relationship can have implications for the 'meaning' of a person's life both for themselves and also for others. The case emphasizes the significance of events such as feeding both in the interpersonal sense and also as symbols in the attempt to make sense of and come to terms with what it means to get older. The implication here is that there is a sense in which one has a relationship both with others and also with one's own life as a whole narrative. But the case also shows that such relationships are not easy and reveals that the decline of one person confronts others too with the fact of their own decline and death and this can make relationships in long-term care particularly challenging.

THE CASE OF EMMI

Emmi is 85 years old and lives in a nursing home, suffering from the effect of two serious strokes. She has always been very particular about her appearance. Even now she continues to wear nice clothes and make-up, despite the weakness in her left side.

Recently she suffered a further stroke which left her with a lasting paralysis of the throat. It has become necessary to change Emmi's diet and to feed her only puréed food. Despite this, the food still often gets caught in her throat. Emmi feels ashamed about this and about the way she appears when eating in company with the others who live in the home.

At a recent staff meeting, one of the workers thought it might help if Emmi could be fed in her room. Other workers felt, however, that she should come out and eat with the others, as not to do so would mean isolating herself. It was decided that the head nurse would speak to the other residents. They said that they thought it was 'disgusting' when Emmi coughed at the dinner table and that she had difficulties with swallowing. The result of this discussion was that Emmi started to sit off to the side and sometimes even to eat in the nursing home's kitchen. For practical reasons, it was not possible for Emmi to eat at a different time to the other residents. The nurses cannot afford to spend any more time over meals than they already do as there are not enough staff. The other residents continue to say that they are disgusted by Emmi.

Emmi's doctor and the nursing home staff are considering using a new artificial and medically assisted type of food provision for Emmi. However, Emmi makes it clear to the nurses that she will refuse any and every form of artificial food and fluid administration.

Commentary on the case of Emmi

Chris Gastmans

Caring should always be considered as an inter-human endeavour. It is not only the nurse, but also the resident, nursing colleagues and doctors, who play essential roles in the caring process. All of these participants have their own ethical and practice-based intuitions concerning the essential meaning of 'good care'. In the case of Emmi, the ethical intuitions of all are being tested. The inter-disciplinary team of doctors and nurses is being challenged to clarify and justify their opinions about 'good nutritional care'.

It is worth mentioning that it is not very common for nurses and patients to talk about problems such as those described in this case. The day-to-day aspects of work in a residential home mean that nurses have very little time available for this kind of activity. There is not much time left for reflection on the human quality of the care provided. Residents like Emmi are often ashamed to ask for more attention from the nurse, and it is therefore up to the nurses to take the initiative and to adopt an attitude that invites confidences within the limits of time and resources available. We would like to give some short suggestions on how to come to an ethically 'acceptable solution' in a case like that involving Emmi.

Firstly, as much information as possible about the case has to be collected. Informing ourselves about the technical and factual aspects of the problem is the first step in the ethical reflection process. If the problem is described in a one-sided, incomplete or even inaccurate manner, then the ethical question itself and the solution we give to the question will be distorted.

Which possible ways are there in which we could help Emmi with her eating and drinking problems? Is there enough competence in the way nurses deal with the difficulties Emmi faces with eating and drinking? Is there enough space and time provided to help Emmi during mealtimes? These and many other questions have to be answered if we are to gain an insight into the real problem described in the case of Emmi.

Secondly, the emotional and intuitive reactions of all those involved in the case have to be clarified. This is important because, whilst ethics is generally represented as a rational endeavour, to see it as such inevitably excludes emotions from the ethical discussion. We want to deny this option. In our opinion, emotions are the 'feelers' with which ethical problems can be detected. The emotional reactions (e.g. disgust) of the elderly residents make clear that there is a (value laden) problem with Emmi. The other elderly people experience the life situation of Emmi as a contradiction to human dignity. Emotions are also important because they prevent hardening, routine behaviour, selective blindness and so on which all tend to prevent nurses from experiencing the ethical meaning of care. Also in the case of Emmi, it is important that the emotions and the quite unclear attitudes about 'good nutritional care' of all people involved can be clarified. What are the real motivations for Emmi's refusal of every type of artificial food and fluid administration? What are the attitudes of nurses towards eating and drinking disorders? Are there any cultural perspectives on meals expressed by Emmi, nurses, doctors and other residents? What kinds of personal experiences have the nurses themselves had with meals?

If this clarification doesn't take place, emotional reactions threaten to dominate or even block altogether the ethical discussion. The ethical debate, however, cannot only be based upon emotions. Emotions and intuitions fulfil an important role in the detection of unethical situations but in the discussion of ethical problems, the emotional level has to be transcended. For, we have to evolve towards the level of rational ethical argumentation.

Thirdly, during the ethical clarification process, various alternative solutions have to be evaluated. This evaluation consists of a clarification of the moral values (advantages) and disvalues (disadvantages) which are inherent in each alternative.

At first sight, two alternative solutions might be distinguished. The first of these would be to force

Emmi to be fed in an artificial (medically assisted) way. This 'solution' possibly brings a higher level of physical well-being for Emmi, which can be seen as a value (a quality which we spontaneously view in a positive way). Nevertheless, ignoring the wishes of Emmi, is undoubtedly a disvalue (something we condemn spontaneously). The second possible solution would be for nurses to continue feeding Emmi in a natural way, despite all difficulties (e.g. isolation during mealtime). As the most important value, we have to consider in this regard the respect for Emmi's autonomy. On the other hand, there is another disvalue which surfaces, namely the disruption of Emmi's chances of a higher level of physical and social development.

ACTIVITY: Stop here for a moment and consider Emmi's case in the light of these comments. Chris Gastmans is keen to emphasize the meaning and the symbolic significance of feeding and interpersonal relations in long-term care. At this point it appears that there are two possible alternative solutions: either to force Emmi to accept artificial nutrition or to continue feeding her as 'naturally' as possible despite the difficulties this presents. What are the arguments in favour of and against each of these 'solutions'. Then go on to read the rest of this commentary in which Chris Gastmans goes on to argue that, in fact, neither of these solutions is acceptable and attempts to offer a third alternative.

After having conscientiously weighed up the values and disvalues which are inherent in both alternative solutions, we have to admit that neither of these 'solutions' is acceptable to us. Moreover, we feel uncomfortable seeing Emmi losing the battle of being right between the doctor and the nurses. The important ethical question is not 'who is right?' or 'who may decide?' but 'what is good for Emmi?'

With that last question, we return to the essence of our case. What should nurses do with Emmi? Should they introduce artificial food and fluid administration or not? The answer to this question has to be the result of an interdisciplinary consultation including all those involved in the case. In our opinion, this case requires an individualized approach. Maximum attention should be given to the development of a relationship based on trust between the nurses and Emmi. They have to search together for the 'most humanly possible' outcome which can be realized in this (not ideal) situation. The autonomy of Emmi should be promoted by maintaining and supporting the natural feeding process. To realize this ethical option in the case of Emmi, a high level of competency, creativity and devotion will be required. It is our opinion that the question of the artificial administration of food and fluids may only be taken into account when the capacity and the will of Emmi to continue the natural feeding process are undermined, and when all medical and nursing means to postpone or avoid the artificial fluid and food administration fail. Emmi unambiguously expresses her will to eat and drink in a natural way. Taking into account her capacity to achieve this, nurses have to analyse the ways in which they might be able to support and even promote Emmi's ability to do things independently as much as possible. In our opinion, supporting Emmi in her natural feeding and drinking behaviour, adopting an attitude of respect and patience, seems to be the most responsible ethical caring behaviour that nurses can show. If nurses do their best to put this ethical option into practice, they consider themselves as persons who are supposed to accept a certain amount of responsibility (moral agents), rather than as victims of circumstances beyond their control (in this case, the shortage of staff).

> ACTIVITY: We would now like you to go on to read another commentary on the case of Emmi, this time by Guy Widdershoven who as you might expect focuses on a relationship-based approach. Whilst you are reading consider the similarities and differences between these approaches.

Commentary on the Case of Emmi

Guy Widdershoven

Eating is an important aspect of life. We often create rituals around eating, and feel good when these rituals are executed. Eating habits are a way of giving meaning to one's life, and realizing central values in life. Eating in one's own personal way is also a way of realizing one's autonomy. This sense of autonomy is also a sense of relatedness; eating always involves relations with other people, who provide the food (even if one cooks oneself, and for nobody else but oneself, the food will be bought from somebody else). Thus, in eating we are aware of both our independence and our dependence. As a ritual, eating is symbolic for life itself.

For people who have few experiences, such as those in nursing homes, eating is a central part of their daily life. The rituals around eating show people that they are cared for, and that they take care of their own life. Eating rituals are evident examples of care, as defined by Joan Tronto and Bernice Fischer:

On the most general level, we suggest that caring be viewed as a species activity that includes everything we do to maintain, continue, and repair our 'world' so that we can live in it as well as possible. That world includes our bodies, our selves, and our environment, all of which we seek to interweave in a complex, life-sustaining web (Tronto, 1993, p. 103).

From this perspective, it is quite understandable that Emmi wants to continue to eat by herself, even if she is no longer able to do this as competently and neatly as she used to. But it is not evident that she wants to eat together with the other patients. Although eating is a social phenomenon (as explained above), this does not mean that eating always should take place in the company of others. Emmi might very well want to eat on her own, and would perhaps rather not exhibit her present lack of skills before others. In that case, eating alone would not mean isolating oneself, but feeling responsible for one's behaviour in front of the others. Actually, this is what she seems to opt for, since she feels ashamed, and manages to eat 'off to the side'. But she evidently does not get much help in realizing her objectives. Would it really take too much trouble to have her sit at a separate table (either in the common room, or in her own room)?

As to the reaction of the other patients, given the importance they will also attach to their eating rituals, one can understand their feelings of disgust. If Emmi actually obstructs their established practice of eating, and thus frustrates a central element in their life, this is probably difficult for them. Yet there are some critical remarks to be made here. It seems unfair that the other patients condemn Emmi for her behaviour, without paying any attention to her intentions. She actually wants to prevent their experience of disgust, and this moral attitude is not honoured at all. Emmi is only seen as someone who intrudes upon their practice, and not as someone with whom one might try to come to a joint practice, an arrangement which is better for all – for instance by giving her more privacy, and thus making everybody happier. The staff, by presenting the issue in the way they do, do not seem to foster any positive attitudes in the other patients towards Emmi, nor do they open a way to a joint solution. Again, one might want a more flexible and responsible approach from the staff.

The option of giving artificial food and fluids may seem the easiest way out, but it totally breaks with any possible arrangement of building up eating habits which are meaningful for all the people concerned. Therefore, the revulsion of Emmi is quite understandable. This option should be postponed as long as possible, and regarded only as part of a worst-case scenario.

ACTIVITY: As we come to the end of this chapter, it is clear that there is a range of ethical questions which occur in long-term care. Guy Widdershoven, Daniel Callahan and others have argued that these ethical questions are, in some qualitative sense, very different from the ones we face elsewhere and that these differences relate in some important sense to

the centrality of the role of meaning in our lives. To what extent do you consider this to be true? Do we really need a new and unique approach to ethical issues in long-term care or are these questions amenable to analysis in the more usual principlist way which emphasizes autonomy, beneficence, non-maleficence and justice? In the final part of this chapter we will go on to consider the question of what is unique about the meaning of old age.

What is special about old age?

Guy Widdershoven has introduced the idea of ethics being to do with the meaningfulness of relationships and he has used the Emanuels' schema as a way of analysing the moral dimension of different types of patient–doctor relationship. In the end he argues that the deliberative model is the best approach because it respects and enhances meaningfulness and meaning-making in some way. By this he means that it allows and enables both patients and physicians to engage in the joint process of 'making-sense'.

One question which has not been addressed directly, though it has been a theme running through this chapter as a whole, is that of the meaning of old age itself and whether this period of life is distinct in any morally significant way. Is there anything uniquely special about long-term care at the end of life which raises particular ethical and moral problems? For an approach which is based on the concepts of the meaning and significance of relationships, it must surely be essential to address the question of the differences (if indeed there are any) between the meaning of different stages of life. For, if there are such differences and they are morally significant, then they must be of importance in the ethics of long-term care.

ACTIVITY: Stop for a moment and consider this question. Do you think that there is in fact a distinct stage of life which we might call 'old age'? Is old age socially constructed or are there features of the later stages of life which make it both unique and universal in important ways? Attempt to write down a list of features of old age which make it different from other stages of life.

How easy or difficult was this activity? As we tried to do this, we felt it to be very difficult, especially in the light of recent changes in the lifestyles of the 'young old', to describe a distinct stage of old age. (As we write this, the pensioner father of one of the authors is in Barbados running a marathon, for example.) However, this need not mean that it is impossible to say anything sensible about this period of life. For, whilst rejecting the idea of a discrete stage we might still agree that there are features of life as it comes to its end which are distinctive. It seems likely that many of us as we reach the latter years of our lives will reflect more on the nature of our decline and death than we did when we were younger and will perhaps begin to reflect increasingly on the nature of our lives as a whole.

It remains the case, however, that we are reluctant to talk about these things publicly. Daniel Callahan, in *Setting Limits*, argues that there is an urgent need for a public discussion of the values and distinctive characteristics of old age. He suggests that modern patient-centred medicine (the bioethics approach described by Widdershoven earlier) has tended to undermine the meaningfulness of old age by its emphasis on individualism and life-extending treatments. He suggests that it is tempting for us to avoid a consideration of the meaning of old age and to be fearful of it. For, modern medicine and modern individualistic society tend to consider old age as if it were an inferior version of earlier stages of life. He rejects this conceptualization and demands that we take the distinctive features and values of old age seriously. He asks,

What kind of sense can be made of old age, of the fact that our bodies change and decline, sicken and decay, and then die? Even if we distinguish between growing old and becoming ill, between becoming old and becoming stale, between chronological and biological age, or between our externally assigned social role and our internal sense of place – even if, that is, we make all

of the distinctions recommended in the professional literature on ageing, in the end death happens, and we exist no more. While old age and death are obviously distinguishable, death comes at the end of old age. How should we prepare for that moment, and what should we think about it? (Callahan, 1987, p. 31)

ACTIVITY: Now read the following three descriptions of the importance and distinctiveness of old age and reflect on how these differ from or reinforce your own view. Finally, consider as you read them what implications each account of the meaning of old age would have for the resolution of the case of Lisa and Martin.

Three pictures of old age

Cicero (44 BC)

Old men . . . as they become less capable of physical exertion, should redouble their intellectual activity, and their principal occupation should be to assist the young, their friends, and above all their country with their wisdom and sagacity. There is nothing they should guard against so much as languor and sloth. Luxury, which is shameful at every period of life, makes old age hideous. If it is united with sensuality, the evil is two-fold. Age thus brings disgrace on itself and aggravates the shameless licence of the young (Cicero, 1951, p. 37, Quoted in Callahan, 1987).

Simone de Beauvoir (1972)

The greatest good fortune, even greater than health, for the old person is to have his world inhabited by projects; then busy and useful, he escapes both from boredom and decay . . . There is only one solution if old age is not to be an absurd parody of our former life, and that is to go on pursuing ends that give our existence a meaning – devotion to individuals, to groups or to causes, social, political, intellectual or creative work. In spite of the moralists' opinion to the contrary, in old age we should still wish to have passions strong enough to prevent us from turning in upon ourselves (de Beauvoir, 1972, p. 28, quoted in Callahan, 1987).

Daniel Callahan (1987)

Old age has to find an integral place in the lives of those who . . . become old. An old age lacking in meaning is not, save for the rarest person, a humanly tolerable condition. Yet, even if there is some agreement that the search for a common meaning would be valuable, it requires the complementary help of a reinvigorated theory of the life-cycle (including old age) . . . Our civilization has repudiated the concept of the whole life . . . A concept of a whole life requires a number of conditions (such as) that life [is seen to] have stages . . . (Callahan, 1987, p. 30).

Aristotle

Callahan's emphasis on the fact that the meaning of old age (or of any other stage) can only be grasped, or worked out within a conception of the life as a whole, follows Aristotle who argued in relation to ethics that,

The good for man is an activity of soul in accordance with virtue, or if there are more kinds of virtue than one, in accordance with the best and most perfect kind. There is a further qualification: in a complete life. One swallow does not make a summer; neither does one day. Similarly neither can one day, or a brief space of time, make a man blessed and happy (Aristotle, 1980, p. 76).

This conception of ethics as both related to meaning and in particular to the meaning of the whole life seems to imply that old age has a very special status in relation to ethics. For, it is **only** at the end of life that we can reflect upon and consider our lives as a whole. Despite this however, and in relation to the quote from Callahan earlier, the fact is that, whilst old age might be ethically special, it is so if at all because we have to come to terms with some very difficult facts about our-

selves and those around us, notably the inevitability of our decline and death. This in itself may mean that not everyone is going to be able to reflect or to engage in narrative and this must be seen as a limitation of the narrative approach which would seem to depend to at least some extent upon a range of cognitive capacities. Nevertheless, the narrative ideal, as expressed by Alasdair MacIntyre below, still has great appeal.

. . . both childhood and old age have [mistakenly] been wrenched from the rest of human life and made over into distinct realms . . . it is the distinctiveness of each and not the unity of the life of the individual . . . of which we are taught to think and to feel . . . The unity of a human life [should instead be] the unity of a narrative quest (MacIntyre, 1981).

> **ACTIVITY: As your final activity of this chapter we would like you to go back to the remaining cases (you've already done this for the case of Lisa and Martin) and to spend some time considering them again in the light of your reading of the chapter. This will enable to revise the key points of the chapter and help you to assess whether the aims and objectives set out at the start of the chapter have been met. As you do so, make a summary of key points in this chapter.**

Suggestions for further reading

Agich, G. (1993). *Autonomy in Long Term Care.* New York: Oxford University Press.

Callahan, D. (1987). *Setting Limits: Medical Goals in an Ageing Society.* New York: Simon and Schuster.

Gilligan, C. (1982). *In a Different Voice: Psychological Theory and Women's Development.* Cambridge MA.: Harvard University Press.

Lindemann Nelson, H. and J. (1995). *The Patient in the Family.* New York: Routledge.

Tronto, J. (1993). *Moral Boundaries: A Political Argument for an Ethic of Care.* New York: Routledge.

Mental health

Introduction

We begin this chapter on Ethical Issues in Mental Health with a case from Italy. We decided to use this case as the starting point both because it raises important ethical issues in itself but also because it brings to the fore ethical questions about mental health more widely. Are there morally significant differences between psychiatric medicine and medicine of other kinds? Are there also such morally significant differences between different types of psychiatric conditions? If so what are the implications of these differences for the practice of psychiatric medicine? Having raised these questions very broadly in the first section, we will then go on to explore them and others in greater depth in the sections which follow.

We would like you to start by reading the case of Mr AB and as you do so we would like you to consider the extent to which you feel that the difficulties which arise in the case are morally significant or 'ethical' and the extent to which they are simply a practical or clinical matter. To what extent do you think it is possible to make such a distinction? Do clinical decisions such as those concerning Mr AB always have an ethical dimension?

Section 1: Ethical conflicts in mental health

THE CASE OF MR AB

Mr AB was a 90-year-old man who suffered from dementia. After several years of being cared for at home by his wife, Mr AB was finally admitted to a Special Care Unit in northern Italy because his wife no longer felt able to bear the demands which caring for her husband placed upon her.

On admission to the Unit, a clinical and multi-dimensional evaluation of Mr AB's condition revealed him to be severely cognitively impaired and to be extremely frail as a result of malnutrition. Mr AB was capable to some limited extent of walking and also of eating but was dependent upon others in virtually every other respect. Although he was able to walk, Mr AB found balance very difficult and needed the support of a carer. The doctors who saw him also recorded that he had severe 'behaviour disorders' associated with dementia, such as anxiety and agitation.

The physician responsible for Mr AB's care designed a walking rehabilitation programme for him and the nurses in the unit tried to improve his nutritional status by means of personal care and attention during meal times and by the use of nutritional supplements. It was also decided to reduce the levels of psychotropic drugs with which Mr AB had been treated while he was living at home.

After 20 days of treatment at the Special Care Unit, Mr AB's cognitive and functional status had improved dramatically and he was now able to walk alone, without help. His behaviour disorders were also less severe and disturbing (especially his anxiety and agitation), despite the fact that his treatment with psychotropic drugs had been reduced.

After 35 days at the unit, however, Mr AB developed a fever and cough which became progressively worse. This was diagnosed as pneumonia. As a result of the pneumonia, Mr AB became much more confused again and was no longer able to walk. He also lost the ability to feed himself. All this resulted in a dramatic and serious decline in Mr AB's health. It was felt that Mr AB's life would be at risk unless his pneumonia were treated and he received some nutrition.

After discussing the patient's condition with his wife, the physician started treating Mr AB intravenously with fluids and also with antibiotics. However, during attempts to administer intravenous drugs Mr AB became very irritable and agitated. He also refused food during assisted meals.

After further consultation with Mr AB's wife, short-term physical restraints were adopted by the hospital staff both during the administration of drugs and during assisted meals. After 2 weeks Mr AB recovered from pneumonia and returned to his previous daily nourishment and drug therapy.

ACTIVITY: Stop here for a moment and consider the ethical questions raised by this case as described. Start off by making a list of the actions taken which you consider to raise ethical questions and those which you consider to be simply clinical. Next to each of these note down your reasons for your decision. Take a few moments to think about the extent to which it is possible to draw a distinction between what constitutes a clinical and an ethical problem. If you think it is possible, what is it which marks the difference? If you think it is not possible, what are the implications of this for ethics and practice?

At first sight the case of Mr AB might be seen to be an everyday one involving a series of relatively straightforward clinical decisions. He entered the unit in a very poor condition and was given a course of treatment which increased his quality of life greatly. This course of treatment was interrupted by his pneumonia which was itself then treated, thereby allowing Mr AB to return to his earlier much-improved condition. From a utilitarian or consequentialist perspective, that is if we judge the morality of actions and choices in terms of their consequences, the treatment seems to have been justified, at least on first inspection. The patient's quality of life was improved greatly both by his admission to the unit and his consequent treatment, including the use of restraints. Nevertheless, the use of restraints and compulsory treatment on a patient clearly raises ethical questions of great importance independently of their short-term consequences. Whilst it is not clear that the patient was actually refusing treatment, its administration was obviously making him extremely anxious and agitated. Under what conditions is it right to override someone's wishes and in fact to physically force treatment upon them on the grounds of an assessment of their 'best interests'?

John Stuart Mill once famously argued that the moral thing to do, from a utilitarian point of view was to respect and uphold the liberty of individuals in so far as such liberty is compatible with the liberty of others and this is a warning to us that we have to think very carefully indeed before we use utility/best interest as a justification for overriding the freedom and wishes of patients.

The main ethical consideration which we felt to be a feature of the case on first sight was this tension between the healthcare professional's duty to respect the choices and wishes of the patients in their care and the complementary duty to act in the patient's best interests. Sometimes, perhaps mostly, these two duties pull in the same direction, i.e. the patient wants to have the treatment which is in their best interest. However in this case the carers felt that this was not the case and that their responsibility to act in the patient's best interests was more important than to respect the patient's 'wishes'. To what extent do you agree with this? One of the features of work with at least some psychiatric patients, of course, is that it is often unclear just what the patient's wishes are, and this throws a different light on the tension between wishes and best interests. Assuming for a moment that the patient was indeed attempting to refuse the treatment, there is clearly a sense in which he is a danger to himself and putting himself at risk by refusing both nutrition and treatment for his pneumonia. To what extent do we have the right and perhaps the duty to physically restrain another person from doing what they want to do (assuming we know what this is), even where we consider it to be harmful to them or to be against their best interests? In most forms of medicine other than psychiatry such a conflict might be interpreted in terms of paternalism (doing something against the patient's wishes, for their own good) vs. the patient's right to choose, but in psychiatry such conflicts tend to be described in terms of the incompetence of the patient. The argument here, put simply, would be that Mr AB by virtue of his confusion, his dementia and his anxiety was incapable of having sufficient understanding of his condition or of the proposed treatment to enable him to make an informed choice, either to refuse or to accept his treatment, thereby 'justifying' the healthcare professional's attempts to act in his best interests despite his protests.

Stefano Boffelli, an Italian old-age psychiatrist, comments on the case as follows.

The patient, after admission, was judged to be incompetent in taking decisions about himself: cognitive status testing showed a severe decline, [which was] also worsened by the heavy psychopharmacological treatment administered at home. The patient was also frail: malnutrition, frequently found in nursing home patients, was the main risk factor for developing pneumonia. However, the patient was not in the end stage of the disease, as was shown by the clinical improvement after rehabilitation. The patient had never written an advance directive about medical treatment before the onset of

dementia. So decisions about rehabilitation and the pharmacological treatment of his pneumonia were discussed with his wife, as a substitute decision-maker.

The decision to use physical restraint (for a short time only) was taken with the caregiver. Both in the doctor's and in the caregiver's view, restraining the patient was judged to be an acceptable process to administer drugs and nourishment. Mr AB's wife said of the outcome, that ensuring his recovery from pneumonia was worthwhile, even if obtained through short-term discomfort. The patient's reactions against the nurses (agitation and irritability) were interpreted as the effects of dementia, not as an attempt to refuse treatment (S. Boffelli, 1999, personal communication).

> **ACTIVITY:** To what extent do you agree with the doctor and the patient's wife that restraining the patient was an acceptable process in order to administer drugs and nutrition? What arguments can you think of against this view? What do you think about the wife's view that the restraint was simply a 'short-term discomfort' for her husband? Although the outcome may have been one which gave the patient a quality of life which was greater than that which he had before treatment and perhaps even saved his life, it is legitimate to ask ourselves, in the spirit of John Stuart Mill, what are the limits to the extent to which we are willing to override the patient's wishes and freedom in favour of what we consider to be their best wishes?

In the case of the treatment of a fully competent patient we would surely consider it unacceptable to restrain a patient in this way in order to forcefully treat them. It is only in cases where we consider the patient incapable of making an informed choice that we even contemplate such things (such as Re W, a case which is explored later in this chapter). Thus it would seem that the physician and the patient's wife are basing their claims upon the argument that there is a morally relevant difference between the practice of psychiatric medicine with patients who are not fully competent and that of ordinary medicine with those who are.

> ACTIVITY: To what extent do you think that this is true? Stop here for a moment and note down any ways in which work with psychiatric patients who are not fully competent might be ethically different from other forms of medicine. It may well be that on reflection you consider the actions of the carers in the case of Mr M C to have been ethically justified and unproblematic. If so, think for a few moments about how the case would have to have differed for you to feel that Mr M C's refusal would have to be respected.

It is important to remind ourselves at this point that, for most psychiatric patients there is no doubt about their competence. Most are fully competent. Most psychiatric patients are seen as outpatients for a wide variety of psychological problems. For this reason and as a result of the variety of types of mental illness, it is important to remind ourselves that psychiatric illness is not a homogeneous category. Indeed, as we shall be going on to see in the next section, the question of competence is still a matter of considerable debate even in the treatment of long-term inpatients.

The competence of psychiatric patients

The case of Mr AB raises, as we have seen, the question of the conflict in psychiatric medicine between the healthcare professional's duty to respect the wishes of their patients and the duty to work in their best interests. This is a particularly acute problem in situations where the patient's competence to make informed choices appears to be compromised. Were it legitimate to claim that psychiatric patients such as these are simply incapable of making informed choices about their treatment as a result of the incompetence associated with their illness, we might be justified in arguing that it is the duty of those who take care of them to make decisions on such patients' behalf, in their best interests. But to what extent is it true to say that patients are either competent or incompetent in any general sense, and to what extent are psychiatric patients actually capable at least sometimes of making such informed choices? One way of answering this question

would be to ask those who work most closely with psychiatric patients, notably psychiatric nurses. In 1996, Maritta Välimäki and Hans Helenius did just this, by means of a questionnaire submitted to 127 professional nurses working on long-term wards in four hospitals in Finland, of whom 117 replied. We would now like you to read through the following extract from the article in which they reported their findings. While you do so, we would like you to consider the implications of this for the account you provided earlier of the extent of the morally significant differences between psychiatric medicine and medicine of other kinds.

The psychiatric patient's right to self-determination

Maritta Välimäki and Hans Helenius

Over half (53 per cent) of the nurses in our survey (n=117) said that they thought that self-determination was very important to the psychiatric patient; 33 per cent considered it rather important; and 4 per cent said it was not so important. Only 1 per cent thought that self-determination was not at all important for psychiatric patients. 9 per cent said that they 'don't know'.

The nurses were also asked to give reasons for their views on the importance of self-determination. Almost half of the respondents(48 per cent) referred to human dignity, self-esteem and equality. Psychiatric hospitals are closed, isolated institutions where it is important for patients to be able to feel a sense of human dignity, as some nurses answered:

If you are not in a position to make up your own mind, you will lose your personal self-esteem.

It's a person's basic right, even for those who are not well!

If I were a patient in a psychiatric hospital, I wouldn't want someone else to make all the decisions for me, to say what is best for me. It's a basic condition of human existence, being able to make your own decisions for as long as possible. A chronic illness does not necessarily mean that you are unable to make decisions.

40 per cent of respondents said that psychiatric patients' right to self-determination was an important condition for successful treatment. For example, if nurses are able to get their patients involved in the process of planning treatment, they will also be better motivated to follow through decisions that they have jointly made.

This could strengthen the patient's positive attitude towards treatment, if he realises that someone else values him as a human being, that he can be trusted, that he is given the opportunity to make it.

When someone is admitted to psychiatric hospital, especially for a long period of time, that person may be deprived to a lesser or greater extent of humanity. Every possible means is important in this situation (to avoid this). We cannot expect good results in treatment if patients are not allowed to look after themselves in hospital.

ACTIVITY: It is clear from the findings of these researchers that the psychiatric nurses questioned felt that respect for the self-determination of their patients was important for two complementary reasons: firstly, they argued that the right to self-determination is a fundamental human right which should be enjoyed by everyone and secondly, they felt that such respect is clinically effective and improves the quality of life and the consequences of the treatment for the patient. Can you think of any counter-arguments or counter-examples which might be used against this position?

According to the authors of the paper however, there were also some nurses who responded negatively to this question and felt that self-determination was not an important consideration in the care of the groups of psychiatric patients they work with because they are not competent to make decisions about their own lives. These nurses felt that in this kind of situation it was the duty of the carer to protect the patient.

In my experience, long-term patients portray an untruthful picture of themselves and their environment and are unable to make decisions about their own affairs.

Realistically speaking, most long-term patients are unable to evaluate their own treatment or to get over their illness. Therefore, the only way they can cope in their everyday life is if they are told what to do.

Certainly it is difficult to see how allowing Mr AB to continue to refuse treatment would have enhanced his quality of life but, as the majority of the nurses claimed, not all cases are like this one. As Välimäki and Helenius argue at the end of their paper,

The important thing to recognize is that, even though a patient is unable to make independent decisions in certain areas of life, that does not have to mean that all freedom and independence in all areas has to be closed down. It is extremely important for patients' self-determination and moral dignity that they are allowed to make at least some decisions, however trivial. It is quite clear that no one can have an unlimited or absolute right to self-determination, let alone the right to harm other people or put them in jeopardy. When principles of healthcare are in conflict, the important thing is to try and strike a sensible, and sensitive, balance.

ACTIVITY: What Välimäki and Helenius are claiming here is that competence and incompetence are not necessarily generalizable attributes which apply to people across all activities and choices. They suggest both that there may be degrees of competence and that people's competence may be fragmented such that they are highly competent in some respects whilst being incompetent in others. Stop here for a moment and reflect upon the extent to which this is true.

When we considered this, we felt it to be an important insight. It is relatively common in writing in medicine to find people described as competent or incompetent as if this were always a general attribute.

The claim that human understanding is by its very nature often both fragmentary and a matter of degree has clear implications for the discussion of competence. It suggests that the assessment of a patient's competence ought to be carried out on a case-by-case basis and that a patient may be competent in some matters to a greater degree than she is in others. (Section 3 of this chapter is on competence, autonomy and advocacy, and we shall be returning again to this point in that section.) The claim that competence is often a matter of degree also implies that, whilst patients may not be able to make an informed choice alone, they may well be able to participate in decision-making with some assistance.

The British Medical Association and most doctors now recognize this.

For people with borderline or fluctuating capacity, their ability varies over time. The ability to make the same decision may vary in relation to whether the subject is tired or bored or anxious to have lunch. The BMA, for example, holds that health professionals have an ethical obligation to enhance capacity where it is possible to do so. Many simple techniques have been developed, such as talking to the patient in familiar surroundings, with a close family member present and in terminology familiar to the person, which can make the difference between the individual being judged competent or incompetent in relation to a particular decision.

But what do patients themselves think about the question of self-determination? As a follow-up to their research into the attitudes of psychiatric nurses, Välimäki and Helenius, along with Helena Leino-Kilpi, carried out some further research into the attitudes of psychiatric patients themselves about the importance of self-determination. As we come to the end of the first section of the chapter we would now like you to read the following extracts from their report of that research in the *Journal of Nursing Ethics* (1996).

Self-determination in clinical practice: the psychiatric patient's point of view

Maritta Välimäki, Helena Leino-Kilpi and Hans Helenius

The right to decision-making

Patients had rather similar views on whether they felt the right to decision-making existed and whether they were in a position to exercise that right. 75 per cent were of the opinion that psychiatric patients do have the right to decision-making while 10 per cent said that they did not have the right; 65 per cent had actually taken part in decision-making, 19 per cent had not.

From the patients' perspective, the most important thing about decision-making was that they were present when the decisions were made. These decisions were manifested in the interactions between patients and nurses in everyday situations, or at special meetings where patients made proposals, asked questions or expressed wishes.

When the patients' rights to decision-making were not implemented, they were not present when the decisions were made and they did not have the opportunity to express their opinions. Some patients felt that decisions were made behind their backs and that they really had no option but to obey the staff. In addition, some felt that the staff knew more about them than they did themselves, but they could not extract that information.

The right to consent

Consent was examined as the right of patients to be asked for permission to treat before treatment took place. Over half (61 per cent) of the patients were of the opinion that psychiatric patients have the right to be asked for their permission, while 19 per cent felt that this is not essential in psychiatric care. About one third (30 per cent) said that they had been asked for their permission, 37 per cent said that they had not. Again, asking permission involved conversations between staff and patients who were capable of voicing their own opinions, making their own decisions, and obtaining information from nurses. When the right to consent was withheld, the staff did not ask for the permission but just went ahead without it.

The right to refusal

The psychiatric patients' right to refuse treatment was the most difficult aspect of the concept of self-determination. Over one third of the patients (39 per cent) thought that this right did exist, but 20 per cent thought that it did not; 13 per cent were unable to answer the question, and 28 per cent were undecided. Almost half of the patients (48 per cent) said that they had not refused treatment or co-operation with nursing staff, but 42 per cent reported that they had refused at some time . . . One patient said,

If this drug makes me feel bad, I feel that I can say no. This doesn't mean I can actually refuse, but I can choose the drug I want. In this sense I can refuse.

> **ACTIVITY: In this introductory section of the chapter we have explored some of the ways in which mental illness raises important ethical questions. We have also explored the tension between the importance, on the one hand, both for patients and for their carers, of patient choice and self-determination and, on the other hand, the risks which such patients can sometimes pose to themselves. The fact that, in some cases, the patient's autonomy, identity and rationality are in question adds a particularly interesting and difficult ethical dimension to work in psychiatry. In the remainder of this chapter we will be going on to explore these and other issues in greater depth. Before you go on to look at Section 2, in which we shall be exploring the issues of consent and compulsory hospitalization, stop for a moment and write down the key issues raised so far about competence and incompetence in a psychiatric patient.**

Section 2: Consent to treatment and compulsory hospitalization

In Section 2 we will look at one set of issues which arise when practitioners in mental health try to take ethical questions seriously: those concerning consent to treatment and compulsory hospitalization. Section 3 concerns a related but separate cluster of questions around the criteria for competence, including dilemmas about rationality and risk.

We would like you to begin this section with a guided reading exercise based on an article by Ron Berghmans, 'Protection of the rights of the mentally ill in the Netherlands'. The Dutch system will also be briefly compared to Italian legislation, which focuses on patients' rights and outlaws psychiatric long-term hospitalization altogether. However, the patient's rights position runs into problems, Berghmans argues, when it allows psychiatric patients to reject treatment aimed at alleviating their mental illness. After looking briefly at comparable Italian legislation we will then contrast the strong Dutch and Italian patients' rights positions with an important English case, *L* v. *Bournewood*, in which patients' rights were quite strictly limited, at least in relation to informal admission to hospital. By thinking about the contrasts between and difficulties in the three nations' approaches to patients' rights, you will be able to work through the practical application of the concepts of autonomy, competence, vulnerability and risk to self which, as the previous section suggested, raise particularly difficult ethical issues in psychiatry. Those concepts will recur in Section 3, which will build on your work in this section.

Now read the first two sections of Berghmans's article.

Protection of the rights of the mentally ill in the Netherlands

Ron Berghmans

Introduction

In my article I will address a number of issues with regard to autonomy and patients' rights in Dutch mental healthcare. Firstly, I will describe a number of developments that were aimed at strengthening and protecting patient rights and autonomy. These developments have led to a reform of the law as well as to the creation of special facilities for the protection of the rights of committed mentally ill patients.

An issue of central importance in this debate concerns the morality and legality of the use of coercion towards the mentally ill, and the limits of the mentally ill patient's right to refuse supervision and treatment.

Protecting the rights of the mentally ill

In the Netherlands, a strong movement for the protection of patients' rights has significantly contributed to a process of law reform, taking place from the start of the 1970s up until the enactment of a law on compulsory admission in 1994.

This new law (officially: the Act on Formal Admissions to Psychiatric Hospitals) can be seen as a political compromise between two competing views with regard to the morality of coercive treatment of the mentally ill. Firstly: the view, based primarily on the moral principle of beneficence, that considers mental healthcare exclusively as a benevolent service to alleviate the suffering of mentally ill people. Central to this view is the idea that the mentally ill are suffering from a mental disease, that their freedom is more or less compromised, and that their capacity to make choices in some or all domains of decision-making is defective.

This traditional emphasis on beneficence is contested by those who adopt a civil rights-based view and focus on the corresponding moral principle of respect for the autonomy of persons. This second view regards persons principally as bearers of rights that deserve respect and, first and foremost considers persons as free and responsible agents. This assumption also applies to the mentally ill, who are considered to have the same civil rights as any other citizen.

Within the first view, that of beneficence, a paternalistic outlook dominates, and the use of coercion and of compulsory treatment in the care of the mentally ill is seen as a necessary element in the provision of mental healthcare. The civil rights view by contrast takes a strong anti-paternalistic position, and considers uninvited beneficence as an intrusion upon the ultimate freedom of persons to live their own way of life (Berghmans, 1996).

ACTIVITY: Stop here for a moment and make a chart of the conflicting concepts and premises associated with the two views Berghmans identifies. The two contrasting views can be characterized in different ways, but we have headed them 'paternalism' and 'civil rights'. Our chart begins like this:

PATERNALISM	CIVIL RIGHTS
Key concept: beneficence	Key concept: autonomy
Mentally ill are different	Mentally ill have the same rights
Patient's autonomy is compromised	Autonomy should be respected
Coercion may be necessary	Coercion is intrusive and wrong

Now read the next paragraphs of Berghmans' paper.

The law

In the Netherlands, a distinction can be made between the informal and formal admission of patients to mental hospitals. The informal or 'voluntary' admission to a mental hospital before 1994 – the year when the new law came into force – was reserved for all cases in which the patient did not object to hospitalization. If the patient objected, a court order was needed (formal admission). Generally, about 85 per cent of patients residing in mental hospitals had the status of informal patient, and 15 per cent the status of formal patient.

The new law has changed this state of affairs dramatically. Under the new law, a formal procedure is necessary if a person 'does not exhibit the necessary willingness to be hospitalized'. This implies that it is not only persons who object to hospitalization, but also persons who do not object and at the same time do not exhibit a willingness to be hospitalized (i.e. certain mentally handicapped persons and psychogeriatric patients) who are subject to formal procedures. Formerly, these groups (the 'non-objecting and non-consenting') were considered to be informal, 'voluntary' patients.

ACTIVITY: In the Netherlands some 85 per cent of patients in mental hospitals were formerly admitted as 'informal' patients, so long as they did not actively object. What are the implications of this fact for (a) psychiatric practice and (b) the definition of consent to treatment?

Our answer to (a) is that abolition of the 'informal' admission procedure will have massive resource implications for practice in any system where informal patients are in such a vast majority. (The percentage of informal admissions for dementia, autism and learning difficulties is even higher in the UK; fewer than 10 per cent of mentally disordered patients in hospitals and mental nursing homes were admitted under the formal provisions for compulsory admissions, although the larger part of the remainder are voluntary admissions – competent patients who have consented to admission.) Formal admission procedures or appeals will entail vast amounts of time. There is also a risk that some patients may fall through the net – not meeting the criteria for formal admission, because they do not have a treatable mental disorder, but still needing help.

Our answer to (b) is that consent to treatment must be active in other areas of medicine; it is simply not good enough to read the absence of dissent as consent. Surgeons who did that would rapidly find themselves the subject of legal actions for battery or negligence. Consent serves two functions: first, it provides the legal justification for what would otherwise be trespass to the person and a violation of the patient's bodily integrity. In clinical practice, second, it creates the basis of trust and relationship between doctor and patient (Montgomery, 1997, p. 227, citing *Re W*, 1992). So, consent is not to be taken lightly; but the practical implications of taking consent seriously in relation to the demented, autistic or learning-disabled patient are tremendous, as our answer to (a) suggested. This is the essential conflict.

Now go on to read the next section of Berghmans.

Under the new law, a person can be involuntarily committed if the following conditions are met:
(a) he suffers from a mental illness;
(b) he is dangerous to himself or others;
(c) this dangerousness is a result of the mental illness;
(d) he does not exhibit the necessary willingness to be hospitalized; and
(e) there is no alternative way to prevent the dangerousness.

After a patient has been coercively committed to a psychiatric hospital, the psychiatrist has the legal duty to negotiate a so-called treatment plan with the patient. The treatment plan aims at the amelioration of the disorder that has led to the danger that the patient posed to himself or others before he was committed. After being informed about the proposed treatment plan, the patient can consent to or refuse treatment. If the patient is considered to be incompetent or decisionally incapacitated, the physician has the duty to discuss the treatment plan with a proxy of the patient. This representative of the incompetent patient also can consent to or refuse treatment.

This implies that a compulsorily (formally) admitted mentally ill patient has the legal right to refuse treatment. The fact that a patient is involuntarily committed in the mental hospital is a necessary, but not a sufficient, ground to overrule a treatment refusal. In other words: the decision regarding compulsory treatment is a separate decision based on grounds other than the decision regarding compulsory admission to the mental hospital.

Compulsory psychiatric treatment (i.e. psychiatric treatment against the will of the patient) can be legally justified under one of the following three conditions:
(a) if a competent patient refuses treatment, and the treatment is absolutely necessary to avert serious danger to the patient himself or others in the mental hospital;
(b) if the proxy of an incompetent patient refuses treatment, and the treatment is absolutely necessary to avert serious danger to the patient himself or others; and

(c) if an incompetent patient refuses treatment, and the treatment is necessary to avert serious danger to the patient himself or others. Thus, in this last case, even if the proxy of an incompetent patient consents to treatment, this treatment of the refusing patient can only take place if necessary to prevent serious danger to the patient himself or others.

As far as the right to refuse treatment is concerned, the Dutch law makes no distinction between the refusal of treatment by a competent patient, and treatment refusal by an incompetent patient.

A refusal of treatment by an incompetent patient may raise serious ethical problems in the practice of mental healthcare. The patient can be formally detained, but unless he becomes a serious danger to him or herself or others, treatment aiming at improvement of the mental condition of the patient cannot take place if he or she opposes such treatment.

ACTIVITY: Berghmans has moved on from the question of informal admission to the patient's equal right to refuse treatment even if he or she satisfies the criteria for compulsory admission. Here too, the paternalistic approach has been rejected in favour of an autonomy-centred strategy. To what extent need it be true to say that an autonomy-based approach means that an incompetent patient who is apparently resisting treatment must not be treated? Compare the rights of the compulsorily detained patient or his/her proxy to refuse treatment aimed at improving mental condition with the procedures prevailing in your own healthcare system. Is there such a right? For the patient? For the relative? Is there a distinction between refusal by a competent and an incompetent patient? Between refusal of psychiatric treatment and of general medical treatment? In the UK this last distinction is made clear by Section 63 of the Mental Health Act: broadly speaking, a compulsorily detained psychiatric patient may not refuse treatment intended to improve his or her mental condition, but retains the right to reject treatment for

physical illness. However, if the physical disorder is caused by the mental disorder, or if physical treatment is part of a plan of care designed to help the mental disorder – for example, in forcible feeding of patients with anorexia nervosa or compulsion to self-harm by refusing food – the distinction is not so clear (B v. Croydon HA, SW Hertfordshire HA v. KB).

Although the Netherlands is well known for its libertarian approach to social policy, you may be surprised to learn that the Italian legislation is even more far reaching. While the Italian system relies heavily on implicit consent in other contexts, spurning the language of rights (Calzone, 1996; Calzone and D'Andrea, 1996) none the less long-term psychiatric hospitalization has been banned entirely in Italy.

The trend in recent years has been to admit patients into psychiatric units in general hospitals only when absolutely necessary, treat them aggressively, and then discharge them to the next appropriate level of treatment (day centres, therapeutic communities, supervision in the community, day hospitals, halfway houses (Mordini, 1997).

As possible rationales for long-term hospitalization, Italian law accepts neither the notion of preventative detention, on the basis of risk to the community, nor of forcible treatment in the patient's best interest, on the grounds of necessity. The former is unacceptable because it constitutes a form of discrimination: no one else can be detained on the basis of crimes which they might commit in the future, but only after the offence. The latter is thought surplus to requirements: sophisticated pharmacology can keep florid systems under control, it is felt, without the need for long-term hospitalization. However compulsory short-term hospitalization is allowed under three strict conditions:

- The patient refuses treatment after all attempts to negotiate have been exhausted.
- No other solutions are available (community care, hostels, or self-help communities)
- The degree of mental illness is so severe as to require immediate intervention. Although the

law does not define this term, there is broad agreement that 'severe' means either that the patient's life is at risk or that his compelling interests are at risk.

It is worth noting – in the absence of these risks – that it is doubtful whether mere evidence that the patient's mental health will deteriorate consitutes sufficient reason for compulsory hospitalisation (Mordini, 1997).

Now read Berghmans's conclusion before going on to the English case of Mr L. As you read that case, think about Berghmans's warning that the 'right to be left alone' leads down a slippery slope to the 'right to rot'. Was this the issue in the L case? Or was it actually more complex?

In conclusion

Coercive treatment and the protection of patients' rights in psychiatry is a complex issue raising a number of medical, legal, ethical and policy questions. Societal developments have led to a strong emphasis on the moral principle of respect for the autonomy of persons. The mentally ill have been given liberty rights which they had traditionally lacked under the guise of paternalistic psychiatric beneficence. In a number of jurisdictions this has led to a right of mentally ill people to refuse treatment. In the Dutch context, a major emphasis was given to the negative right of the mentally ill to be left alone. Respecting the autonomy of the patient first and foremost is interpreted as a duty not to interfere with the affairs of the mentally ill person.

Recognizing a 'right to be left alone' may be devalued to a 'right to rot' if communities and mental health professionals use this liberal principle to legitimate indifference and lack of compassion. On the other hand, psychiatric coercion, although generally motivated by good intentions, involves *prima facie* a morally offensive action. In particular in mental healthcare, interventions may deeply intrude into the physical and mental integrity of the subject. In these cases moral reasons reaching beyond the presumed best interest or benefit of the patient are needed to provide an ethical justification of coercive treatment.

THE CASE OF MR L

What does it mean to respect autonomy and the right to give consent in the case of demented or otherwise incompetent patients? This question was thrown into sharp relief in England and Wales when the Court of Appeal ruled in December 1997 that Mr L, a severely autistic man, has been unlawfully detained by Bournewood Community and Mental Health NHS trust. Although the case was subsequently overturned by the House of Lords, it raised serious issues of law and ethics for practitioners. One of the Law Lords, Lord Steyn, expressed his concern that 'The general effect . . . is to leave compliant incapacitated patients without . . . safeguards,' even though he felt he had no alternative but to rule against Mr L under existing law. 'The only comfort,' he continued, 'is . . . that reform of the law is under active consideration.'

Before the *Bournewood* decision, psychiatrists relied heavily on informal admission for patients like Mr L, rather than use of the formal procedures under the Mental Health Act 1983. For patients admitted informally, legality of treatment depended on the general rules relating to consent under common law (judge-made law, rather than statutes like the Mental Health Act). There are, in fact, some limited protections in the Mental Health Act for informal patients, e.g. no psychosurgery or hormonal implants without consent, and section 131 of the act does concern procedures for informal admission. But according to the decision in the Court of Appeal, under both that section of the MHA and the common law, only those patients who are competent to decide whether to consent can do so. This is the crux of the difficulty: those incompetent to consent cannot give meaningful consent under common law, but if admitted informally, their civil rights are not protected by the Mental Health Act.

This was the case with Mr L, an autistic man of 48 with profound learning disability and complex needs requiring 24-hour care. He had a history of fits, and temporal lobe abnormality. Unable to speak, with no ability to communicate consent or dissent to hospital admission, Mr L was admitted informally to the mental health behavioural unit at Bournewood hospital in Surrey after agitated behaviour at his day centre.

Although the foster carers with whom he lived could control his behaviour, they could not be contacted at the time. Mr L was at risk of serious self-harm, banging his head violently and repeatedly against the wall. The centre had to be evacuated to avoid possible risk to the safety of other patients. A local doctor administered a sedative, and he was taken by ambulance to the Accident and Emergency Department of Bournewood Hospital. As the sedative began to wear off, he became agitated again, and was seen by a staff grade psychiatrist, Dr Perera, who recommended that he should be transferred for inpatient treatment at the hospital's behavioural unit.

There the consultant who had been treating him since 1977, Dr Manjubashini, decided to admit him on an informal basis: she considered detaining him under the provisions of the Mental Health Act, but came to the conclusion that his apparent compliance rendered that unnecessary.

Perhaps because Mr L had previously been a patient at Bournewood for 30 years, or perhaps because he continued to be sedated, he made no attempt to resist admission or leave the hospital once he was there. His carers, Mr and Mrs E, with whom he had lived for four years as one of the family, were not allowed to see him while his needs were being assessed, on the grounds that he might attempt to leave with them before he was fit for discharge. The carers applied to the High Court for judicial review of the trust's decision to detain Mr L, seeking a declaration that his detention was unlawful, and asking that he be released forthwith.

Although the High Court found in the hospital's favour, the Court of Appeal judgement (2 December 1997) held that Mr L had indeed been unlawfully detained. Informal admission requires active consent, not the mere absence of open resistance, it was stated. A person who lacks the capacity to consent or dissent must be admitted under the statutory procedures of the MHA. As an informal patient, Mr L had been wrongly denied the safeguards and civil rights which are built into the Act (e.g. the right to apply to an independent tribunal for discharge).

After the initial Appeal Court hearing, and pending the actual judgement, the Trust had thought it prudent to formally detain or 'section' Mr L under Section 5 of the Mental Health Act. Following the Appeal Court Decision, hospitals throughout England and Wales (the judgement did not apply to Scotland) were advised to do the same by the NHS Executive, the Royal College of Psychiatrists and the Department of Health. It was estimated that as many as 48 000 extra patients a year would have to be sectioned (that is admitted under a section of the MHA). They would now have the right to appeal to mental health review tribunals, with cost implications in terms of staff time. The resource implications extended to Social Services as well: formally detained patients have a right to free aftercare under Section 117 of the MHA.

So, it was with relief that many psychiatrists heard the highest court, the House of Lords, reverse the Appeal Court decision. The Court of Appeal had held that doctors could not treat Mr L under the principle of necessity – the principle which allows emergency admissions to casualty wards to be treated without consent. There was no need to use the principle of necessity when there was a perfectly valid statute ready and waiting to be used instead. In their judgement of June 1998, the Law Lords disagreed. Lord Goff's opinion noted that 'the decision of the Court of Appeal has caused grave concern' in the profession and that 'it was obvious that there would in the result be a substantial impact on the available resources,' although the case was on a point of law and not overtly, at least, on resource issues. The questions on which the final judgement centred were whether Mr L had not been unlawfully detained after all, and whether the principle of necessity could in fact apply. These were two separate issues, in the opinion of Lord Steyn: one a matter of fact, the other of pure law.

The Law Lords disagreed over whether Mr L had

in fact been detained against his will. Lords Goff and Lloyd found that Mr L had not been wrongfully detained without his consent, although he had been physically taken to Bournewood Hospital, and although the duty psychiatrist made it plain that she would detain him under the MHA if he resisted admission. The issue was the wrong (or 'tort') of false imprisonment, for which there must be a complete deprivation of the patient's liberty, in actual fact. Mr L had been accommodated on an unlocked ward and had never attempted to leave the hospital. Although the psychiatrist intended to restrain Mr L if he did try to leave, and to consider compulsory detention under Section 3 of the Act, he did not in fact try to do so, and so there was no tort of false imprisonment. This reasoning was rejected by Lord Steyn as 'stretching credulity to the breaking point': L had been sedated, physically conveyed to hospital, sedated again in hospital, barred from seeing his carers on grounds that he might try to leave with them, and closely monitored by nursing staff, even though the ward was unlocked. 'The suggestion that L was free to go is a fairy tale,' Lord Steyn stated categorically 'In my view L was detained because the healthcare professionals intentionally assumed control over him to such a degree as to amount to complete deprivation of his liberty.'

Lord Goff added that Mr L had never been finally discharged from Bournewood Hospital, only sent to live with Mr and Mrs E on a trial basis. Therefore, the Trust remained responsible for his treatment, and any steps taken to 'detain' him were in discharge of their duty of care. Whether or not Mr L had in fact been detained was a separate matter from the justification for detaining him, in terms of the Trust's duty of care. It could actually be rightful to detain him for that purpose, and indeed part of the hospital's responsibility, as Lord Nolan argued.

This leads into the second ground, which the Law Lords gave for overturning the Appeal Court decision: the psychiatrists were justified in their action by the common-law doctrine of necessity. That is, they were justified in taking measures they judged to be of therapeutic benefit and in his best interests, so long as it was not practicable to communicate with him and the actions taken were those a reasonable person would take in the circumstances. It was against this common law background, according to Lord Steyn's opinion, that the mental health legislation must be understood. The Percy Report of 1957, which laid the basis for the Mental Health Act 1959, marked a shift from the older 'legalism' under which all patients had to be 'certified' before being admitted, to a situation in which patients would be received 'informally'. There should be 'the offer of care, without deprivation of liberty, to all who need it and are *not unwilling to receive it'* (emphasis added).

Here, then, is the basis for the practice of equating lack of resistance with active consent to treatment. Compulsion was to be regarded as a measure of last resort, so that as many patients as possible would be treated, and treated without the stigmatization of formal procedures. In the name of the patient's best interests – an essentially paternalistic criterion – the Mental Health Act 1959 incorporated this philosophy in Section 5(1) on the informal admission of patients, which noted that 'Nothing in this Act shall be conceived as preventing a patient who requires treatment for mental disorder from being admitted to any hospital or mental nursing home in pursuance of arrangements made in that behalf and without any application, order or direction rendering him liable to be detained under this Act.' The 1983 Act reproduced this section verbatim as Section 131(1). In other words, this is a sort of mopping-up clause which allows a patient to be admitted informally and treated under the doctrine of necessity, if that is judged to be in his best interests, regardless of whether or not doctors choose to invoke formal procedures. Despite his view that Mr L had been unlawfully detained, and his strong fears that informally admitted patients are denied the safeguards afforded to compulsorily detained patients, Lord Steyn was forced to conclude that the Court of Appeal had erred. 'The conclusion cannot be avoided that Section 131(1) permits the admission of compliant incapacitated patients where the requirements of the principle of necessity are satisfied.'

> **ACTIVITY: In the case of *L* v. *Bournewood*, English law briefly flirted with the patients' rights approach epitomized by the Dutch law on informal admissions before reverting to a more paternalistic stance. Was this the right decision, do you think? Make two lists of the ethical arguments for and against the practice of informal admission for patients who are not fully competent to consent to treatment. Try to distinguish the ethical arguments from the practical ones, such as shortage of resources.**

So far we have mainly considered the practical and resource arguments in favour of informal admission, but an ethical argument can be made for the practice, too. The most obvious argument would be based on beneficence, doing good, which Berghmans identified as the underpinning principle of paternalism. If patients cannot be admitted informally, but only under the provisions of the Mental Health Act, many will fall through the treatment net because they do not have a treatable mental disorder, although they still need help.

A not uncommon clinical example is admission for establishment of diagnosis and aetiology of cognitive impairment without evidence of risk to the health or safety of the patient or others. If such a patient cannot provide consent and does not fulfil the criteria for the Mental Health Act, do we deny them admission and investigation? That would be ethically wrong according to the principle of beneficence, which emphasizes the patient's best interest (Shah and Dickenson, 1998).

Even if the prospective patient does have a treatable mental disorder, relatives may be reluctant to give permission for admission under Section 3 of the Act, as is required. There is still a stigma attached to mental illness and psychiatric hospitalization.

But we could also argue in favour of informal admission from the viewpoint of the patient's rights – rather surprisingly, in terms of Berghmans's scheme. This would be a more sophisticated version of the argument from

autonomy, running something like this. Does requiring active consent to psychiatric treatment enhance or threaten the autonomy and dignity of patients with dementia, learning disability and autism? If such patients are incapable of giving meaningful consent, they cannot be admitted informally, even if they would benefit. Is this a formalistic interpretation of patient's rights which does nothing for the dignity and welfare of vulnerable people without real capacity to consent? Would their autonomy actually be enhanced by treatment that made them better able to live a more normal life?

A further distinction can be made between positive and negative rights, a distinction commonly made in political philosophy. Negative or liberty rights concern freedoms from arbitrary power; positive or welfare rights are rights to enjoy certain benefits. Suppose we think of psychiatric patients as having not just the negative right to be free of compulsory hospitalization, but also the positive right to treatment which will benefit them. Then the distinction between the paternalistic model and the patient's rights view begins to look less fixed and firm.

But, even if this is true, we might still have qualms about equating the absence of resistance with active consent. We have no evidence from Mr L's lack of active resistance that he was really trying to exercise his positive right to beneficial treatment. Is it condescending and paternalistic to take a patient's absence of resistance as consent to informal admission? This would be the more obvious kind of patient's rights argument, and it could be backed up by an argument about discrimination and injustice.

It is particularly disturbing that cognitively impaired people are treated very differently from everyone else. In effect, the agreement of the nearest relative is sufficient for informal admission; yet English law upholds individual autonomy strictly in formal situations by refusing to recognize proxy consent (such as giving consent to an operation where the competence of the patient is in doubt) where competence is not obvious (e.g. in the case of comatose patients,

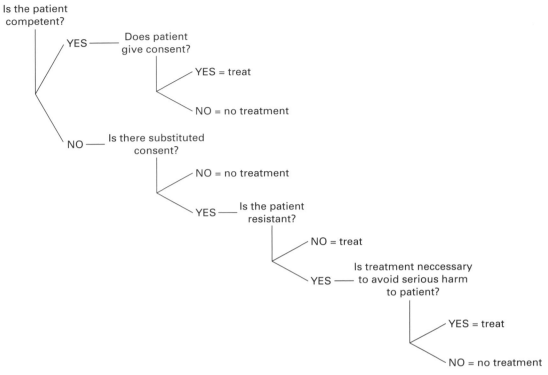

Fig. 6.1. The Welie diagram.

whose life-sustaining treatment cannot be withdrawn simply on the say-so of a relative). People with dementia, learning disability or autism are therefore treated as 'beyond the pale' of English law's general unwillingness to let others consent on a patient's behalf.

ACTIVITY: To review your work in this section, please look at Fig. 6.1, which was drawn up by a Dutch academic lawyer, Sander Welie, as a flowchart for when interventions may be undertaken (Welie, 1996). As you look at the diagram we would like you to consider whether the 'yeses and 'noes' are in the right place, by trying to use the diagram in relation to (a) the case of Mr L, and (b) your own practice. As you do so, and before you move on to the next section, take a few moments to make a list of the key points raised by this section.

Section 3: Competence, autonomy and advocacy

In the previous section we concentrated on a case in which the patient clearly lacked capacity to make treatment decisions: Mr L was profoundly mentally handicapped and autistic. Although people with dementia, autism and learning disability constitute a large proportion of informal admissions and a sizeable percentage of psychiatric patients, our discussion has so far said little about cases in which incompetence is not so obvious. That will be the focus of Section 3. What are the criteria for competence? Are they universal, or do we need to bear in mind the risk of multicultural misunderstandings in assessing rationality? What is a competent psychiatric patient able to refuse? What about competent minors? And how can a patient of borderline competence be helped, perhaps through patient advocacy, to exercise enhanced autonomy and make treatment decisions? – rather than have them made for her on a paternalistic basis.

We have seen, in relation to informal admission of patients lacking capacity, that English law tends more to the paternalistic side of the patient's rights – paternalism spectrum. Perhaps we might expect it to err on the sceptical side in assessing the competence of mental patients as well. Can a patient with serious psychiatric disorders ever be said to be competent to refuse treatment?

THE CASE OF MR C

C, a 68-year-old patient suffering from paranoid schizophrenia, developed gangrene in a foot during his confinement in a secure hospital. He was removed to a general hospital, where the consultant surgeon diagnosed that he was likely to die imminently if the leg was not amputated below the knee. The prognosis was that he had a 15 per cent chance of survival without amputation. C refused to consider amputation. The hospital authorities considered whether the operation could be performed without C's consent and made arrangements for a solicitor to see him concerning his competence to give a reasoned decision. In the meantime, treatment with antibiotics and conservative surgery averted the immediate threat of imminent death, but the hospital refused to give an understanding to the solicitor that in recognition of his repeated refusals it would not amputate in any future circumstances. There was a possibility that C would develop gangrene again. An application was made on C's behalf to the court for an injunction restraining the hospital from carrying out an amputation without his express written consent. On behalf of the hospital it was contended that C's capacity to give a definitive decision had been impaired by his mental illness and that he had failed to appreciate the risk of death if the operation was not performed. (Re C (adult: refusal of medical treatment) [1994]).

ACTIVITY: Do you think that Mr C should have been allowed to refuse the amputation? Make a list of the arguments for and against his right to refuse.

Now consider the following additional facts: Which, if any, is relevant?

- Mr C had emigrated from Jamaica in 1956, with his passage paid by the woman with whom he had lived since 1949. He stabbed her after she left him in 1961.
- Since that time Mr C had been confined either in prison or in a secure hospital.
- For the past six years he had been accommodated in an open ward and was described as having 'mellowed', having become more sociable and even-tempered.
- Mr C was very adept with finances; he had saved all of his earnings during his 30 years' time in the secure hospital.
- However, when his solicitor asked him to whom he intended to leave his savings, he replied 'I'll leave it for myself, for when I come back'.
- Mr C's delusions included the belief that he was a world-famous vascular surgeon who had never lost a patient.
- Mr C also believed that his doctors were torturers.
- Mr C's refusal of amputation reflected his religious convictions, although not part of a formal creed.

Rather than simply revealing whether Mr C was, in fact, allowed to refuse amputation, we will ask you to work through the legal and ethical implications of the facts of the case. Let's begin with the question of Mr C's Jamaican origins. The high percentage of psychiatric patients of West Indian ancestry has often been remarked on, but opinion is divided on the extent to which their comparatively high rate of psychiatric diagnosis reflects actual pathology, or simply an ethnocentric tendency in psychiatrists to 'pathologize' behaviour which would be quite normal in another culture. It is important to recognize that psychiatric diagnosis is itself an ethical problem, as is assessment of rationality and competence; unwitting discrimination against members of another culture is all too easy in a diagnostic process which is sometimes said to be more vulnerable to inconsistency, poor reliability or cultural bias than in the 'harder' branches of medicine (Reich, 1998). But conversely, we have to be careful about 'psychological relativism'. : 'the abandonment of universal principles of mental disorder . . . [with the result that] cure of mentally ill ethnic minority patients [becomes] impossible except within a totally culture-specific model of therapy. . . . This approach makes every human being a mere reflection of his community, an individual without identity or uniqueness, completely subordinated to his ethnicity' (Benhabib, 1997). Mr C had been sentenced to prison, and then transferred to a secure psychiatric hospital, because of an assault, which would be a crime in any culture. His psychotic delusions also seem quite profoundly embedded, including the beliefs that he is a famous vascular surgeon and his doctors are torturers. So multicultural issues do not seem particularly relevant to assessment of competence in this case. (His religious convictions raise similar problems about relativism: is it right to take a 'hands-off' attitude to cure because of them?)

What about Mr C's delusions, then? – as possibly affecting his competence. One of the consultant psychiatrists involved in the case, Nigel Eastman, believed that Mr C's delusions did affect his belief in what the doctors told him: that he had only a 15 per cent chance of cure without amputation. This seems plausible: if Mr C thought his 'rivals' were jealous of his 'medical reputation', he probably would have discounted their opinion, particularly if he also believed that they were inflicting another form of torture on him by proposing to cut off his leg. One might also argue that his delusions created the crisis in the first place: because he thought the doctors were torturers, he did not report his leg infections until it was dangerous. If so, there would be an argument that Mr C should not be allowed to refuse the amputation – even though that was treatment for a physical rather than a mental disorder. In the UK a distinction between refusing psychiatric treatments and other interventions is made by Section 63 of the Mental Health Act: as we have seen, a compulsorily detained psychiatric patient may not refuse treatment intended to improve his or her mental condition, but retains the right to reject treatment for physical disorder. One could certainly argue that Mr C's physical disorder was related to his mental disorders in its origins, although it is less clear that amputation will actually have a beneficial impact on his mental disorder.

On the other hand, despite his delusions, Mr C was competent in other areas, such as finances. Does this extend to competence to refuse medical treatment? It is important to remember that there is a presumption of competence in adults, and that a finding of mental disorder does not automatically undermine that presumption. In the court hearings expert witnesses testified that Mr C's preferences were shared by many other people with vascular disease, whose competence was not in doubt. Refusing to get on the treadmill of possible repeated amputations is common in such patients. Mr C had strong views that he would prefer to die with two legs than survive with one. These, too, have been expressed by other people facing or experiencing amputation, and have nothing necessarily to do with psychotic delusions. In a letter written after his leg was amputated following his misadventures in Africa, the French poet and traveller Arthur Rimbaud wrote:

If someone in this condition asked my advice, I'd tell them this: never let yourself be amputated. Let them butcher you, flay you, slice you in pieces, but never allow anyone to amputate you. If it means death, this will always be better than living without one of your limbs. Many have made this choice, and if I had another chance I would make it too (letter to Isabelle Rimbaud, 15 July 1891, quoted in Nicholl (1998), p. 294).

In the end Rimbaud died anyway, a possibility which could not be ignored in Mr C's case either. Although the emphasis has so far been put on the 85 per cent chance that he would die without amputation, chronic vascular disease and the possibility of renewed gangrene meant that there was no guarantee that Mr C would necessarily survive in the long run even if he accepted the procedure. Indeed, the consultant vascular surgeon, Dr Rutter, did testify that below-the-knee amputation carries a 15 per cent mortality risk. This raises questions about rationality and risk preferences. It is always tempting for clinicians to reject patients' treatment decisions which do not correspond to the doctors' own evaluation for the best chance of success. But patients are entitled to their own risk preferences; refusing a procedure which the doctor thinks likely to succeed is not in itself proof of irrationality.

Prima facie, every adult had the right and capacity to decide whether or not he will accept medical intervention, even if a refusal may risk permanent injury to his health, or even lead to premature death. Furthermore, it matters not whether the reasons for the refusal were rational or irrational, unknown or even non-existent *(Re T [1992], All ER 649)*.

The criteria for competence, as enunciated in the case of Mr C, are functional; they concern the ability to make this particular decision, not 'rationality' in the abstract. The touchstone is whether mental disorder had reduced the patient's understanding of the nature, purpose and effects of the proposed intervention to such an extent that he or she is incapable of making this particular decision. It could be said that even a patient whose delusions are plainly irrational may be competent to make a treatment decision if he or she fulfils the following criteria:

(a) Comprehending and retaining information relating to the decision
(b) Believing the information
(c) Weighing it in the balance when making a choice.

This is a functional test of competence: it measures competence to make this particular decision. It is not a measure of general competence. On the basis of these criteria, Mr C was found competent to refuse the proposed amputation, discounting the finding of his principal consultant psychiatrist, Dr Ghosh, that his was an open-and-shut case of incompetence, not even borderline. Even Dr Eastman, who had suggested the three-stage criteria, was of the opinion that C had achieved

the first stage but not the second: he did not believe what the doctors told him.

What was important, according to Mr Justice Thorpe's opinion, was Dr Eastman's testimony that C did not believe the doctors had actively caused his condition, even though he believed that they were torturers. 'Plainly, C's capacity is reduced by his mental illness. But for him [Dr Eastman] the decision as to whether it is sufficiently reduced remains marginal in the absence of any direct link between the persecutory delusions and his present condition.' That C was able to meet the third criterion, weighing the information, was shown by his acceptance of the possibility that he might yet die as a result of refusing amputation, although he expressed faith that God and good medical/nursing care would see him through. Overall, Mr Justice Thorpe wrote in his opinion, 'His answers to questions seemed measured and generally sensible. He was not always easy to understand and the grandiose delusions were manifest, but there was no sign of inappropriate emotional expression. His rejection of amputation seemed to result from sincerely held conviction. He had a certain dignity of manner that I respect *(Re C, 823)*.

> **ACTIVITY: Stop for a moment and consider whether these three points are the things you would want to know about a patient's competence. Are there any other factors? Think back to other cases you may have heard about. Then make a chart for yourself, a kind of protocol, of the factors which you will want to consider in future, drawing on the C case and your own reflections.**

One point, which may have occurred to you in doing this exercise, is that we have been speaking of competent/incompetent as if they were clear polar opposites. We need to qualify this oversimplification:

It may not be a case of capacity or no capacity. It may be a case of reduced capacity. What matters is whether at that time the patient's capacity was reduced below the level needed in a refusal of that importance, for refusals can vary in importance *(Re T [1992], 664)*.

There are two additional points worth noting in relation to the case of Mr C.

Firstly, the case established that the hospital could not operate without C's express written permission even if he became incompetent in the future; for example, if he became comatose in the event of a serious relapse. This is the principle of the living will or, more properly, advance directive, which states in advance what treatments a patient would want to accept or refuse. The C case established that advance refusals are broadly valid in law, although no court has yet, at the time of writing, determined the validity of an advance directive made by a patient who is now incompetent. (Montgomery, 1997, p. 445). (Mr C did not actually become incompetent, and so there was no need to activate an advance directive, nor did he die: he survived, with the 'dry' form of gangrene in a useable but 'mummified' leg.)

Although the C case did not go so far, it leads to interesting speculation on whether a mentally ill person, who is still competent, should be allowed to formulate wishes in advance regarding involuntary hospitalization (Savulescu and Dickenson, 1998; Berghmans, 1992 and 1994; Brock, 1993).

In a psychiatric advance directive (PAD), a mentally ill person can formulate his or her wishes with regard to psychiatric hospitalization and/or treatment in case, in a future situation, he or she becomes incompetent. As incompetence is neither a necessary nor a sufficient condition for involuntary psychiatry hospitalisation or treatment, incompetent mentally ill persons cannot be hospitalised or treated unless they consent. Unless they are considered seriously dangerous to themselves or others, as a result of the mental illness, coercive hospitalization or compulsory treatment cannot take place . . . In my view, from a moral perspective, a PAD strikes a responsible balance between the moral principle of beneficence and respect for patient autonomy. Through the use of PADs it would be possible for mentally ill persons who are competent, with their disease in remission, to give prior consent to treatment at a later time when they are incompetent, have become noncompliant, and are refusing treatment. This prior consent justifies overruling of the paternalistic overruling of the patient's current wishes (Berghmans, 1997b).

Secondly, the case illustrates how active advocacy can improve a patient's functional competence to make healthcare decisions. The involvement of a strongly patient's rights-minded solicitor, Lucy Scott-Montcrieff – who also acted for Mr L – allowed Mr C to make his convictions felt. The judge, Mr Justice Thorpe, can also be seen as a kind of patient advocate in that he interviewed C in hospital, actively soliciting his testimony. More frequently, the role of patient advocate falls to nurses and sometimes to doctors. Alternatively, there may be governmental ombudsmen charged with this duty – particularly in Scandinavia. In the Netherlands, the same legislation which we discussed in Section 2 also makes it obligatory for all mental hospitals to have a patient advocate, whose tasks are to advise and inform patients, to act as intermediary between the patient and healthcare professionals.

The patient advocate has an open ear for all questions and complaints of patients with regard to their relationship to the hospital (i.e. admission, care, treatment, supervision, discharge). Every complaint is taken seriously, even in cases where the healthcare professional tends to attribute the complaint to the mental illness of the patient. The patient advocate identifies with the patient, and sees the patient's interests as the patient evaluates his interests himself. This implies that the patient advocate is not impartial: he takes the point of view of the patient as his leading view. The advocate has an independent position: although he works within the confines of the institution, he is not an employee of the hospital. The patient advocate is employed by an independent body that is financed by the government (Berghmans, 1997b).

> **ACTIVITY:** Before moving on to the next section, stop here for a few moments and note down what you consider to be the main key points of this section.

Section 4: The mental health of children and young people: presumed incompetent?

In Section 3 we saw how fundamental the presumption of competence is in relation to adults. Even Mr C, with profound psychotic delusions arguably related to his physical disorder, was found competent to make decisions relating to that illness, although the result might have been his death. In this section we will begin with an example which illustrates how the opposite applies to children and young people. This is the case of a 16-year-old girl with anorexia nervosa, a life-threatening condition – like Mr C's – and again on the borderline between the purely physical and the purely mental.

THE CASE OF W

W, aged 16, was orphaned at the age of 8, when her mother died of cancer. Three years earlier, her father had died of a brain tumour. Together with her brother and sister, W was taken into the care of the local authority; her aunt, who had been named as testamentary guardian, was unable to care for the children. After a foster placement broke down, she was moved to a second family, but her new foster mother developed breast cancer. Her grandfather, to whom she was very attached, died shortly thereafter, when W was 13. A few months later W began losing weight; she had been suffering from depression and a nervous tic for some time before, and she was referred for her eating disorder to the same clinic which had been treating her other conditions. But sessions with a clinical psychologist at the clinic did not really resolve the problems, and shortly before her fifteenth birthday W was admitted on an inpatient basis to a specialist London residential unit for children and adolescents. Here she began injuring herself by picking at her skin and other forms of self-harm. A few months later her condition had deteriorated to the point where she had to be fed by nasogastric tube, to which she consented; her arms were encased in plaster to prevent her picking at her skin.

The local authority decided to move W to another treatment unit, to which W was opposed. She had developed a good relationship with staff at the first centre, she argued – although it was also true that she had occasionally been violent towards staff there. However, the original treatment centre wanted to continue working with W and opposed the move. Her weight was now stable at about 7 stone. In March 1992 W reached the age of 16 and exercised her right to be represented by a solicitor of her own choice. Under the provisions of the Family Law Reform Act 1969, which treats the treatment choices of 16- and 17-year-olds as equally valid to an adult's, it appeared that W would have the right to refuse the transfer. The authority made a formal application to the High Court to test whether this was so, requesting leave to move W to a named treatment centre without her consent, and to give her whatever treatment the new centre deemed necessary, also without her consent.

The High Court ruled that W was competent, with Mr Justice Thorpe – also the judge in the C case – stating: 'There is no doubt at all that [W] is a child of sufficient understanding to make an informed decision.' This was consistent with the evidence of Dr G, a consultant psychiatrist specializing in anorexia nervosa, who noted: 'I am convinced that she has a good intelligence, and understands what is proposed as treatment'. It might seem, therefore, that because W was competent, she would be allowed to refuse both transfer to the second centre and the 'blank cheque' which the authority was seeking for her treatment there.

One could certainly argue that the treatment at issue in W's case, the possibility of further artificial or even forcible feeding, is medical treatment rather than psychiatric treatment, and that she should have been allowed to refuse it, in the same way that Mr C was allowed to refuse amputation. But because there is a presumption of incompetence for minors under eighteen, this was not the case. W had no right to say no, it was held in both the High Court and the Court of Appeal.

The effect of the W case is that young people under 18, even if found competent, are not allowed to refuse consent to treatment so long as someone with parental responsibility consents. (In W's case the local authority had parental responsibility.) The case of W went beyond an earlier judgement, that of 'R', which held that a young person of fluctuating mental condition was not competent to refuse treatment (in R's case, antipsychotic drugs). W was found competent but denied the right to refuse treatment none the less.

Whereas in the case of Mr C the court was impressed by his dignity of manner and self-control, in W's case her attempt to control her environment, carers and body itself were viewed as pernicious. Lord Donaldson called W's desire for control a pathological symptom of her condition: 'One of the symptoms of anorexia nervosa is a desire by the sufferer to 'be in control', and such a refusal [of treatment] would be an obvious way of demonstrating this' (*Re W*, p. 631). This looks particularly odd compared to the C case (although the W judgement predates C). It seems quite likely that Mr C's refusal was a manifestation of his schizophrenic delusions – giving rise to his patho-logical distrust of the clinicians – even if it was also a desire held by other sufferers from vascular disease. Lord Donaldson argued that W's anorexia undermined her 'Gillick competence', the formu-lation laid down in an earlier case establishing that the test is ability to understand the nature and purpose of the proposed treatment. The test in the *Gillick* case (1985) was whether the child had 'sufficient understanding and intelligence to enable him or her to understand fully what is pro-posed' (*Gillick*, p. 423). None the less, Lord Donaldson, in the Court of Appeal, declared that this was not enough in W's case:

What distinguishes W . . . is that it is a feature of anorexia nervosa that it is capable of destroying the ability to make an informed choice. It creates a compulsion to refuse treatment or to accept only treatment which is likely to be ineffective. This attitude is part and parcel of the disease and the more advanced the illness, the more compelling it may become. Where the wishes of the minor are themselves something which the doctors rea-sonably consider to be treated in the minor's best inter-ests, those wishes clearly have a much reduced influence (Re W, p. 637).

W had broken unit rules at her current treatment centre with impunity, it was noted. A judgement in her favour would merely be another form of capitulation, reinforcing her sense that she, not the clinicians, was in control. Throughout the judgement the language of discipline, control and hierarchy is evident. Whereas the judge in C seems to regard Mr C as his equal, the judgements in W are given from a paternalistic position. Thus the W case reinforced the important principle in UK law that children and young people are pre-sumed incompetent to refuse treatment, although they may give consent. This is the limit to which their competence can extend.

ACTIVITY: Do you agree with the judgement in the W case? What would you have done?

It may well be that, in the particularly pressing circumstances of W's case, you would also have erred on the side of paternalism. This is an under-standable interpretation of professional respon-sibility in the context of a life-threatening emergency: W's weight was just over five stone at the time the judgement was given – although it is also worth pointing out that her weight only began to drop so radically when the court pro-ceedings began, having been stable at 7 stone before that.

You may also feel that it is perfectly reasonable to require a higher 'tariff' for refusal of consent than for acceptance of treatment. The conse-quences of treatment refusal, some argue, are generally more severe, because treatment would not be suggested unless it were of benefit (Buchanan and Brock, 1989). Against this, one might argue that this wrongly assumes the doctor's opinion about the probability of treat-ment succeeding is always correct (Devereux et al., 1993).

It may also depend on whether the proposed

treatment is life-saving. What happens when forcible treatment cannot be justified on the basis that it could save the patient's life? – as the court accepted in the W case. One such difficult example is electro-convulsive therapy without consent, in adolescents. We would now like you to read brief excerpts from an article by Melissa Oxlad and Steve Baldwin on 'ECT administration with children and adolescents: review of ethical considerations.' As you read, ask yourself whether the practices described by Oxlad and Baldwin are simply atypical and bad practice, or whether they are more representative than that. Have you encountered anything like this in your own practice?

ECT administration with children and adolescents: review of ethical considerations

Steve Baldwin and Melissa Oxlad

Internationally, the administration of ECT to children and adolescents remains an area of unresolved controversy in contemporary psychiatry. ECT proponents have advocated no distinctions between the client group of children/adolescents and adults; minors have been viewed as merely another clinical sub-grouping, for whom benefits after ECT are believed to occur. Detractors have attempted to proscribe all ECT administration with minors, on clinical, moral, ethical, legal and philosophical grounds.

In the UK and Channel Islands, children and adolescents have been given ECT as a psychiatric intervention for a range of clinical problems. These have included: mood disorder, thought disorder, eating disorder and other more specific clinical conditions such as Tourette's syndrome and learning disability (Jones and Baldwin, 1992). A 1993 survey of UK child psychiatry services by the Royal College of Psychiatrists produced more than 60 cases where ECT was administered to children/adolescents during the 1980s. However the survey was restricted to data obtained via questionnaires from a small sub-sample of statutory health services, and therefore true prevalence rates were underestimated. Documented rates based on multiple case sampling of 217 instances from the USA, UK and Europe have been reported in a previous publication (Baldwin and Oxlad, 1996). Accurate prevalence rates of ECT administration in the USA and UK have been difficult to determine.

Elsewhere in Europe, the true prevalence of ECT administration with minors is unknown. In France, administration rates traditionally have been low, with a traditional focus in both psychiatry and psychology services on psychoanalytic perspectives. Similarly in Germany, although reliable data are presently unavailable, prevalence rates are believed to be low, due to restrictions on clinical freedoms since psychiatric legislation reforms. Likewise, in the Netherlands, ECT administration even with adults is uncommon in the 1990s. Due to protective mental health legislation, ECT with minors is virtually unknown.

Throughout Italy, since the mental health service reforms of psychiatria democratica, ECT administration with adults has declined in popularity. With a contemporary focus on psychosocial interventions, ECT with children is unknown. Recent public scandals in Romania (i.e. during the Ceaucescu regime) and Greece (e.g. Leros) have revealed the extensive use of physical treatments such as ECT and pharmacotherapy with minors in psychiatric services. Despite considerable efforts, however, accurate and complete data sets have been impossible to obtain. Since the internal reforms in the former Soviet Union, conditions in psychiatric services are reported to have improved; the appalling record of human rights in Russia seems to have been partly reversed. Throughout Scandinavia, use of ECT with children and adolescents is almost unknown, due to a primary focus on psychosocial interventions, mental health legislation reforms, and a strong user/consumer voice in advocacy services.

Informed consent for children and adolescents who have been given ECT is a complex ethical theme. According to Cook and Scott (1992) the

American Psychiatric Association (APA) has not yet agreed upon appropriate consent procedures; these authors also have reported that more extensive research on the use, possible benefits and effects of ECT on children and adolescents is needed. The APA (1990) has, however recommended: 'that ECT should never be used as a primary treatment for children and adolescents'.

In a review of ECT with minors, Bertagnoli and Borchardt (1990) also stated that there has been scant ethical discussion about 'consent' for children and adolescents. These authors suggested that it is 'probably appropriate' for parents to provide consent for pre-adolescent children, but asserted that the issue of adolescent consent was more complicated. Bertagnoli and Borchardt (1990) recommended that consent should be given both by the adolescent and their parents.

ACTIVITY: Stop here for a moment and consider whether the legal case, *Re W* would justify giving ECT to a young person on the sole consent of someone with parental responsibility. In what circumstances, if any, do you think that ECT is justifiable for minors? Would you require the young person's consent? Make an informal protocol for your own practice in relation to ECT, other invasive psychiatric therapies (e.g. psychosurgery), and drug prescription. Then compare your own protocol with that given by Carlo Calzone, an Italian child psychiatrist, in your final reading of this section.

Drug treatment in child psychiatry

Carlo Calzone

Psychopharmacotherapy in childhood and adolescence raises three types of ethical issue:
(a) The lack of certainty on the outcome of treatment as concerning risks and benefits
(b) The relationship between psychoactive drugs and personal freedom
(c) The rights of non-autonomous patients

(a) The lack of certainty on the outcome of treatment is related to the following aspects:
(i) We cannot transfer onto children the results of experiments on adults because of the uncertain response to drugs of an immature central nervous system. The paradoxical effects of many drugs on this age group, e.g. stimulants and benzodiazepine, are well known.
(ii) With under-age subjects, experimental protocols need to be more stringent. In Italy, for example, drugs and placebos cannot be compared and this obviously limits research.
(iii) Individual variance, a well-known phenomenon in pharmacology, is much higher in children and adolescents because of interfering development processes and of the social–psychic context in which they take place.
(iv) In developing subjects, untoward effects, also long-term ones, can be especially unpredictable and serious (e.g. late dyskinesia caused by antipsychotic drugs).
(b) The use of psychoactive drugs can be seen as a limitation to personal freedom because:
(i) Some drugs, such as benzodiazepine or SSRI, can induce addiction.
(ii) Pharmacotherapy actually changes the patient's personality. Think, for example, of the changes that can be induced by drugs in manic-depressive or schizophrenic patients.
(iii) The elimination of symptoms, albeit accepted as socially useful, can be felt by the patient as a loss. In this sense, I would like to mention the case described by Oliver Sacks of the patient with Tourette's syndrome, who discontinued his therapy with haloperidol in non-working days, because he wanted to revert to his own 'Tourette personality'.
(c) The lack of autonomy in under-age patients can be ascribed to various factors, such as:
(i) Physical and cognitive limits
(ii) Emotional dependence on adult figures
(iii) Economic dependence
(d) Legal limitations, varying from one country to the other, such as the age of majority or the concept of liability of adolescents

These three factors are not independent and start a vicious circle that discourages many clinicians from prescribing psychoactive drugs in childhood and adolescence. A careful work methodology and an ethical evaluation of each case can help child psychiatrists in the choice of using drugs according to the principle of benefits accruing to the young patient.

The following vignettes illustrate two opposite cases of damage to the child because of opposition to drug treatment and damage due to a careless prescription.

VIGNETTE 1 (AM, AGED 11)

Family and school referred AM to a psychiatrist requesting drug therapy for unstable and aggressive behaviour. When she was 5, AM was diagnosed with psychotic-type personality disorder with dissociative manifestations and obsessive rituals. Since 6 years of age she has been undergoing psychoanalytical therapy. Her therapist always refused drugs because she fears they can interfere with therapy. Given the worsening of symptoms, the child's family decided on a new consultation in view of a drug therapy. After a few interviews neuroleptic drugs were prescribed along with continuation of psychotherapy. After one year, AM showed improvement in behaviour and school performance. It is unfortunately impossible to evaluate possible long-term untoward effects.

VIGNETTE 2 (S, AGED 15)

When 5 years old, S was seen for delayed psychomotor and language development. On this occasion, evidence was found of physical abuse by his mother. The mother decided to undergo psychiatric treatment, but discontinued care for her son. Later the parental couple divorced and S now lives with his father and younger sister, but sees his mother every day. After having completed grammar school, his father took S to see a child psychiatrist. The boy shows mild cognitive retardation, behavioural inhibition with serious impairment of social competence, night enuresis and occasional encopresis. He

had been taking neuroleptics and carabamazepine for two years, prescribed by his mother's neurologist. After the original prescription, no control or examination followed. The psychiatric team diagnosed Munchausen syndrome and suggested support psychotherapy, social activity and discontinuation of drugs.

Below is a suggested protocol which may help to avoid the extremes of both these cases.

The path of drug prescription

Clinical approach	Complete psychiatric evaluation of child and family
	Clinical interviews
	Psychological tests
	Behaviour observation
	Medical tests
Diagnosis	According to DSM IV or ICD 10
	Psychodynamic or structural diagnosis
Choice of drug	Negative
	Symptomatic
	Aetiological
Agreed treatment plan	
Parents' and patient's informed consent	Discussion on: nature of complaint
	Nature and duration of treatment
	Risks/benefits
	Therapeutic alternatives
	Prognosis with or without treatment
Progressive dosage increase	Physical examination
	Standard laboratory tests
	Specific tests
	Clinical observation
	Scoring (Connors, AIMS, etc.)
	Low initial dosage
	Progressive increase
	Maintenance dosage
Initial controls	Evaluate: compliance
	Untoward effects
	Benefits
	Perform blood tests
	Clinical observation
	Scoring (Connors, AIMS, etc.)

The path of drug prescription (*cont.*)

Periodic controls   Every 6 months check possible
                        discontinuation of drug
                       Evaluate: compliance
                       Untoward effects
                       Benefits
                       Perform blood tests
                       Clinical observation
                       Scoring (Connors, AIMS, etc.)

It is however advisable to observe the following general indications:

- Evaluate a possible drug treatment as support for each patient, recording reasons of choice.
- Do not use a drug as last resort after failure of other treatment plans.
- Use a limited number of well-known drugs and systematically collect data on cases.
- Choose whenever possible a single therapy rather than a multiple therapy in order to control positive and negative effects of each drug.
- Always use better-known drugs as first choice.
- Read and analyse carefully manufacturers' instructions on commercial prescriptions.
- Always obtain the parents' informed consent, to be kept with other records, since very often authorised therapeutic indications do not allow many drugs to be used on children (for Italy see Law n. 161 of March 25, 1996, Urgent provisions concerning experimenting and use of drugs, *Official Gazette* n. 73 of March 27, 1996).
- The preceding path solves some of the problems related to the therapist's discretion in drug treatment in favour of the young patient, but it leaves some important questions that I would like everyone to reflect upon:
- What specific limitations should be observed for experiments on under-age children?
- Can information provided by mass media direct patients' and clinicians' choices on these issues?
- How can better informed consent be assured?

ACTIVITY: Before moving on to the next section take a few moments to make a list of the key points raised in this section.

Section 5: A different voice in psychiatric ethics

Until now in this chapter, we have contrasted two approaches to psychiatric ethics: the rights-based view and the paternalistic model. It is probably fair to say that the analysis so far has tended to be critical of medical paternalism, particularly in the UK, and more supportive of the patient's rights approach, as exemplified in recent Dutch legislation. However, we have also focused on the limitations of that approach, for example in Berghmans's critique. But you may still be left with the feeling that although analysing the differences between the models helps to clarify your thinking, the two approaches impose an artificial straitjacket on actual clinical practice. Is there room for another approach?

The chapter has also concentrated on legal cases, which provide a good basis for contrasting analyses and which have direct parallels in clinical practice. However, it might be argued that we have not talked very much about ethical theory, beyond the principles of beneficence and autonomy (with a brief mention of justice in relation to Mordini's argument that Italian law rejects preventive detention as unfair discrimination against the mentally ill). In this final section we provide a more extended, exploratory discussion of ethical theory, in an article written by a practising clinician, a forensic psychiatrist with a particular interest in medical ethics and ethical theory: Dr Gwen Adshead, consultant psychiatrist at Broadmoor Hospital and the author of the following extract, 'A different voice in psychiatric ethics'. In the article Adshead argues for what has come to be known as an ethics of care approach. (Autonomy, and alternative models to it in new theories such as this, are considered at greater length in the 'Autonomy' chapter.)

The idea that it is possible to build an approach to biomedical ethics around the concept of care is one which has become increasingly popular particularly among nurse and theorists of nursing, as well as among some feminist bioethicists. But just what is meant by the ethics of care? Before you go on to read the paper by Gwen Adshead, we would like you to read the following extract from a paper by Peter Allmark (1995) in which he provides an outline of this approach.

Amongst nurse theorists the idea of an ethics of caring is especially popular. Nursing has long sought to gain an identity separate from medicine and some writers hope that care may be the key to finding this identity. Caring has roots in the work of Carol Gilligan (Gilligan, 1982). The key idea is that the detached, impartial observer ideal of morality, characteristic of ethics since the enlightenment, is flawed and inappropriate, particularly for women. In its place is recommended an approach stressing involvement in the situation, with an attitude of care for others also involved. As such, the importance of relations between people in their practical reasoning is highlighted rather than the more common approach stressing abstract principles.

. . . Blum (1988) lists what he sees as some of the differences between 'impartialism' and the ethics of care. (a) The care approach is particularized. It does not abstract from the particular situation and attempt to see, for example, which principles are operative, or what is the ethical framework. Gilligan and Noddings (Noddings, 1984) have both criticized Gandhi for his 'blind willingness to sacrifice people to truth', that is, some form of abstract truth. (b) The care approach is involved. It does not see the person making moral decisions as a radically autonomous self-legislating individual. Rather she is tied to others. Autonomy is not seen as some kind of ideal. Involvement with the person on whom one acts draws on capacities of love, care, empathy, comparison and sensitivity. This dimension of moral understanding is ignored by the 'impartialist' approach. (c) For the care approach, moral reasoning does not involve rationality alone but an intertwining of emotion, cognition and action. Noddings quotes Hume with approval. It seems that for both, 'Reason is, and ought only to be the slave of the passions'. (d) The care approach is not concerned with universalistic right action. Gilligan talked instead of situationally based responses based on the 'cognisance of interdependence'.

ACTIVITY: Bearing this description in mind, we would now like you to go on and read the paper by Adshead, listing as you do so the features of this approach which you consider to be its strengths and those which are weaknesses.

A different voice in psychiatric ethics

Gwen Adshead

Introduction

In this section, I will argue that the perspective of an ethic of care is of particular relevance to psychiatric treatment, where therapeutic relationships are themselves the vehicle of treatment. The limitations of a rights-based, or justice-based vision alone, will also be discussed.

Different voices in bioethics

There are multiple theories of ethical reasoning in healthcare, including those based on interpersonal relating (Beauchamp and Childress, 1994). In relation to psychiatry, the dominant discourse has been one of an ethic of justice/rights, with considerable debate about the rights of vulnerable people to treatment, to be protected from coercion, and competing rights of public safety and personal freedom (Fulford & Hope, 1994).

Within psychiatric ethics, concern for rights and justice must be important because patients are made vulnerable by their mental illness, and are also vulnerable to abuse by others. Using case examples, I will suggest that ethical debates in psychiatry which focus solely on conflicts between two principles, and set up ethical dichotomies (e.g. respect for beneficence or respect for autonomy) cannot address the complexity of the lives of individuals, and the relationships in which they are embedded, both in the past and in the present. A rights/principles account that does not consider the patient within a matrix of relationships runs a risk of over-simplifying the patient's autonomy, and thus not doing justice (an appropriate word) to the complexity of the dilemma for this person.

THE CASE OF MISS A

Miss A suffered from borderline personality disorder. In childhood, she had experienced prolonged and extensive sexual abuse by her father. As a result, she suffered from depression, and intermittent feelings of loathing towards her own body which resulted in acts of deliberate self-harm and episodes of self-starvation. She was admitted to a psychiatric hospital and over a long period of time developed a reasonable relationship with her male psychiatrist, who was concerned for her welfare.

During one admission (after a period of years), Miss A's weight began to drop so dramatically that her doctor threatened to force-feed her in order to save her life. She went to court to get an injunction to prevent him from doing so. The dilemma here for both the patient and the doctor is obvious. Respecting her autonomy may result in her acting so riskily to herself that she suffers harm, and dies.

It may be relevant when contemplating this dilemma to consider how force-feeding is a symbolic re-enactment of the original abuse (she was subjected to forced fellatio over a period of time). The experience of child abuse frequently leaves individuals with real concerns about the extent to which they are in control of their own bodies even if retaining control incurs risk.

A relevant issue is that of Miss A's self-concept, i.e. her attitudes of herself towards herself (Attanucci, 1988). Her own ambivalence about herself ('I don't matter . . . I do matter') was mirrored in the attitudes of staff, who alternatively saw her as incompetent to care for herself, and needing to be force-fed; or as manipulative and trying to bully them. This mirroring also replicated the relationship between herself and her parents. Legal argument focused on her competence to make decisions and refuse help (but that will not be examined here).

On a rights/principles perspective, or even a utilitarian analysis, there is a tension between Miss A's view of what was right for her, and the staff's view. A broader view of her welfare, which included thinking about her past, and present relationships with caretakers, might understand the dilemma as part of the concern that abused adults have about their control over their own bodies. By supporting her at these times when she was at her most self-destructive, it might be more possible to understand her self-destruction (and thus her ethical conflict with staff) as a response to her own previous experiences of abuse. Time could also be offered to staff to explore their feelings about Miss A, which might help to reduce the tension between them, and help them to feel less threatened by Miss A's expression of autonomy.

THE CASE OF MISS B

Miss B seeks psychotherapy for depression. She recalls, in her therapy, a history of abuse and neglect especially from her mother, with whom she is still in contact. Miss B becomes very dependent on her therapist, who responds warmly and empathetically. At Miss B's request, the therapy sessions become more frequent, and take place outside the clinic, because 'it feels too impersonal and frightening there'.

Miss B and the therapist become closer, and one day during one stormy session, the therapist offers physical comfort in the form of a hug; which turns into an embrace. Miss B and her therapist become lovers; the therapy sessions continue. The therapist becomes anxious at the turn of events have taken, and abruptly terminates therapy. Miss B takes an overdose and threatens to kill her therapist. In such a case, the relationship between the therapist and the patient is crucial to an understanding of how an ethical principle (that of not exploiting a patient) was violated. The principles approach would argue that the principles of beneficence and non-maleficence were breached. The therapist might counter with the argument that she did as the patient wished by ending the therapy sessions, by responding to the embrace and that the patient consented to become sexually involved with her. To this it might be counter-argued that Miss B was not competent to exercise her autonomy to make that kind of decision. One might also argue that Miss B was harmed by the therapist's failure to maintain boundaries, even though she had requested that they be breached; and Miss B is also wronged because she is treated as a means to the therapist's pleasure.

What is then set up is a conflict between the therapist's understanding of Miss B's autonomy, and her vision of professional beneficence. Miss B's own view is in danger of being lost, and is to some extent replaced by the therapists' own view of what has been going on. The relationship between them has changed, and with it, the therapeutic perspective which is part of the duty of care. There seems to be no way out of the dilemma, except to conclude that there should be an absolute bar to sexual contact between therapists and patients. However, the justification for such a conclusion may make more sense if a relational perspective is taken. Then we may try and understand how the therapist may have mistaken her personal feelings of wanting to respond to Miss B's neediness as a professional duty. The therapist may well be encouraged to ask herself why she feels the need to make reparation for past wrongs and whether, indeed, that is possible or even desirable. In this case, the therapist may not have taken seriously her own attachment to the patient, or the patient's to her.

A shift in the nature of the relationship, from professional to sexual, means that there is a shift in the management of power relationships within the therapeutic setting. The feelings of the therapist may complicate the feelings of the patient, and make it difficult for work to proceed. It arguably also gives the patient an extra problem to contend with; that of the therapist's feelings. Rather than justifying a ban on therapist-patient sexual contact from an absolutist position (as suggested by the Hippocratic Oath), a relational perspective, which includes attention to both duties of care and patient rights, can offer a more coherent justification for prohibiting therapist–patient sexual relationships.

Such a perspective may also offer a way forward in managing the aftermath of such an event. A professional response would be to look at the relationship between the two parties and reflect on the way the therapist is feeling; if not with the patient, then with a supervisor. In such cases it is common for the therapist to be quite aware that she is doing something 'wrong', but she could be unable to think about it. Thinking about how one 'should' behave in the context of an ongoing connection is the very substance of a notion of the duty of care.

Autonomy and relationship

One of the limitations of a rights-based or a principles approach rests on the definition of autonomy. Rights-based accounts of autonomy provide a rather static atomistic picture of autonomy which allows little flexibility and disallows the importance of connections between persons (Christman, 1988). What is needed is a more complex notion of autonomy within a relationship; a synthesis and dynamic of independence in in-dependence. The reality is that most of us, but especially those who are made vulnerable by physical or mental disability, actually need connections with others in order to act freely. The case of Mr C demonstrates the impact of physical disability on psychological autonomy, and also the importance of family relationships when making assessments of harms and benefits.

THE CASE OF MR C

A 21-year-old young man was maimed by a truck at the age of 10, leaving him disabled. His persisting disability provides a caring role for his mother. He allows his mother to do things for him which he is capable of doing; he is also ambivalent about going out, expressing concerns about others' response to his disability. His mother supports him in his reluctance, and suggests that it is too difficult for him to go out. Attempts to increase his opportunities for socialization (money for taxis, identification of peer groups) are met with verbal aggression by his mother, and benign sabotage on the part of the patient. The young man's family appears to be connected together by his disability so that attempts to rehabilitate him out of the house, which would indeed do him 'some good', seem to cause distress within the family system. Active interventions to motivate him may actually do him harm, in the sense that they disarrange a complex family dynamic.

Changing that family dynamic requires a subtle assessment of harms and benefits, and an understanding of the relationships between all members of the family. A less subtle analysis of harms and benefits, which focused on only the young man's physical context, and not his emotional one may lead to difficulties, and clinical failure. Such failures are not uncommon, particularly in the area of psychiatric care in the community; and may reflect the lack of training which clinicians receive; both about the scope and nature of their ethical duties, and the nature of relationships between people (Carse, 1991).

Discussion: psychiatry and relationships

There are many types of healthcare relationships within medicine, and not all are equivalent in terms of time, mutuality and complexity. Relationships characterized by brief discrete episodes, where the patient's independence or self-esteem is not threatened, are arguably different from those where the condition is life-long, wide-ranging in terms of effects and causes substantial disability. In this situation, the patient forms a complex system of relationships with all his carers, including healthcare professionals (Agich, 1990). Feelings arise on both sides of these relationships, which affect the perceptions of responsibilities and are an important aspect of any empathic connection between carers and patients.

Such a broader contextual vision of psychiatric illness addresses the impact of the illness on a patient's relationship, both towards himself and with his carers. The patient's self is understood as construed in terms of relationships with others, with knock-on effects for understanding his capacity for agency, and the exercise of autonomy. Sutton (1997) describes the ethical difficulties presented by adolescent patients with mental health problems, whose autonomy is not only interconnected but also developing. Understanding the self in the context of dependent relationships allows for a dimensional understanding of the capacity

for agency in psychiatric patients; from those whose capacity is more limited by psychotic or dementing illnesses, to those whose capacity is less limited by neurotic disorders.

It is perhaps in the field of neurotic disorders that the issue of relationships becomes more prominent. Healthy relationships appear to be important for normal adult mental health, insofar as they may protect against mental illness (Mullen, 1990). People suffering from neurotic depression or anxiety (such as Miss B) frequently describe failures in relationships as their presenting problem. Both depression and anxiety encourage people to withdraw from relationships, which increases a sense of isolation and anxiety.

The importance of relationships is even clearer in relation to the so-called 'personality disorders' (such as Miss A's). The conceptual status of these disorders has long been debated; particularly whether they can be considered 'illnesses'. What is clear is that their essential feature lies in an inability to make and sustain relationships. For example, a significant feature of antisocial personality disorder is an increased capacity to be detached from other people and the lack of empathy in connection with others (American Psychiatric Association, 1994). One of the defining criteria of 'borderline personality disorder' is instability of relationships, which are characterized by intense positive attachments followed by quick rejections and fluctuating attachments (American Psychiatric Association, 1994).

Therefore therapeutic relationships within psychiatry have a number of significant features. Firstly, the patient and their psychiatrist (and/or GP) are likely to be involved in a developing relationship over time, where the psychiatrist has to manage the patient's dependence, while facilitating his independence. Secondly, the illness itself may have profound influence on the relationships that the patient forms; with his doctor, and with his other carers, and those important to him. Thirdly, the ability to make relationships may be affected by the illness.

Lastly, the contribution of the psychiatrist is just as important to the relationship as any other aspect of treatment. This is particularly true in the context of those specifically psychotherapeutic relationships, where there is a high degree of dependence on the therapist which is developed by a regular consistent meeting over a long period of time. The psychiatrist contributes either by a direct impact on the patient, so that changes in the psychiatrist given can actually have an effect upon mental health of the patients (Persaud and Meus, 1994); or indirectly by the effect of her feelings on therapeutic decision-making.

The inequality which is a traditional feature of the doctor–patient relationship may be in some circumstances analogous to the inequality of power and knowledge in parent-child relationships. The therapeutic relationship can also be said to echo two aspects of effective parenting; namely care and containment of distress. A supportive approach by psychiatrists to decision-making by the dependent patient will (hopefully) be different from usurpation of judgement, or strong paternalism. Present-day ethical dilemmas may reflect difficulties in past relationships with parents, who may not have been able to let the patient be themselves. A failure to appreciate this may mean that important emotional influences are left out of the ethical reasoning process.

Conclusion: four principles and psychiatric relationships

The three cases outlined above (drawn from real cases, but not based on any individual patient) show the complexity of relationships that have to be considered in the management of ethical dilemmas that affect psychiatric patients. Miss A's case highlights how an ethical dilemma may be understood in terms of the relationships between a patient and the multidisciplinary team. Miss B's case shows how the relationship with an individual therapist can become complex over time, and thus generate ethical tensions which were not there at the start of treatment. Mr C's case demonstrates how difficult it can be to delineate harms and benefits in the case of patients who are chronically dependent on others; and where their

interests may have a direct bearing on the interests of the patient.

> **ACTIVITY: Here is a comment about this paper by one of our critical readers, Win Tadd. As you read it think about whether you agree with the point being made and about how Adshead might respond.**

I'm not sure what Adshead is claiming in the case of C. I assume her to be arguing that simply to focus on C's 'dependence' or his 'lack of autonomy' when considering his case, as she claims the principlist approach requires of us, would be to overlook many other important ethical considerations. In relation to this case I think that Gerald Dworkin's (1988) account of autonomy would avoid many of her concerns. He argues for example that any theory of autonomy should not 'imply a logical incompatibility with other significant values' and therefore, 'the autonomous person [should] not be ruled out on conceptual grounds, from manifesting other virtues or acting justly'. In C's case it might be the case that he truly values and understands his mother's need to feel 'needed' and therefore, as a consequence, 'autonomously' decides to allow himself to be dependent upon her (W. Tadd, 1999, personal communication).

> **Now continue with your reading of Adshead.**

'Bare' principlism, which addresses ethical dilemmas in psychiatry only in terms of competing principles (such as beneficence vs. autonomy) may not do justice to the complexity of the relationships and feelings that may be involved between the psychiatrist and the patient, and between the patient and his family. Too strong an emphasis on competing principles may cause clinicians caught up in ethical dilemmas to ignore important relationships in the patient's life, which are ethically significant (Jinnet-Sack, 1993).

The issue of respect for justice also needs careful consideration in relation to psychiatric patients. Real concerns about the abuse for psychiatric patients led to an undoubtedly valuable trend towards de-institutionalization and an emphasis on individual human rights. Nevertheless, the lack of services, care and the presence of stigma in the community has meant that patients could sometimes be abandoned with their autonomy respected; 'dying with their rights on'. Such outcomes seem to suggest an understanding of justice as having an 'all or nothing' quality. It also seeks justice in an adversarial form, where A is pitted against B. In cases where A is a dependent member of the same society as B and where A and B are not as different as they may seem, then a more complex analysis is needed.

Principles theory needs to be supplemented, developed and enriched by other perspectives, including the ethic of care (Pellegrino, 1994; Robertson, 1996). This would appear to be particularly true in the practice of psychiatry and psychotherapy. This approach is also likely to have *some value in other settings where patients suffer from long-term disabilities, and where relationships with others are both a significant part of their problem, and part of the approach to treatment.*

ACTIVITY: What do you consider to be the strengths and weaknesses of an approach based on the ethics of care? In his paper in the *Journal of Medical Ethics*, Peter Allmark argues that the concept of care used in this context is hopelessly vague because it lacks either normative or descriptive content. By this he means that it does not enable us to make a distinction between times when we are caring for the right things or the wrong things and it cannot tell us whether we are expressing our care in the right way. In short, he argues that 'care' is used by ethics of care theorists as if it is always and inevitably a good thing. This, he argues, is to leave the concept seriously under-examined. Do you agree with this? If so, why? How does this criticism bear on Adshead's article?

In order to consider this question and the relative strengths of this and the other approaches we have discussed in this chapter we would now like you to look at an extract of a report on this issue by the Danish Council of Ethics. As you read through it we would like you to consider just how far this rights-based approach is compatible with the ethics of care.

Rights and care in psychiatry: the Danish situation

In 1998, the Danish Council of Ethics produced a report on *Conditions for Psychiatric Patients*. In it they proposed, after much discussion, a set of rights for psychiatric patients. In summary the rights they proposed were as follows:

1. The right to good hospital standards

The Council of Ethics feels, in principle, that anyone admitted to a psychiatric ward should have the possibility of staying on a private ward. There should be no compulsion to place mentally disordered admissions on multiple-bed wards unless it reflects the patient's wishes or is in some other way deemed appropriate for the sake of the person concerned. The Council then, does not feel that the right to a private ward (as argued by the Kallehauge Committee below) . . . should be confined to cases where it can be said to be medically indicated.

In their report, the Council refer to the Kallehauge Committee who argued for five rights relating to good hospital conditions: (a) the right to stay on a private ward, where medically indicated; (b) the right to stay in modern structural conditions; (c) the right to a suitable offer of employment and teaching; (d) the right to at least one hour in the fresh air daily; and (e) the right to go out accompanied, as and when desired.

2. The right to differentiated offers of treatment

In principle the Council of Ethics considers it essential for safeguarding psychiatric patients' personal integrity and achieving the best possible relationship of trust between the psychiatric patient and the treatment system that the Psychiatry Act provide clarification and assurance that, as far as possible, treatment will consider the patient's own perceptions of his or her own symptoms, paying the greatest possible heed to the patient's own wishes with regard to choice of treatment forms. Only a tiny minority of patients are totally incapable of relating to their own condition and to what is happening to them.

3. The right to a continued stay on a psychiatric ward

As a working basis, the Council of Ethics feels that the hospital authority assumes special responsibility for the health and well-being of a mentally disordered person the instant that person is subjected to coercive measures. In the Council of Ethics' opinion, therefore, there is also a concomitant obligation to ensure that patients who have been subjected to coercion in connection with admission are not discharged until there is a reasonable likelihood of their being able to cope outside of the psychiatric ward. The Council of Ethics therefore feels that, for such patients, introducing a right of continued stay on the psychiatric ward should be considered until such time as they are deemed fit for discharge and the requisite extra-mural measures are in place.

4. Limits on the use of coercion

There is scarcely any way of avoiding the use of coercion on the mentally disordered in some cases. However, it must be maintained that using force is a serious intervention and every effort should therefore be made to try and restrict such measures wherever possible . . . The Council of Ethics therefore feels that restricting the use of coercion as far as possible must be upheld as a central and vitally important objective in organizing mental health treatment.

5. The right to a patient counsellor in cases of involuntary treatment

The Council of Ethics holds the view that, for the sake of patients' civil rights, a provision should be introduced whereby involuntary measures must be added to the ward's coercion records and trigger the right to a patient counsellor. Doing so would also enable these patients to complain about certain measures.

6. The right to complain and to appeal

The Council of Ethics feels that the right of appeal should be organized in such a way as to make it as easy and manageable as possible.

> **ACTIVITY:** For your final activity of this chapter we would like you to apply the Danish rights to the three cases described by Adshead. Do you get different outcomes? What does this mean for Win Tadd's claim that the rights based and the ethic of care are not necessarily incompatible.
>
> Before you move on to the next chapter, make a list of the key issues raised in this chapter.

Suggestions for further reading

Bloch, S. and Chodoff, P. (1993). *Psychiatric Ethics*, 2nd edn. Oxford: Oxford University Press.

Edwards, R. (1997). *Ethics of Psychiatry.* New York: Prometheus Books.

Fulford, K. W. M. and Dickenson, D. (2000). *In Two Minds: Case Studies in Psychiatric Ethics.* Oxford: Oxford University Press.

Holmes, J. and Lindley, R. (1991). *The Values of Psychotherapy.* Oxford: Oxford University Press.

7

Children and young people

Introduction

States parties shall assure to the child who is capable of forming his or her own views the right to express those views freely in all matters affecting the child, the view of the child being given due weight in accordance with the age and maturity of the child. . . . The child shall in particular have the opportunity to be heard in any judicial and administrative proceedings affecting the child, either directly or through a representative or an appropriate body, in a manner consistent with the procedural rules of national law. ((Article 12) UN Convention on the Rights of the Child (1989))

To whom does the childcare practitioner have responsibilities? Working with children and young people brings with it ethical responsibilities which may be different from those involved in work with adults. One answer to this question emphasizes the importance of listening to what children have to say. To a certain extent this child-centred approach can be said to reflect medicine's more general concern (particularly in northern Europe and the United States) with patient-centred care. It is commonly felt that practitioners ought to weigh up the value of a medical intervention solely in terms of the benefits and risks it is likely to have for the patient in front of them, in relation to that person's autonomy, and quite apart from the wishes of others such as the patient's family.

The patient-centred approach defines the relationship between the patient and the practitioner

as the arena of care and hence of moral concern. The moral agents in such cases are assumed to be the patient and the doctor or other healthcare practitioner. But this approach does not resolve all of the particular difficulties faced by practitioners in their work with children. For, even from the perspective of children's rights, it is often possible in such cases to ask oneself, 'Where do my responsibilities lie?' 'Who is the patient?' Is it the child, is it the child's family and parents, or is it some combination of these? Patient-centred care will have different meanings and different implications for practice in each of these cases.

Section 1: The child in the family

ACTIVITY: Before going on with the chapter, stop here for a moment and, in relation to your own experience, think about the practical and ethical implications of different possible answers to the questions raised above. What, for example, ought to happen in cases where there is or appears to be conflict between the practitioner's perception of the child's best interest and the parents' perception?

Please read the following case study from Austria and consider what ethical issues it raises about working with children and their families.

THE CASE OF PETER

Peter, aged 12, was admitted to hospital after a severe beating from his father; his mother had called the police. The events which led to Peter's hospitalization were only one chapter in a long history of physical abuse, stemming from the boy's inability to meet his father's demands for high grades and perfect behaviour. The immediate trigger to the beating, however, was Peter's theft of a wallet belonging to his school principal. In fact, Peter had been engaging in petty shoplifting and theft with a gang of other boys for some time.

The family were referred to a child psychiatry centre for therapy. Because the physical chastisement of children is illegal in Austria where Peter lives, Peter's father had little alternative but to comply; otherwise he might have faced a sentence of up to 3 years' imprisonment.

At the first family therapy session, he was subdued and submissive, as was Peter's mother, who felt guilty for having called the police. The parents were warned that their relationship with Peter might well become more openly conflictual during the course of psychotherapy, and reminded that their co-operation would not automatically preclude further action by the courts or social services. Nevertheless, they consented both to therapy for Peter and to parallel therapy sessions for themselves.

Peter was nervous about what therapy might entail, but co-operative. He was given an opportunity to explore his feelings about what he could achieve through psychotherapy and to say freely what he feared. A good initial therapeutic relationship was established between Peter and the psychotherapist; Peter stopped shoplifting, which the therapist had interpreted as an unconscious rejection of his father's demands, and began standing up to his father in a more positive manner.

ACTIVITY: In the account of Peter's case above, the therapist believes that he obtained informed consent for the therapy to continue. To what extent do you agree with this? Has consent really been obtained and if so, from whom? This inevitably relates to another question: to whom is the psychotherapist responsible in this case, and who is the patient?

When all is going well, it is easy to forget these questions because all interests seem to pull in the same direction. These issues become central, however, when things start to go badly. Then conflicts can arise between the various parties and the practitioner's responsibilities can seem to pull in different directions. Think for a moment about what kind of conflicts are possible in this kind of situation. Then go on to read what happened next in Peter's case, bearing these questions in mind.

THE CASE OF PETER (cont.)

Three months after therapy began, the family were informed by social services that no further action would be taken against them. Peter's father immediately stopped coming to therapy. His mother continued for a time, in a state of ambivalence; she complained that 'the family's peace' was being threatened. Eventually she, too, ceased attending.

Peter continued with his therapy, but now his father began demanding that the therapist should reveal the content of these sessions to him. The therapist refused, on grounds of patient confidentiality. Peter's mother tried to prevent him attending any further sessions. Finally, he stopped coming altogether.

Some weeks later Peter visited the therapist alone, during school hours. He said that his parents had flatly forbidden him any further contact, but he had come to say good-bye. Without a stable therapeutic alliance with the entire family, Peter's therapist did not feel any more could be done, although he encouraged Peter to call him whenever he needed help or support.

ACTIVITY: Do you think that the therapist has fulfilled his responsibilities to Peter? To Peter's father? To his mother? Should he perhaps have tried to build more on the independence which Peter had begun to develop? After all, Peter did show a good deal of independent-mindedness even in coming to say goodbye, when he had been forbidden any further contact at all. Has the therapist provided Peter with enough support for the future? Why was a stable therapeutic alliance with the entire family so important? Would it be equally important in other areas of medicine?

The quotation from the UN Convention at the start of this chapter suggests that listening to the child's voice ought to be central to work with children. But is the patient-centred approach a realistic or workable model in all work with children? Surely, to view the child solely as an individual is to exclude a large and important part of the child's world. It means leaving out those others who would seem to have a legitimate interest in the outcome of any intervention; such as the child's parents, siblings and other relatives. Whilst it is important to some extent for us to consider the child as an individual, being an individual is at most only part of what any of us are. We are also social beings defined by relationships and social interactions. The implication of this is that, in at least some cases, account will need to be taken of people other than simply the child and the healthcare practitioner.

To focus solely on the one-to-one relationship between practitioner and patient, in this case the child, is to ignore the fact that both patient and practitioner are inevitably part of wider social networks which are of crucial moral significance. In the case of children this often tends to mean their family and in particular their parents. There is usually a variety of interested parties in any case and surely these others ought to have their importance recognized. This is particularly the case with children and their families.

It should not be forgotten that the child's interest [tends to] depend upon his well-being within his family. In this regard children teach us wisdom. They often minimize the conflicts of opposition. . . . A child who is hurting does not easily submit to treatment, particularly if this hurts his parents! (Hattab, 1996).

Hattab seems to be arguing here that when considering ethical questions relating to working with a child, it is essential to be aware not only of the child herself, but also of the social context in

which she lives. A child may accept or refuse a particular medical intervention, but what will the effects of the intervention be upon the child's family or other social relationships? If it will be in the child's interests in the short term but will destroy the family in the longer term, is it in the overall interests of the young person? It is also important to remember that the child is often, but not always, a member of a family, and that parents or guardians have a special form of relationship with and responsibility for the child.

ACTIVITY: What do you think about this point? Is there something special about the child's social location as compared to the adult's? To argue both that decisions about the treatment of children must take into account their location in relationships and at the same time to argue, that in the case of adults, the important principle is the respect of their informed choices is to rely upon the existence of a morally significant difference between the two cases. What might this be? One way of responding to this is to claim that the distinction is one based on the different levels of competence of children and adults. What other arguments might there be? We shall be returning to the question of competence in Section 4 of this chapter. For the moment, however, we want to continue with our consideration of the role of the child's location in a family.

Hattab's idea that the child is always the child in the family raises important questions. One of these is once again the question of where the healthcare practitioner's responsibility lies in work with young people. Who is the practitioner treating, the child, her parents or the family as a whole?

Is it always the case that the preservation of the family unit is in the child's best interests? In the case of Peter, for example, the family unit was preserved. Do you think that Peter's best interests were served in this case? If not, what are the ethical implications of treating him differently? Can you imagine circumstances in which a child ought to be treated without his or her parents' consent?

What do you see as the risks of seeing children as part of a family? Why might it be important to focus on the needs and wishes of the child as an individual rather than as a family member?

Hattab suggests that, in practice, children often place the stability of their family above their own immediate well-being. Can you think of any reasons why this might be? Peter's case seems to illustrate Hattab's point. He tries to lessen the conflict within his family.

In this case Peter himself wanted treatment but his parents did not. Below is another case, that of Sean, in which conflict is also a feature of the relationship between the parents and the child but in quite the opposite direction. Please read the case and consider the ethical questions raised by this kind of conflict.

THE CASE OF SEAN

Sean is 15 years old. He lives at home with his parents and a sister who is 12. His father is a senior civil servant and his mother is a healthcare professional. They live in a small town in an affluent part of Ireland.

When Sean's father first made contact with the therapist, he said that he was looking for help for his son because the boy seemed to have a 'chip on his shoulder' and was always in trouble. He said that he had persuaded Sean to see someone. They arrived together for the first session but Sean was seen on his own.

Sean was anxious and uncomfortable, uncertain why he was there. He felt that he was being blamed for the tension that existed between his parents. It seemed that there had always been conflict between father and son; when Sean was younger, he was frequently beaten for what he saw as minor misdemeanours. He said that his father would hit first and possibly listen later. Sean felt that he could not rely on his mother to protect him from his father's anger. Sean had harboured fantasies for at least the last 6 years of 'getting his own back' by beating his father. He also constantly talked about wanting to be away from home.

Sean says that he has always felt that he is not good enough, that he has not achieved enough

and is a disappointment to his parents. The transition from junior to senior school was a difficult one for Sean. In the senior school he associated with the boys in his class who smoked and took time off school. He felt that one teacher in particular was against him, because he constantly reprimanded and punished Sean for being cheeky. Two years ago there was a disagreement between Sean and the teacher during which Sean hit the teacher. Sean was then expelled from school.

His parents were very angry with him and immediately sent him away to boarding school. Sean was very distressed and refused to go but he was forcibly taken to the school and left there. In the first few weeks he was bullied by the other boys and ran away. He was apprehended by the police and returned to school where he continued to be subjected to frequent beatings. A little later he ran away again and managed to avoid being found by hiding in a derelict building. He then returned home, where he was surprised by his parents' acceptance that he did not want to return to the boarding school. Instead, he was to attend as a day boy at a school nearby. Since then there had been no further conflict at the school he does attend.

Disagreements continue at home, however. Sean feels that his parents, his father in particular, are constantly spying on him. He is never allowed to be in the house on his own. Sometimes he is allowed to go out with his friends, but sometimes this is refused. He has continued to get into fights with other youths in the town and on one recent occasion was seriously assaulted. He feels bitter that his father did not find the youth and beat him up. He is nervous when he goes into town and recently has started to drink very large amounts of alcohol. This has caused more arguments at home, but Sean feels that his father has been hypocritical because he also drinks heavily on occasion.

Sean is confused about why he should need to see a therapist. He feels that his father is the cause of all his problems and is trying to offload the blame onto him. Sean's father wants his son to settle down to work at school so that he can go to university. He feels frustrated and angry about his son's behaviour and hopes that a few sessions with the therapist will 'sort him out'.

> **ACTIVITY: What do you think the therapist should do in Sean's case? In the light of the case study itself and your own experience consider the following questions.**
> (a) **What do you think are the practitioner's duties and responsibilities in cases such as the one above? Clearly, Sean doesn't want to be in therapy, though it might be said that he does appear to have a reasonably good understanding of why he is there. If you were the practitioner in this case, where would you see your responsibilities?**
> (b) **If the best interests of the child are to be identified with remaining in the family, does this mean that the practitioner ought to follow the wishes of parents, even when the young person does not request or accept treatment? Think of any cases from your own experience for a moment. Where would you as a practitioner place your responsibilities?**
> (c) **Is it in fact always the case that the cohesion of the family is best obtained by respecting the wishes of the parents? Is it possible that, by respecting parents' wishes, a practitioner may not achieve it? Can you imagine a situation in which this might be the case?**

The cases of Peter and Sean demonstrate how hard it is to say just where the practitioner's responsibilities lie when the child's voice collides with parents' preferences. In such cases we might want to say that the real responsibility is to act according to the best interests of the child or young person. 'Best interests' seems to be a middle position between uncritically accepting the 'child's voice', on the one hand, and equally uncritically, assuming that the child is always best served by respecting the parents' wishes, in the interests of family unity.

Now read the following two statements.

The interest of the child, a consideration which appears in the Conventions and in other international instru-

ments drawn up during the last 40 years, is more than just a recurring theme, it is a true fundamental and universally shared idea (Magno, 1996).

In all actions concerning children whether undertaken by public or private social welfare institutions . . . the best interests of the child shall be a primary consideration' (Article 3) UN Convention on the Rights of the Child.

> **ACTIVITY: What does the idea of the best interests of the child mean? The idea is framed in the UN Convention and in the national laws of many countries, but what does it mean in practice? In some ways these two statements might be seen to be on the same side of the fence, but in themselves and in the light of our consideration of the questions raised by Sean's and Peter's cases, they appear too simplistic.**
>
> The cases we have considered above exemplify the ways in which our sense of our responsibilities as practitioner to children and to their families or guardians might pull in opposite directions. But might we not also be pulled in other directions by other responsibilities such as those we have to other practitioners or to the law?
>
> Take a moment to consider the various other responsibilities which might impinge upon the work of a practitioner in relation to children and young people.

For example, in England and Wales the paramount principle in deciding all questions about the child's upbringing, including health decisions, is the *child's welfare*. This is a form of the 'best interests' principle. The other two principles, the *child's voice* and *family cohesion*, are considered to be relevant to the child's welfare, but may be overridden.

In the Children Act 1989, 'welfare' is not explicitly defined, but courts are directed to apply a 'welfare checklist' of relevant factors. The 'ascertainable wishes and feelings' of the child – expressions of the child's voice – are one factor, and in fact they come first on the list (s1[3][a]). But the checklist also directs health and social care practitioners to consider the child's physical, emotional and educational needs; the likely effects of changes in circumstances (which would presumably include any changes undermining family unity); harm which the child has suffered or is at risk of suffering; the child's age, sex and background. Another factor in the checklist also allows family unity to be overridden if that is in the child's best interests: 'how capable each of his parents . . . is of meeting his needs'.

So the Children Act, the most all-embracing legislation on Children in England and Wales, tells practitioners that their main responsibility is to uphold the child's best interests. But what sort of guidance does this provide in difficult clinical decisions? In the next section we will look at this question in greater detail.

> **ACTIVITY:** Before moving on to the next section, take a few moments to note down the key points raised in this section.

Section 2: Consent to treatment and the child's best interests

In Section 1 we looked at three possible interpretations of the practitioner's principal responsibility:

- to listen to the 'child's voice',
- to maintain 'family unity', or
- to think first and foremost of the child's 'best interests'.

The example of Sean in the previous section showed some of the difficulties in knowing what is in the child's best interests when his assessment of his or her own welfare conflicts with that of his parents. In addition, there is the physician's own assessment of the child's best interests to consider. Perhaps the doctor disagrees with both the parents and the child; perhaps he or she agrees with one parent more than the other. In Peter's

case, for example, there were some indications that the mother had a less rigid view of what was in Peter's best interests than the father, who was particularly strict; but when 'push came to shove', her willingness to accept the therapist's view of Peter's best interests took second place to her strong desire for family cohesion.

It is, perhaps, possible to argue that the crucial question here is not so much 'what treatment is in the child's best interests?' but 'who decides what treatment is in the child's best interests?' A related question is this: who has the ultimate power to give or withhold consent to treatment?

> **ACTIVITY:** Please read the following case study. As you read, ask yourself these questions:
> (a) How does this case compare with Peter's?
> (b) What conflicting interpretations of the child's best interests are illustrated by this case? Who has the ultimate power to give or withhold consent, based on their interpretation of the child's best interests?
> (c) How does the child psychiatrist in this case interpret his responsibilities?

THE CASE OF EMILIA

Emilia, aged 4, had been brought to a child psychiatrist because she had regressed in her behaviour and speech. Since her parents separated, on the grounds of the husband's alleged physical violence against his wife, Emilia had been living with her mother. However, she had seen her father on regular access visits.

Clinical examination of Emilia revealed high risks of psychopathological disorders, but no current identifiable pathology. Emilia's mother was concerned that the child's condition was worsening, and she attributed the child's problems to stress induced by fear of her violent father. She asked the psychiatrist to support her application for a court order discontinuing the father's access visits. The psychiatrist refused, stating that 'It is part of the therapy to side with the child rather than with either parent.'

After an initial period during which Emilia regularly attended therapy sessions, with reasonably good results, the mother renewed her request to the psychiatrist for an expert opinion to back up her court application. The psychiatrist again refused. There was no overt confrontation, but the mother stopped taking Emilia to the therapy sessions.

There are interesting parallels between Emilia's case and Peter's: in both cases, parents refuse consent to treatment on behalf of a child – although, of course, Emilia is much younger, so that the 'child's voice' is perhaps less relevant. Since these parents are already divorced, unity of the family is not really an option. So, this case turns more clearly than Peter's on conflicting interpretations of the child's best interests.

In both cases, however, a parent's interpretation of the child's best interests clashes with that of the clinician. Emilia's mother feared that regular access visits were harming the child; that harm, she judged, was the real cause of Emilia's speech and behaviour problems. She has the ultimate power to withhold consent to treatment on Emilia's behalf, but her power may seem rather hollow to her because it is only negative. It does not extend to success in persuading the psychiatrist to give expert testimony against the access visits, which she views as the step most likely to advance Emilia's best interests.

The psychiatrist thought that therapy was progressing favourably, and that the child's best interests lay in continuing it. He viewed the mother's refusal to continue therapy for Emilia as motivated by annoyance at her failure to win him over to her side in the court case, not by concern for Emilia's best interests. Yet, in stating that 'it is part of the therapy to side with the child rather than with either parent,' was the psychiatrist ignoring his responsibilities? There might be times when 'therapeutic neutrality' is not really in the child's best interests, either. If the mother was right – and she had reason to think that the father was violent, at least in her own case – perhaps the access visits really were the underlying cause of

Emilia's problems, and no amount of therapy would work unless the underlying problem was removed.

In Emilia's case, there was no possibility of forcing the mother to continue taking Emilia to therapy, it seems. But, in other sorts of cases involuntary treatment does arise. In the extreme case, that might mean treating the young person against his or her will. Yet with adults, at least, consent to treatment is fundamental in most legal systems. In English common law, for example, intervention in the absence of consent constitutes battery. What is true of common law in England – judge-made law, relying on precedents set down in earlier cases – is true of statute or constitutional law in other European jurisdictions. Article 32 of the Italian Constitution, for example, states that no one can be given treatment against his or her will, although in the case of minors the right to be informed is legally vested in the parents (Calzone, 1996).

Sean's case illustrates a comparatively mild example of treating the young person against his or her will. Sean is uncertain about whether or why he needs psychotherapy, and he feels scapegoated by his father. That raised issues about who was the 'real' patient: was the clinician in Sean's case responsible primarily to Sean or to his father? However, Sean doesn't actually have to be forced to attend therapy – although there was a strong element of compulsion in his being made to attend boarding school by his parents. That, however, is not involuntary medical treatment. Indeed, because both Peter and Sean were being treated by 'talking' cures, it's hard to see how forcible treatment could be illustrated in either case.

ACTIVITY: What sorts of psychiatric treatment might require actually forcing the child or young person against their will?

Drug regimes, injections or force feeding are the most obvious sorts of cases. In general practice there might be a wider range of issues than in psychiatry. You may have been able to think of other sorts of treatments. Across different countries there are likely to be further differences in what treatments physicians and psychiatrists are willing to consider in the absence of overt consent to treatment from the child or young person.

The notion of treating children against their will can arise because in many legal systems, children are presumed incompetent to consent to treatment, whereas adults are presumed competent. As we saw, the Italian legal system vests the right to be informed in parents rather than children, assuming that children are less than fully competent to give or withhold consent to their own treatment. Different legal systems may accord different possibilities for minors to prove that they are capable of giving or refusing consent to treatment. But whereas adults' refusal of treatment is generally taken at face value, that of children and young people may not be. Even where a child or young person consents to treatment, perhaps we ought to think about this question: what does it mean for a child to give consent, if a child cannot legally refuse treatment? In other words, can a child genuinely consent?

It's especially important to consider cases of involuntary treatment, against the child's expressed wishes but in the name of his or her best interests – because they raise in the starkest form the conflict between the child's autonomy and the physician's duty to act in the child's best interests of beneficence. What are the practitioner's responsibilities if the child refuses treatment?

> **ACTIVITY: Stop here for a moment and think what sorts of cases these might be. Have you encountered any in your own experience? Have any come up in your national press? If you can think of more than one case, were there any common threads? Then read the following case study from England.**

THE CASE OF W (revisited)

W, a 16-year-old young woman suffering from anorexia nervosa, was accepting psychological treatment in a specialist residential unit for her condition, keeping her weight stable, but low. She was in the care of her local authority following the death of her father when she was 5 years old, and of her mother when she was 8. Therefore her local authority had what is called 'parental responsibility', giving them the same rights and duties of deciding what was in her best interests as her parents would have had. The local authority decided that W was not doing as well in her treatment centre as she might in another centre, where it was possible that she would be subject to compulsory feeding. But W did not want to leave the first centre, where she felt that she had established a good relationship with her therapists.

The local authority sought a court order requiring W to change to the second centre. During the long drawn-out court hearings at both trial and appeal level, W's weight dropped by about 8 kg; now her life actually was in danger. The Court of Appeal finally held that W should be required to accept transfer to the second centre, partly on the grounds that W's condition, anorexia nervosa, made it impossible for her to give a reasoned judgement. In fact, it went further, holding that even a competent young person under 18 could not refuse treatment so long as someone with parental authority consented.

> **ACTIVITY: How does the case of W differ from those of Sean or Peter?**

We've already noted that Sean and Peter were undergoing 'talking cures', whereas an issue in W's case was the possibility of artificial nutrition and hydration. There are several other differences which might have occurred to you.

(a) In W's case the conflict is not between the young person and the parent(s), but between the young person and one set of clinicians. The therapists at the first treatment centre were on W's side. This raises difficulties about what is therapeutically best for the child; that is a matter of dispute between clinicians. Is this often the case, do you think? If so, then there is no longer a neat dividing line between what is obviously clinically indicated and what the child or young person may want. That is, there may be more than one clinical interpretation of what is really in the child's best interests; 'best interests' is not an objective, agreed criterion that puts an end to all dispute. And, to the extent that the young person is more likely to comply with a treatment regime that fits her own wishes, 'best interests' and 'the child's voice' converge.

(b) In Peter's case, and to a lesser extent in Sean's, the therapist was very concerned with keeping the family together. This itself was thought to be a therapeutic goal, as well as an ethical one, consistent with the 'family unity' approach. That raised the question of who the patient was: the young person or the family. But in W's case, as in Emilia's, the family unit has already broken down; this time the parents are entirely absent, and the child is in local authority care. Are the clinician's responsibilities different in that case? We no longer need to consider the family, it seems. But, if the child's interest does not then depend on her well-being in the family – as Hattab claimed – what does it depend on?

(c) W's case raises life and death issues in a way that those of Sean and Peter do not. Does this mean that the responsibilities of the practitioner are more serious in W's case? Should practitioners automatically give preference to the treatment which has the best chance of keeping W alive, even against her wishes? What could be more truly in the child's best interests than keeping her alive, after all? However, it is not at all clear that W was deliberately risking death; she was accepting treatment which was keeping her weight low but stable, although she was not gaining any weight.

But what about a young person who refuses treatment on religious grounds, such as a Jehovah's Witness? Jehovah's Witness parents would not see their child's 'best interest' as mere continuation of life, but as eternal salvation. Because blood transfusions are regarded as an offence which carries the risk of eternal damnation, the real 'best inter-

ests' of their child, they might argue, lie in refusing consent to transfusions – even if that means death.

ACTIVITY: Now please read the following Dutch case study, which we looked at briefly in Chapter 1, concerning a 12-year-old Jehovah's Witness boy with cystic fibrosis. As you read, ask yourself these questions:

(a) Was this child competent to give or withhold consent to treatment?
(b) How relevant is the child's age in this case?
(c) What would have been the consequences of taking custody of the child away from the parents and imposing treatment in the name of the child's best interests?

THE CASE OF JW *(revisited)*

JW was a 12-year-old boy who had cystic fibrosis. Since his condition had been diagnosed, JW had been visiting the same hospital and physicians regularly for many years. Both he and his family were well known to the staff there and enjoyed a good relationship with them. In recent months, however, the boy's condition had become very serious. He had developed extensive varices of the oesophagus, which brought with them an accompanying risk of serious bleeding which would put the boy's life in danger.

When the doctor informed the family that the seriousness of the boy's condition might require a blood transfusion in order to save his life, both the boy and his family refused to consider such an option because of their faith. The whole family were devout and active Jehovah's Witnesses.

The paediatricians involved in the case disagreed about how they ought to proceed and asked a child psychiatrist to assess the child's competence to make the decision to refuse treatment. One possible option which was considered was to make an application for a court order to take custody of the boy away from his parents in order to allow the transfusion to take place.

The psychiatrist reported that the boy was intelligent and sensitive, that he was in no sense emotionally or socially disturbed and that he had a good relationship with his parents. He also had a clear understanding of his illness and of the treatment and was conscious of the consequences of his decisions to refuse a blood transfusion. He stuck to his decision and said that his parents had exerted no pressure on him. He simply wanted to live according to the principles of his faith.

After also interviewing the parents, it seemed clear that they cared very much for their son and indeed for all of their children. On the whole, they were rational about the decision to refuse the transfusion and appeared, as the boy himself had said, not to have put any explicit pressure on the boy to refuse the treatment.

It seemed clear that this was a caring family who, in the light of their religious beliefs had come to a reasoned decision to refuse this particular form of treatment.

In this case the child's competence appears quite plausible, so that the 'child's voice' arguments appear well founded. But, although the child did seem able to judge the consequences accurately, he was still young enough to be very dependent on his parents and their opinion. They, in turn, were not entirely autonomous, but perhaps under pressure from their religious community. So, the 'child's voice' and 'unity of the family' positions both argue in favour of allowing the boy to refuse transfusions; but should they take precedence over the child's 'objective' best interest in longer life? That question is complicated in this case by the boy's cystic fibrosis. Although cystic fibrosis sufferers whose condition is detected and treated early in childhood do now survive into adulthood, late adolescence was frequently their lifespan in the past. So there is no straightforward contest between extended life and religious belief in this case; it may well be that the boy's long-term survival is doubtful in any case.

English law allows adult Jehovah's Witnesses to refuse blood transfusions, but does not extend the same right to young people. There has been at least one case *(Re E)*, however, in which a

Jehovah's Witness boy with leukaemia, whose refusal of a transfusion had been overruled when he was 15, elected to refuse further transfusions as soon as he turned 18, and then died.

It is worth bearing in mind when considering cases involving Jehovah's Witnesses that the question of acceptable surgical techniques is changing quite rapidly (e.g. the use of cell-savers). This is reflected in the increased interest taken in this matter by specialized journals, for example, *The American Journal of Surgery*, Vol. 170. No.6a suppl. December 1995 and that, whilst such cases are useful for raising ethical questions, practice in these cases and the view of the Jehovah's Witness community is more subtle than is usually assumed.

Now please read the following article by John Pearce.

Ethical issues in child psychiatry and child psychotherapy: conflicts between the child, parents and practitioners

John Pearce

Children are not given the same freedom as adults to give consent to treatment and to make ethical decisions. These are not simple decisions. In fact, the distinction between what constitutes a child and what makes an adult different from a child is extremely blurred. Every adult is also somebody's child. And all children have similar qualities of character, mental function and physical activity to those that adults have. What differences there are between children and adults are concerned almost entirely with maturation and development – with quantity and complexity.

Another example of the difficulties in making decisions is that, although rights and responsibilities are often thought of as quite distinct and separate from each other, they are in fact inextricably linked. If a person's rights are assumed to be separate from his or her responsibilities, problems and conflicts inevitably arise unless somebody somewhere takes on the responsibility for that individual's rights. In the case of infants and young children, the responsibility associated with the exercising of their rights is taken on by the parents or legal guardian.

A decision about what is ethical and what is not might suggest that an absolute distinction exists and a line can be explicitly drawn between the ethical and the unethical. However, thinking about these complex issues in terms of absolutes is absurd and even dangerous. For example, there is no such thing as absolute informed consent about drug treatment, because to be fully informed would require a complete awareness of all the possible effects and side-effects of the drugs which would require extensive knowledge of psychopharmacology. Most lay people would find it difficult to form a balanced view about the risks in taking a potentially life-saving drug, based only on the information in the medical formulary. Likewise, there is no absolute definition of what a child is. Whatever age is decided upon to distinguish between childhood and adulthood will always be open to debate. In any case it is more appropriate to use a child's stage of development rather than the chronological age when making this decision.

In spite of the problems that arise from thinking in terms of absolutes, a line does have to be drawn somewhere and ethical decisions have to be made. Nevertheless, there will invariably be scope for disagreement as to exactly where or how the distinction should be made, and conflicts between children, parents and clinicians may be difficult to avoid. One way in which people have attempted to resolve conflicts about ethical issues in relation to children is to make decisions that are always in the best interest of the child. This sounds ethical and inherently right. However, there is still plenty of scope for disagreement and conflict even with this praiseworthy goal in mind. For example, in the case of an emotionally abused child – is it best to remove the abusing parent from the home or the child, or the child from the abusing and rejecting home?

Although it is clearly difficult to make ethical decisions and avoid conflict, a good starting point is to clearly recognize that making absolute distinctions will inevitably give rise to problems and confusions. The process of ethical decision making will be enabled and the likelihood of conflict will be reduced if the following factors are taken into account:

(a) The child's stage of development

It is essential to recognize the ever-changing needs of children that are influenced by the stage of development that they have reached. Thus a knowledge of child development is central to ethical decision-making in relation to the clinical treatment of children.

(b) Relationships between children and significant others

Decisions about clinical treatment and the ethical issues that arise must be considered in the context of the relationships that the child has with significant figures such as their parents, their clinicians, relatives, teachers and peers. The child who has a poor relationship with his or her parents may reject a recommended treatment merely to make the parents angry and upset. This can present the clinician with the ethical dilemma whether or not to override the child's refusal to consent to treatment. Positive relationships make conflicts in clinical decision-making much less likely to occur.

(c) Taking time to make decisions

Because children's needs are constantly changing, it is usually best to take time before arriving at treatment decisions involving ethical issues where there is the likelihood of conflict between the child, the parent or the practitioner. It takes time to assess the stage of development that children have reached and the nature of their relationships, as well as to gain an adequate awareness of their various needs. A child who has refused to consent to a particular treatment on one occasion may reverse that decision several days later, in the context of their developing awareness or their changing relationships.

(d) Rights and responsibilities must be considered together

If children are given rights without considering who takes the responsibility associated with these rights, this can easily lead to children being exposed to having to make decisions for which they are not in a position to take responsibility. Although every human being has equal rights, they may not have equal responsibilities. The responsibility for babies' rights or the rights of the person with learning disabilities has to be taken by the primary care giver. In clinical practice these responsibilities are shared between the child, the parents and the clinicians. A recognition of this shared responsibility for decision-making is probably the most important factor that can reduce conflict in ethical decision-making.

In conclusion, the conflicts that arise in clinical decision-making between children, parents and therapists are firmly rooted in the natural tendency to think in terms of absolutes with a clear line drawn between opposing views. Such polarization of opinions puts children at risk of inappropriate and possibly dangerous decisions being made. The chance of harmful conflict can be reduced by an awareness of the central importance of child development and supportive relationships. Agreement on clinical and ethical issues is much more likely if sufficient time is allowed for a decision to be made.

Pearce concludes by warning against 'the natural tendency to think in terms of absolutes with a clear line drawn between opposing views'. This is a useful reminder at our current point in this chapter. For clarity in analysing decisions, we've separated out best interests, the child's voice or rights and family unity. Pearce, however, reminds us that the effective making of ethical decisions involving children must involve all three.

In Section 1 we looked at Magno's idea that 'the interest of the child . . . is a true fundamental and universally shared idea'. That may seem attractive at first, perhaps intuitively true. But trying to work out what the child's best interests mean *in practice* is a great deal more difficult, even if we accept that the child's interest is the primary concern and even if it is clear that the child is the 'real patient'. As Pearce says, the balance is hard to achieve. A further case study from Finland illustrates some of the problems.

> **ACTIVITY: Please read the following case study about 'Pekka'.**

THE CASE OF PEKKA

The Finnish Act on the Status and Rights of Patients (enacted 1993) offers a minor who is mature and capable enough the chance to make decisions about his or her own treatment, but in practice parents make decisions for children under 12. According to Finnish mental health legislation, at 12 a child can himself appeal against a compulsory treatment decision to an administrative court; the parents also have a parallel right to make a complaint. A child is an independent subject in his or her own right; the child's interests can be separate from, and even contrary to, the interests of his or her parents. For example, Section 7 of the Finnish Act on the Status and Rights of Patients states that:

The opinion of a minor patient on a treatment measure has to be assessed with regard to his/her age or level of development. If a minor patient . . . can decide on the treatment given to him or her, he or she has to be cared for in mutual understanding with him or her.

This strong line on children's autonomy goes beyond law and practice in other Scandinavian nations, such as Sweden. However, while a child is said to be a subject in his or her own right, children usually lack resources and means to put their own rights into practice. At worst, the 'independence' of the child is merely a slogan which entitles the state to intervene into family life.

Despite this strong 'child's voice' stance, a 1995 case illustrated that these legal criteria are sometimes flouted. A boy of 11 – call him 'Pekka' – was treated under compulsory psychiatric order for 10 months, against his and his mother's wishes. She managed to arrange his escape from the institution where he was being treated and sent him to live secretly with relatives in Estonia. He only returned after his twelfth birthday, when by law his own opinions had to be heard. Even more important than the legal position, however, were institutional rules. The psychiatric hospital where the boy had originally been treated did not take children of 12 and over. The institution for young people over 12 diagnosed the boy as normal, and he now lives with his mother and attends a normal school.

ACTIVITY: In Pekka's case, it might be argued that the state intervened against the wishes of both the child and his mother, despite the emphasis in law on the child's voice. Stop now for a moment and think about what you know of comparable legislation in your own country. Is there a similar requirement to take the child's own wishes into account in devising a treatment plan? What are the provisions governing involuntary committal of minors?

Do you agree with the interpretation given above of the case of Pekka? Are other interpretations possible?

Tony Hope, one of our critical readers, argues in response to this case that there are a variety of other possible interpretations which might be made (without further information about the case). He points out that any of the following might also be true: (i) the original diagnosis might have been wrong; (ii) Pekka might have got better as a result of maturing; (iii) the 10 months in hospital might have helped Pekka a great deal; or (iv) he is now in very bad psychological shape and would benefit from more enforced treatment. What this reminds us usefully is that it is important not to jump to conclusions about a case on the basis of limited information.

If we accept the interpretation above, however, Finland appears to set a high value on the auton-omy of young people, in conformity with a pattern more typical of northern than southern Europe – at least in the usual stereotype. But, although there are real differences, sometimes the 'autonomy-minded North' is not really very good at protecting children's rights. Despite the emphasis in Finnish law on the minor's voice in making treatment decisions, the number of young people given involuntary treatment actually nearly doubled in 1991–1993. So it sounds as if 'Pekka's' case is increasingly typical, despite the ostensible emphasis on the child's voice.

ACTIVITY: Now please read the following extract (adapted from Launis, 1996). As you read, ask yourself why you think this situation has arisen, and whether there are any lessons.

Moral issues concerning children's legal status in Finland in relation to psychiatric treatment

Veikko Launis

The Finnish Mental Health Act, which came into effect at the beginning of 1991, sets down a different criterion for the involuntary treatment of patients under 18 than for adults. Minors can be given compulsory psychiatric in-patient treatment not only on grounds of mental illness, but also because of a 'serious mental disorder'. That is, personality disorders, not normally sufficient grounds for the compulsory treatment of adults, are enough reason to hospitalise a minor. More precisely:

The child may be sent into psychiatric hospital care involuntarily if, due to a serious mental disorder, he is in need of care, so that failure to commit him to care would significantly aggravate his illness or seriously endanger his health . . . (Section 8).

There are two different sets of questions which arise from this discrepancy between the treatment of adults and young people: ethical and practical. Each one in turn entails two more questions.

The child holds a special place in psychiatric ethics for at least two reasons. First, the child's actions are normally regarded as the responsibility of his or her parents. Consequently, psychiatric intervention in diagnosing or treating the child inevitably involves the parents. Second, the child's capacity for autonomous decision-making is not fully developed (Graham, 1981). However, we must ask whether and to what extent the content of the child's decision should be taken into account in evaluating his capacity to make autonomous decisions. According to a substantive conception of autonomy, some particular decisions (e.g. a person's decision to commit suicide or to use addictive drugs) cannot qualify as autonomous, no matter how they are made. A more formal conception of autonomy denies this, claiming that any given decision, regardless of its content, can qualify as autonomous – so long as it is made in the appropriate way (Husak, 1992, p. 83; Dworkin, 1988).

In practical terms, the first question concerning the Mental Health Act's application to young people concerns the high level of involuntary treatment to which it has led. The level of compulsory treatment of minors of Finland has nearly doubled since the Act came into force, and a large proportion of this is accounted for by the tripled rate of committal under the new criterion, 'serious mental disorder' between 1991 and 1993 (Kaivosoja, 1996, p. 200). This makes one ask whether at least some of these young people should have been helped through less severe measures to decrease the risk of stigmatization and medicalization of disorderly but otherwise normal conduct.

Secondly, the same study indicates that in 1991–3 only 50 per cent of minors treated against their will were treated in units for minors only – despite the provision in Section 8 of the Act on the Status and Rights of Patients that 'Minors shall be cared for separately from adults, unless it is considered in the child's best interests not to do so.'

The Finnish example illustrates the difficulties of reconciling the three approaches to practitioners' responsibilities towards children: to listen to the child's voice, to maintain family unity, or to act in the name of the child's best interests. Legislation which explicitly values the child's opinion is further advanced in Finland than in many European countries, but in practice children and their families actually seem to have fewer rights against compulsory psychiatric treatment than they had before. Nor is it clear that 'best interests' criteria are really being met, when children are being treated in adult facilities so frequently: it is hard to believe that this is really in their best interests 50 per cent of the time. The example of Finland shows how difficult it is, even in a small and homogeneous country, to put a legally and ethically coherent policy concerning children and compulsory treatment into practice.

Summary

In Sections 1 and 2 we began with cases involving young people's consent to psychiatric treatment but broadened the discussion to include other examples primarily involving somatic medicine, such as those of the anorexic girl or the cystic fibrosis boy. Three possible interpretations of the practitioner's responsibility were examined:
- to listen to the child's voice,
- to uphold family unity, or
- to serve the child's best interests.

These three views relate to the question of 'who is the patient?'. Although listening to the child's voice is an important responsibility, enshrined in European and UN conventions, difficulties arise because it is not the only voice to which practitioners must respond. The demands of other family members, the requirements of the law, and 'purely medical' best interests must also be considered. But these, too, are rarely uncontroversial; even medically defined best interests are usually open to disagreement among clinicians. These conflicts come to a head in the example of involuntary treatment, based on the debatable but often legally valid assumption that children and young people are not fully competent to consent.

Section 3: Confidentiality and conflicting responsibilities

The Finnish Act on the Status and Rights of Patients also gives the under-age patient the 'right to forbid the disclosure of information about his health and care' (Section 9). That is, children are entitled to the same standard of medical confidentiality as adults. That implies a 'child's rights' or 'child's voice' approach to looking at confidentiality as well as at consent to treatment. This, too, raises possible conflicts with what is really in the child's best interests, or with what the family think is in the child's best interests. We saw in Peter's case that the clinician resisted pressure from Peter's father to reveal what Peter said in the treatment sessions. There the doctors' duty of confidentiality to the child patient seemed exactly the same as it would have been to an adult patient. It seemed an important part of Peter's treatment to maintain his trust, and that depended in turn on confidentiality.

But consider instead the situation where a clinician withholds information about child abuse or neglect for reasons of confidentiality. There confidentiality seems to protect the abuser rather than the abused child. So, in a way, in this kind of case we're back to the question of to whom does the clinician's primary responsibility lie? Confidentiality itself does not tell us the answer to that question.

Instead. we have to know who deserves the first claim on our sense of responsibility in order to know who deserves confidentiality.

THE MONTJOIE AFFAIR

Until the early 1980s most professionals working with abused children in France would invoke the 'Law of Silence'. In this era of silence abuses of discretion abounded. It was difficult to evaluate the number of ill-treated children, or even of fatal cases of abuse. The percentage of abuse cases reported to the judicial authorities was very low. Yet the law did make it plain that doctors were to be released from their normal professional duty of confidentiality when, in the course of their work, they came to know of abuse and neglect of children under the age of 15.

In the early 1980s, however, a public campaign was organized around the slogan, '50 000 children are abused every year; speaking out is the first step.' Interministerial circulars of 1983 and 1985 informed practitioners of their responsibilities and specified procedures for hospital admission in cases of suspected abuse. This was followed up by legislation on the prevention of child abuse, in May 1989.

But, difficulties about confidentiality remained. There was a basic discrepancy between an article of the criminal code which respected professional confidentiality and another article which allowed the criminal prosecution of anyone who 'having knowledge about abuse of a child under the age of 15, does not report the case to the administrative or judicial authorities'. While it was clear that the doctor may report the case of an abused child without fear of criminal proceedings for breach of confidentiality, it was less clear whether he or she had an active responsibility to report cases of abuse encountered in the line of professional practice. Doctors were free to report abuse, but were they obliged to do so?

In December 1992 these dilemmas came to a head in the 'Montjoie affair'. Damien, aged 7, and Mickael, aged 18, had been placed together in a foster family, but Damien's foster parents informed Mickael's educational psychologist that Damien had complained of being abused by Mickael. The psychiatrist on the team, Dr Bernard Chouraqui, was informed 2 days later that the psychologist wished to separate the two boys immediately, sending Mickael to another foster family. After discussion, the team decided to wait 10 days before informing the judicial authorities so as to allow constructive therapy for Mickael, who was thought to be on the verge of a breakdown, which would be worsened by the threat of prosecution. The clinical team felt that he needed to be prepared to face the judicial consequences of his act.

The juvenile court was duly informed 2 weeks after the abuse had first been reported. In January 1993 the investigating judge charged the educational psychologist and the social worker on the team with not having reported the abuse. On the same day, the psychiatrist, Dr Chouraqui, appeared before the juvenile court of his own free will to explain the situation. He was immediately charged with the same offence and imprisoned, together with the educational psychologist. Dr Chouraqui was not released to await trial for another 2 weeks; at his trial 10 months later, however, he was acquitted.

Naturally there was a furore in the medical world. As a result of the outcry over the Montjoie affair, the dilemma about whether doctors were obliged to report abuse or merely free to do so was resolved in favour of the latter interpretation. The new Criminal Code, enacted in March 1994, makes it plain that delayed reporting of abuse cases, or even complete failure to do so, no longer carry penal sanctions. Doctors now know that they are not breaking confidentiality if they report abuse of children under the age of 15 (Art. 226–14) but reporting abuse is a personal decision. But isn't doctors' responsibility all the greater now that it is a personal, ethical decision, rather than a legal requirement?

> **ACTIVITY:** Think about this last sentence. Are ethical responsibilities greater than legal ones? Try to think of other areas in which practitioners' responsibilities are primarily ethical rather than legal.

The Montjoie affair represents an unusually fierce conflict between the clinician's ethical duty of care, as he interpreted it, and the law. Dr Chouraqui thought that it was in Mickael's best interests to give him some time to prepare for the idea of a court action. But, the investigating judge charged him with failure to report the abuse immediately, and under the criminal code he was actually imprisoned.

This is an extreme instance; imprisonment is rarely at issue in conflicts between practitioners and the law. But it does raise in a very graphic way the question of responsibilities under and to the law, and also to other members of the clinical team: it was only after team discussion that the decision was taken to postpone reporting the abuse, so in a sense all members of the team were mutually responsible. Crenier adds that although 'the law of secrecy' no longer prevails in public, the confidential deliberations of clinical teams may constitute another form of 'abuse of discretion'. 'The doctor must feel free to share his doubts and uncertainties with other professionals without having his professional competence questioned. Ultimately, going back to the issue of professional secrecy, one could examine the idea of "secret" remaining such when shared within a professional team.'

So far, we have mainly considered responsibilities to the child and to the family, but at this point we might stop and draw up a checklist of responsibilities to consider in making ethical decisions. Remember that these responsibilities may well conflict.

> **ACTIVITY:** To whom or what am I responsible?
> (a) To my actual patient, the child
> (b) To the parents and other members of the family
> (c) To the law

> (d) To other members of the clinical team and perhaps we should also add:
>
> (e) To my own sense of good practice, my professional standards
>
> Can you think of any less extreme examples from your own experience? What responsibilities did you feel to the child? To the family? To the law? To others in the clinical team? To your own professional standards?

In a child abuse case, it may well be the rightful function of the law to be very sceptical about confidentiality. Child protection must come first. But what about more general questions of confidentiality in working with children? In this chapter we have looked at confidentiality in the psychiatric treatment of children. As a spokeswoman at the British Medical Association points out below, questions of confidentiality and the conflict between the wishes of the parents and those of children are common throughout medical practice.

Professional guidance in the UK says that young people's confidentiality should be respected, unless there are very convincing reasons to the contrary – to protect somebody from serious harm or because a serious crime has been committed. Ideally, however, decisions about their care should be taken by young people with the help and support of their families. Doctors often worry that, by agreeing with minors to exclude parents from some of the potentially life-changing health decisions that are made at times of crisis, opportunities for families to experience proper support and closeness are lost. The BMA finds that doctors are sometimes concerned that maintaining young people's confidentiality arguably deprives parents of an opportunity to carry out their moral duties. At the same time, however, maintaining confidence is vitally important to encourage young people to seek medical advice, and to build a trusting relationship with their doctor. They need to be sure that they can approach their doctors about even the most sen-

sitive of health matters, including treatment for STIs and addiction rehabilitation.

These areas of treatment are an increasing area of enquiry to the BMA, and for many years the Association has had enquiries about young people asking for contraception or abortion without their parents' knowledge. Doctors sometimes have to go to extreme lengths to try and trace minors who, for example, fail to return to the surgery to collect a positive test result for pregnancy or STI. Whether there is a duty 'to pursue' is a difficult question where the patient is an adult, but even more so with minors with whom contact is usually through a parental address. Agreeing a 'safe' way to contact the young person can be helpful.

As with adults, young people's confidntiality should only be breached where this is necessary for the protection of their health or safety, or that of others. Wherever possible, young people should be involved in decisions to disclose information and encouraged to disclose voluntarily. Requests for contraception or abortion can raise a multiplicity of dilemmas. In some areas, local child protection rules try to oblige doctors to report any of their patients' under-age sexual activity, however voluntary the relationship, but the BMA advises that doctors should comply with local guidelines only where these concur with guidance from professional and regulatory bodies.

Drug testing young people is another common query. Sometimes parents who believe that their child is using drugs ask doctors to test. Some schools ask parents to agree to drug testing before a child can be admitted. In any such case, doctors must only comply if they believe that testing is in the young person's best interests and he or she agrees.

Sterilization of young people with learning difficulties used to be a frequent area of enquiry to the BMA, but better awareness of young people's rights and alternatives for managing menstruation and fertility mean that it is less often considered for these patients. Parents may consent to therapeutic interventions for their children, so if sterilization is a side-effect of essential life-prolonging therapy, it will be within the scope of parental consent. Sterilization for contraceptive purposes, however, requires the authorization of a court, which will scrutinize the reasons for the request and require evidence concerning the inappropriateness of other options.

> ACTIVITY: Stop here and spend some time trying to find out what professional or legal guidance there is available on confidentiality and children. Under what kinds of circumstances ought one to be allowed to breach confidentiality? Under what circumstances does one have a duty (ethical or legal) to breach confidentiality? Look for example, at the General Medical Council's guidance for British doctors in Duties of a Doctor.
>
> Before moving on to the next section make a list of the key points raised by this section.

Section 4: A question of competence?

The idea that competence marks a morally significant difference between adulthood and childhood, and is therefore a justification of different treatment, has arisen several times already in this chapter. We would now like to consider this question in a bit more depth by means of a reading exercise around a paper by Donna Dickenson.

> ACTIVITY: Please read the paper and as you do so consider how the issue of competence is relevant (or not) to the cases you have already looked at in this chapter.

Consent in children

Donna L. Dickenson

Introduction

The 'best interests of the child' constitute the traditional test for whether or not a particular procedure or research project can go ahead. In this view, the parents are the formal guardians of those interests, but the clinician is best placed to judge them on the basis of medical criteria. This view is under challenge on several fronts: from developmental research suggesting that children are maturing earlier, from major decisions on such matters as HIV testing which increasingly have to be made involving children and young people, and from an autonomy-centred view such as has made great inroads in the area of adult rights. But what are the rightful limitations of children's consent to medical treatment?

Recent general trends in law, policy and research

There is an ongoing dichotomy between legal trends which increasingly restrict young people's rights, and research emphasising greater involvement of children and young people in making their own healthcare decisions. In the first camp we can set the English court cases Re R and Re W, which continue to define the legal position as one in which even competent young people under 18 cannot refuse treatment so long as someone with parental responsibility consents to it. A similar trend in the United States is indicated by the requirement in most states of mandatory parental involvement in abortion decisions by minors (Ellertson, 1997), despite the evidence that the main effect of such legislation is not to lessen teenage pregnancies or, conversely, to result in more live births, but merely to delay minors' abortions past the eighth week and to drive pregnant minors over the borders of the next state, if there is no mandatory parental involvement there. Other evidence of a 'hard line' towards young people is provided by the national trend in the United States of lowering the age at which children can be transferred from juvenile to adult courts, even though a huge majority of young people in a South Carolina study were found to lack sufficient understanding for meaningful participation in their trials (Cooper, 1997). In the UK the age of criminal responsibility remains similarly out of kilter with that for autonomy in medical decision-making (Dickenson, 1994).

However, there is also evidence of movement towards greater acceptance of children's decision-making capacity on very major matters indeed, in reports from professional bodies such as the Royal College of Paediatrics and Child Health (RCPCH, 1997). While stressing that the child's best interests remain the fundamental concern, the committee behind this report included the case in which the child and/or family feel that further treatment of progressive and irreversible illness is more than can be borne, as one of five situations in which withholding or withdrawal of curative medical treatment could be considered. A much-cited letter in the *British Medical Journal* from a practising clinician in child and adolescent psychiatry argued that children should be presumed competent from the age of 5, rather than presumed incompetent until the age of eighteen (Paul, 1997). This recommendation built on the position paper published in 1996 by the Institute for Public Policy Research, and written by Alderson and Montgomery, who have been among the most active voices in the UK for giving children a greater part to play in decisions about their own healthcare (Alderson and Montgomery, 1996; Alderson, 1990, 1994). They suggest a statutory description of competence focusing on the child's ability to understand the nature and purpose of the proposed treatment, its principal benefits and possible harms, and the consequences of not receiving treatment. Parents should not be excluded from the discussion, however, they stress, and in this respect both this argument and the Royal College guidelines are consistent with a family-centred approach to decision-making.

ACTIVITY: The fact that children of similar ages are judged, on the one hand, to lack sufficient understanding to participate in a trial, and, on the other hand, to have sufficient understanding to make end of life decisions is an indicator of the degree to which there is disagreement on the question of just when children and young people are competent. Stop here for a moment and attempt to draw up a list of the kinds of criteria which mark the distinction between competence and incompetence. To what extent is it true to say that the transition from incompetence to competence in young people is a general phenomenon rather than one which may vary even in one person between different activities and decisions depending on experience? Now continue with your reading of Dickenson.

This conflict continues to trouble practitioners, who have moved beyond simple paternalism but often cannot readily see an alternative which maintains professional standards and personal accountability. In adolescent mental health practice, '[t]he aspiration is towards responsibly defining areas of authoritativeness or lack of it; the greatest pitfalls lie in being irresponsibly unauthoritative (an abdication of responsibility) or authoritarian' (Sutton, 1997).

ACTIVITY: To what extent is this a valid point, that it is possible to go too far along the road of assuming children are competent and end up avoiding one's responsibility for the child? Can you think of examples?

Withdrawal of treatment or refusal of active interventions

Anonymized cases from clinical practice and highly publicized cases from legal disputes both figure in recent literature, with a common focus on refusal of life-sustaining treatment by adolescents and even younger children. The dilemma lies in reconciling the autonomy of children and young people with best medical interests and parental wishes for treatment, in cases such as that of an 11-year-old with osteosarcoma who has had an arm amputated and now refuses aggressive chemotherapy for metastasis of the cancer. The aim is to develop a treatment plan that does not simply follow the parents' wishes (which would entail forcible treatment, upsetting to nursing staff) but nevertheless affirms their responsibility for the child's care. If a child has a stable set of values, gained from experience of chronic illness, that should be taken into account, together with more cognitive criteria for decision-making capacity (Harrison et al., 1997; Dickenson and Jones, 1995; Parker, 1995).

Three very public cases involving adolescents between 15 and 16 all involved refusal of life-prolonging medical therapy with serious adverse effects; in two of these cases, police intervened to enforce treatment against the wishes of both parents and adolescent patients (Traugott, 1997). Adolescents whose decisions are overridden may take drastic steps to avoid treatment – such as running away from home. Even in the absence of such active resistance, young people may simply not comply effectively with long-term treatment if their wishes are ignored. There are both practical and ethical reasons for involving young people in treatment decisions, even if the ultimate decision is to refuse aggressive treatment. In practice, consensus is developing that where burdens of treatment are very great, and benefits uncertain or very limited, the best interests doctrine may be stretched to accommodate greater autonomy for adolescents to refuse (in re E.G., 1989; in re Crum, 1991; Knapp v Georgetown University (DC Cir 1988); Bonner v. Morgan (DC Cir, 1941)). The difficulty is how to strike a balance in a particular case, even if this general principle is accepted. An additional problem in UK law remains the differential 'tariff' for consent and refusal, whereby young people under 18 may be found competent to consent to treatment under the Gillick criteria (Gillick v. W.Norfolk and Wisbech AHA, 1985), but may be barred from refusing treatment if someone with parental responsibility consents. Most UK legal and ethical opinion condemns this distinction as making meaningful consent impossible (Montgomery, 1993, 1997; Devereux et al., 1993),

but there is some support for it among practitioners on the grounds that the consequences of treatment refusal are likely to be more serious (Pearce, 1994). Other clinicians think that cases of overt conflict between a young person and someone with parental responsibility are less frequent than media attention might indicate, particularly if practitioners follow principles of good practice which bring emphasis involving both children and parents in decision-making (Rylance, 1996). As one surgeon defined children's capacity, 'True competence is to answer me back and query things.' (Alderson, 1992).

> ACTIVITY: If children are not considered competent to refuse treatment, how valid is their consent, given that they are considered competent to do this?

Mental health and mental disability

Special difficulties arise in the case of children and young people whose competence to consent or refuse is in doubt because of possible mental illness. Compulsory treatment under UK mental health legislation may be exercised over young people by anyone with parental responsibility, overriding the right to refuse which many commentators had thought the 1989 Children Act had created (Bates, 1994; Re K, W and H, 1993; Children Act, 1989). However, invoking the Mental Health Act may actually be seen as treating the young person more as an adult and as affording more protections (Elton et al., 1995). Conversely, clinicians in other areas of medicine are sometimes all too ready to call in the psychiatric emergency service to deal with a 'suicidal' adolescent on a compulsory basis, when the so-called 'suicidality' actually consists in refusal of treatment (Scotland, 1997). Eating disorders raise particular difficulties about competence to consent, disease status of the condition, and appropriateness of treatment under mental health legislation (Honig and Bentovim, 1996; Birleson, 1996).

For young adults with learning disabilities, the division between adult and child worlds at 18 is as arbitrary as for mature minors who may well be competent at an earlier age. An advocacy model has been suggested and tried out as a more appropriate way of involving intellectually disabled adolescents and young adults in making decisions about their own healthcare than the traditional guardianship model (Carney and Tait, 1997).

Genetic and HIV testing for children and adolescents: who decides?

Nowhere are the limitations of the 'best interests' model more relevantly demonstrated than in the area of HIV and genetic testing of children and adolescents. Clinicians have no monopoly on deciding what the child's best interests are, and treating accordingly, when there is little which can be done by clinical means, as with adult-onset incurable genetic disorders.

Earlier guidelines and research had focused primarily on the case of parents unilaterally requesting testing of very young children, leading to a general prohibition on testing of anyone under 18 (International Huntington Association and World Federation of Neurology Group on Huntington's Chorea, 1989; Clinical Genetics Society, 1994; Genetics Interest Group, 1994; Wertz et al., 1994). Recently, however, older adolescents have been requesting the test for themselves, although most units refuse to test minors. In some cases refusal has resulted in feelings of suicidality, raising ethical questions about whether harm is being done to these young people by deeming them incompetent to be tested (Scourfield et al., 1997) – although the opposite argument is that no good can be done by testing for incurable conditions. Against the older view that genetics tests without immediate medical benefits should never be performed on adolescents, it was also argued that concerns about possible misuse of genetic information, as by insurers and employers, should not hinder more widespread genetic screening of young people, although this claim was contested (Motulsky, 1997; Spiegler, 1997; McCabe, 1996; Mitchell et al., 1996).

ACTIVITY: What are the ethical issues raised when a young person requests a genetic test for a non-treatable, adult-onset genetic disorder such as Huntington's disease? What arguments might be made in favour and against giving them the test? (See the chapter on genetic testing for more on this.)

As in genetic testing on request by adolescents, HIV testing of minors is often prohibited unless parents consent, at least in the majority of US states (Meehan et al., 1997). But in Connecticut a group of adolescents mobilized a campaign to alter such restrictive legislation, claiming the right to be tested and treated, if necessary, independent of parental approval. The number of visits to testing centres and decisions to have the test by high-risk minors tripled after the new legislation. Imposing barriers to young people's access appears to be a 'moral panic' measure which backfires; removing such barriers actually improves testing rates and encourages responsible behaviour, enabling safer sex and prudent decisions about reproduction to be made on the basis of knowing one's serostatus (Hein, 1997). Adolescents are more willing to communicate with and seek help from physicians who assure confidentiality where possible (Ford et al., 1997).

Both genetic and HIV testing focus on the case of young people who consent to a procedure but who are refused it – unlike the cases discussed above concerning refusal of life-prolonging treatment. In light of the English doctrine that minors may consent to treatment but may not refuse where someone with parental responsibility consents, the ongoing prohibition on testing adolescents seems odd, and a British Medical Association working party is expected to report with new guidelines later in 1998.

Is consensus possible?

If best interests, the traditional paternalistic criterion, are no longer viewed as the sole prerogative of parents and clinicians to decide, does that mean that conflict will be endemic between doctors, families and young people? That would be unnecessarily pessimistic. Adolescents do not necessarily assert their rights at the expense of everyone else: the majority of both adolescents and parents agree that parents should be involved in deciding whether young people should partici- pate in minimal risk research studies, although there is a greater perceived need for parental consent among parents than among young people in studies involving more invasive procedures and more sensitive topics (Sikan et al., 1997). In the study of mandatory parental involvement in abor- tion decisions referred to earlier (Dickenson, 1994), 66 per cent of adolescents had voluntarily involved at least one parent.

It is vital for clinicians to understand both that ethics comes into small, everyday decisions in dealing with parents and children, for example, in creating a climate of openness and free discussion on the paediatric intensive care unit (Nelson, 1997). This can create genuine consent by both children and parents, rather than mere deference to the physician's technical ability in the hope of saving the child. Voluntary and informed consent should be seen as a mechanism for conflict reso- lution in adults, not a recipe for increasing conflict, and the same reasoning applies to adolescents. How realistic this prescription is in light of time pressures may be doubted, but clinical ethics com- mittees should also be viewed as another resource – not another restraint. It is also important to remember the particular difficulties which have been identified in involving minority ethnic fami- lies in obtaining meaningful consent, and the con- tinued tendency among clinicians to initiate distressing 'heroic' measures rather than to offer sensitive palliative care (Larcher et al., 1997).

Conclusion

Clinicians and ethicists seem increasingly to be of the same mind regarding children's consent to treatment, rather than on opposite sides of the debate. What is more discouraging is that public policy and case law have not caught up, and indeed have slipped backwards, under the pres- sure of 'pro-family' campaigners and moral panic

over such issues as HIV testing. It is to be hoped that professional task forces will ignore those politically motivated demands and continue to create new codes of practice which involve chil- dren and young people as active agents in making decisions about their own healthcare.

ACTIVITY: In her paper Dickenson indicates that not listening to children and young people and not taking what they have to say seriously may have very unfortunate consequences. In the following section of this chapter we shall be going on to look at some of these consequences in a social context and the related ethical issues. In the meantime, stop here for a moment and list the key issues raised by this section.

Section 5: The child in society

In the first sections of this chapter on the ethical issues involved in work with children and young people, we have explored a wide range of ethical conflicts which can arise in this type of work. We have explored the conflicting responsibilities practitioners feel to the child and to the child's parents or guardians. We have also explored a variety of different ways in which these conflicting responsibilities might be expressed: as the duty
- to 'listen to the child's voice';
- to 'maintain family unity';
- to 'think first and foremost of the child's best interests'.

We have addressed the question of who is to decide what is in the child's 'best interests' and have explored the responsibilities practitioners might have outside of the family, to the law, to others in their clinical team and to their own prac- tice. In this section we will begin to look more closely at how one might begin to develop ways of resolving such conflicts in good practice. The section will take the form of a reading exercise around a paper by Michael Parker on the conflicts which arise when healthcare and other practitioners come into contact with homeless minors. This is a particularly interesting problem in relation to this chapter because it is one in which practitioners can sometimes be faced with all these conflicts at the same time. The aim of this section and the one which follows it is to take us forward, from the recognition of certain ethical problems, towards their resolution in practice.

We would now like you to read the first part of the paper.

Ethical aspects of working with homeless minors in London

Michael Parker

The problem

The rising incidence of homelessness in the countries of Western Europe and the United States, together with the fact that among the homeless the very young are increasingly highly represented, raises a number of ethical and social issues which must be confronted by the whole community: by the homeless themselves, by their relatives, those professionally involved and by the public at large (Shelter, 1992). The effect of homelessness upon the lives of very young children is of particular concern and also where the ethical issues are at their most intense. Despite the substantial and growing number of children who currently run away from home or from local authority care, going on to become homeless, there is no consensus about either the rights of the children themselves or about the allocation of responsibility for their protection (National Children's Home, 1992). Indeed, I shall be going on to argue that this lack of consensus is itself one of the causes of the increase in homelessness among children. For it allows children as young as nine or ten to 'fall through the net' and to end up living on the streets of major cities or, increasingly, rural towns and villages.

Homelessness enters most people's lives through their television screen, their newspaper or perhaps, if they live in one of our larger cities, because they meet homeless people on the street. The rising incidence of homelessness means that few people can be unaware that it exists and that it is an aspect of their own community and the way of life of those around them. In this sense youth homelessness presents itself as an issue of concern and a problem for the whole community.

On the face of it, a good solution to the problem of homelessness might be seen to be one which simply got people off the streets. This certainly can be a worthwhile activity and the British Government's Rough Sleepers Initiative was a positive move in this sense (Strathdee, 1992). However, the question which needs surely to be answered is why it is that so many children are ending up on the streets in the first place, and this question retains its importance even when an emergency shelter is substituted for the street. Clearly, every homeless child has his or her own story to be told. However, in my experience, homelessness has less to do with the details of the individual's circumstances, tragic as these may be, than it has to do with what happens as the tragedy unfolds. For it is ambivalence about the resolution of certain central questions of responsibility which constitutes the 'hole in the net' through which children at risk fall, ending up on the street. It should not seem strange therefore that I begin my consideration of homelessness not with people on the street but by looking at the breakdown of the relationships between children and those who are responsible for their welfare. For this is where homelessness begins.

In most cases children live and grow up with those family members who take responsibility for them from birth. This usually means a member, or members, of the child's biological family, or perhaps a step-parent. A significant number of children, however, will spend their childhood in the care of foster parents, social workers or those by whom they have been adopted. Whichever of these is the case, under normal circumstances, children usually remain the responsibility of their 'family' throughout their childhood, this relationship of dependence ending naturally, though not without difficulty, as the child becomes an adult and achieves something like independence. The first step on the way to a child becoming homeless inevitably involves the breakdown of these forms of 'support' and there are three general ways in which this might come about. These are: (i) when the child runs away from the family home. Approximately 30 000 children aged 17 or under ran away from their family home in England and Scotland in 1990. Or, (ii) when the child runs away from care. In 1990, 13 000 children ran away from care in England and Scotland. Or, (iii) when the parent or legal guardian evicts the child from the household (National Children's Home, 1992).

Most runaways cite arguments within the family as a significant reason for running away from home (Strathdee, 1993). Most are in their mid-teens. This is inevitably a time of transition and some conflict for most children as they move toward independence and adulthood. The conflicts which occur at this time are not all, however, of the kind that lead children to leave home and most get resolved one way or another within the family itself. There are times when as a teenager it is tempting and natural to want to run away but probably wrong to do so. Few children would leave home because they hadn't got the gift they wanted for Christmas or because they had been told to be in by 10 o'clock at night. But there are times, it seems to me, when it clearly is right for a child seriously to consider running away from home or from care. Recent accounts in the news of cases of the sexual and physical abuse of children and of their severe neglect by parents, and indeed by social workers, often make one wonder why the children concerned hadn't run away sooner than they did.

The difference in importance between the kinds of reasons a child might give for considering leaving home or care is clear in the cases I have described but there must also be borderline cases; perhaps where a child feels that she is being restrained unreasonably from doing what she wants to do or where she has been beaten for breaking a house rule and is unsure whether she is at risk in the longer term. In such cases it must be incredibly difficult for a child to decide whether to stay or run away. In general, children find it hard to leave home even when their mistreatment has been extremely serious, often staying in an abusive situation for many years before gaining the courage, or perhaps sufficient fear, to leave. Family loyalty, fear of homelessness and the threat of punishment, even in abusive families, are often so powerful that it is reasonable to assume that if a child does run away and stay away there is almost inevitably something wrong even if it is not in fact abuse. Research by the National Children's Home (NCH, 1992) suggests that just over three-quarters of those children who do run away from home or care return of their own accord within 48 hours, but there is also research showing that of those who turned up at one particular shelter – that of Centrepoint in London – 31 percent said that they were running from abuse (See 'Children Who Run'. Radiance Strathdee, published by Centrepoint, London in 1993, for other related research and statistics). If one takes into account the difficulty involved in talking about such things to strangers, it is possible that the numbers are actually higher than this.

ACTIVITY: Parker reminds us that conflict between parents and children is virtually a defining feature of adolescence and the transition from childhood to adulthood. If this is the case, how realistic is it to look for agreement and consensus between children and their parents in work with teenagers? Clearly, this will be achievable in some cases but not in others. Are there morally significant ways in which the period of adolescence is different from other periods of life? Would you agree with Parker when he claims that there are times when it is morally right for a child to run away from home? Most of us would think that leaving home was almost always the wrong thing to do for a young child, but what about for adolescents? Under what conditions would you say it was morally right for a child or young person to run away? Is it never right? If not, what are the moral consequences of this?

The question of when it is right for a child to run away from home or care is not one that admits of a general and conclusive answer. The decision about whether or not to leave can ultimately only be the child's. It will tend to be based upon something like the extent to which she feels that she is a genuine participant for herself in her relationships with those who are responsible for her, measured against the degree to which she feels she is no longer a participant in this sense but rather the victim of an abuse of power on the part of those who are her 'carers'. Children run away because they have been denied the opportunity to participate in defining their own identity and the nature of the relationships they have with those around them. That they have run away is sufficient ground for concern. For they have chosen the dangers of the street over those of home.

When children run away, most stay in their local area but all are clearly at serious risk (National Children's Home, 1992). One can imagine the places in which they end up sleeping and the dangers they face in so doing; these dangers are increased by the fact that they will know that if they present themselves at a police station or at a nightshelter they run the further risk of being returned to the 'care' of those from whom they have run. Perhaps they have run away before and this has happened. For this reason runaways have, aside from their age, been at particular risk. The reason for this added risk has been that until recently, under Section 2 of the Child Abduction Act 1984, it has been an offence for anyone to take away or detain anyone under 16 years of age and this has meant that agencies working with runaways have faced the risk of prosecution and have had to turn them over to the police. A consequence of this has been that those children who are afraid of going home or afraid of the police, have commonly ended up on the street and in this sense have fallen through even the safety net provided for other (older) homeless people by the voluntary organizations.

ACTIVITY: Parker is claiming here that the law has created a situation in which its consequences are the exact opposite of its spirit. A law designed to protect the young and the vulnerable has had the consequence of making a group of these people more vulnerable still. How common is this? Can you identify examples in your country or which relate to your own practice? In the next section of his paper Parker goes on to set out a range of ethical tensions which arise in work with children. Although he is describing work with the young homeless, it is clear that many if not all of these dilemmas arise in all work with young people. While you are reading this section through, we would like you to make a list of the ethical tensions Parker identifies. If, during the course of your reading, you think of any additional ones from your own practice, add them to the list also.

One of the practical aspects of working with such vulnerable children is that when they arrive at a hospital, shelter or hostel, they are often frightened and tired and tend to have very little reason to believe that adults are to be trusted. The balance between staying with unknown adults in a hostel and sleeping rough on the street may be extremely fine, given the child's experiences. This means that, in a one-off interview or even within the space of a day, hostel workers are often unlikely to hear the child's account of why she has run away let alone any details of where she is from or who she is. The child's fear at this stage may simply be the result of nights on the street or of experiences she has had since she left home, and it may turn out that the reason she left home is insufficient ground for her not to be returned home fairly promptly. She may, however, have been subjected to years of horrendous abuse by those responsible for her welfare and may have been terrified into keeping her secret. If the child is saying nothing, or perhaps nothing other than that she does not want to go home, what ought hostel or health workers to do? In practice, the immediate physical and emotional welfare of the child will provide a priority and this will involve an assessment of what is in her longer-term interest, to be arrived at on the basis (partly) of what the child herself reveals as she comes to trust those who are working on her behalf. But, such a process inevitably takes time, and for this there must be a 'safe place' where a child might be helped to feel at her ease and encouraged to tell her story in her own time to people she could come to trust. Section 2 of the Child Abduction Act 1982, however, has meant that, in the UK, such places have until recently been illegal.

Notwithstanding the legal context, the existence of a 'refuge' of this kind clearly raises all sorts of ethical questions about the rights of parents and other agencies. For, whilst it seems sensible that the primary and immediate responsibility of those who come into contact with runaways ought to be the child's safety, they must also be subject to responsibilities in addition to those they have to the child. The professionals involved are, in addition, responsible to a wider community which includes the police, the social services and, indeed, the child's parents or guardians. In many cases, if not all, these responsibilities will pull in opposite directions and this tension creates a number of practical ethical problems for those who come into contact with homeless runaways. To what extent then, given that the child has in fact chosen to run away, ought parents or carers to continue to be allowed access to the child? Ought the parent or carer ever to be able to demand that the child is returned home immediately and, in cases where this is ruled out, ought the parent to know where the child is and be allowed to have contact? There will be occasions, say in cases where a child is making accusations of sexual abuse, when the question of the parent(s) right to manage their own affairs and the lives of the children concerned will have to be given very serious consideration. The details of any particular case can only be assessed in the light of the facts of that case but it could be argued that, in these more serious cases, the parent or carer ought not to be allowed, at least in the short term, to see the child. For, in such cases, it may be important to keep her location a secret from them in order to prevent her once again from becoming a victim. On the other hand, it also seems clear that there

may well be occasions, certainly not in all cases of abuse but perhaps in cases of other kinds of mistreatment, when the family ought to be able to maintain a certain amount of contact and possibly after some counselling, acquire the right to be reunited. There may, further, be far less serious cases of disputes where the child ought to be returned to the family or carer as a matter of course.

In the short term, however, having discovered a particular child at risk, it may well not be possible to decide quickly which of these descriptions applies, and this poses a dilemma. For, if it is argued that families ought only to lose their right to manage their affairs, in this kind of case, if there is evidence that members of that family have been mistreated and if, as is often the case at this early stage, there is no actual evidence of any kind (other than the fact that the child has run away from home), should not the hostel's primary responsibility be to return the child immediately to his or her family? For the child's parent or carer, the right to have the child returned to them if nothing incriminating comes out is the least that can be demanded. Having come indirectly into contact with the hostel, they have a broader and more general right to be treated fairly in its work. Their right to be contacted and told that the child is well and in safe hands is, then, beyond dispute but should they have any rights in addition to these? This is the other horn of the dilemma. For the claims of parents and carers, important as these may be, need to be weighed against the fact that there may well be reason to believe the child to be at risk from her family. There may also turn out to be some serious criminal consequences, for the parents or social workers, of the child telling her story. How are we to balance the child's need for refuge against the rights of the parent or carer?

The need for a resolution of this dilemma and of these ethical questions is clearly of great urgency. For the consequence of the current ambivalence is that children, fearing that they will not be taken seriously and fearing that they will be returned to those from whom they have run, are avoiding contact with those who, under different circumstances, might be able to help them. In this way, this very ambivalence can be said to be a contributing factor to the problem of runaways who are homeless and consequently at risk.

ACTIVITY: In the previous section Parker has outlined a range of ethical and practical tensions with which practitioners are confronted such as those between their responsibilities to the child, the parents, to other practitioners, to the law and so on. Many of these will be familiar to you both from your own practice and from the cases which we have asked you to read earlier in this chapter. In the section which follows, Parker goes on to look at what ethics can usefully have to say about how these tensions might be resolved. Before you go on to read this, take a few minutes to consider this question yourself.

When we thought about it we realized that, more often than not when ethics is discussed in relation to healthcare, it is usually to raise problems, doubts and concerns. Where ethics has traditionally been weaker in relation to healthcare and medicine (perhaps in contrast to the law), is in relation to the practical resolution of such problems. Parker's approach is, as we shall see, very much oriented towards this but first he addresses the question of the role of ethics and of philosophy in medicine. Now continue with your reading of the paper.

It is clear at the outset that solutions to the problem of homelessness can, in the end, only come about as a result of concerted practical and political measures. Nevertheless, finding the right practical measures depends upon first laying open the unspoken ethical and conceptual assumptions which inform our understanding of particular social problems, thereby making policy decisions, if not easier certainly more clearly delineated. It is here that philosophy is able to make a distinctive contribution. Philosophers are essentially concerned with the use of argument and the pursuit of clarity. Many of the arguments in everyday use are bedevilled by a lack of clarity, much of which

springs from the ambivalence of key concepts. This ambivalence often has practical consequences as in the present case when ambiguities about rights and responsibilities compounds the problems of runaways.

ACTIVITY: In the section that follows, Michael Parker attempts to show what a philosopher can contribute to the debate about ethics in work with children and young people. He starts by asking what it means to say that someone is the member of a community and what duties and rights does this membership bring with it.

I have throughout this paper, referred to homelessness as a problem for 'communities' and before moving on to look at homelessness itself, a little needs to be said about just what is meant by a 'community' here. When asked by a philosopher, such a question is sometimes a demand that one steps back from one's social embeddedness but the definition I have in mind here is a practical one and one with which I believe most people would identify. One's 'community', in the sense in which I shall be using the term in this paper, is to be loosely defined as being constituted by all those people with whom we have to work out meaningful ways of living together. The nature of these negotiations may vary both in form and in intensity, but the existence of negotiation of some kind is fundamental to the possibility of social, and ultimately of individual, life itself. This 'negotiational' account of community allows for the sense of degrees of community or identification which we all tend to feel. Within the family, people enter into complex and extended negotiation about a whole range of aspects of how to live meaningfully together (or separately) as a family. There is often a great sense of reciprocity here, even in disputes, and feelings of community within the family are often by far the strongest sense of community many people are likely to experience. Even within the family, however, decisions about communal life cannot be isolated from the individual's sense of also belonging to a wider community. This might be a matter, for example, of deciding whether to recycle our refuse in response to our concern for future generations or in contrast, it might be a matter of dealing with accusations of abuse when social workers and police arrive on the doorstep in the middle of the night to take our children away. In the modern world, via television, there is also a sense in which, for example, homeless children on the streets of Soho become de facto members of our community. Do we join a charity, give a donation, worry about the safety of our own children or simply ignore the problem? Any of these responses may be meaningful ways of dealing with a newly arrived-at sense of being human beings together – of sharing in a community or rather in a range of communities.

ACTIVITY: It is common for communities to be defined in terms of groups of people sharing certain attributes, interests or location, but Parker defines community in terms of reciprocal relationships, negotiation and so on. To what extent do you think that this conception can handle what we usually think of as our community? It seemed to us that it did have certain advantages in that, for example, it is capable of explaining why we might feel more of a sense of community with people (such as our extended family) who are distant from us than we do with our neighbours. Can you identify any weaknesses of an approach to ethics based upon a concept of community and of relationships rather than rights or duties or consequences?

A common difficulty faced by accounts of ethics which are based in notions of 'community' is that they tend to have difficulty explaining just what would be wrong with, say sexual abuse, were a particular community, or family, universally to see it as right. The problem arises because 'communitarian' approaches tend to see the community as the primary source of notions of goodness and the rights of individuals as secondary to the maintenance of communal life.

It seemed to us that Parker must be right on this point. For, one of the problems with community- or family-based ethics (as many feminists have

argued) is that, whilst on the one hand it enables us to respect the values which sustain families and communities, it is also, on the other hand, unable to recognize the damage which families and communities, can themselves pose to individuals.

It seems to me that, in general, such criticisms of communitarianism are valid. For, any useful ethical approach must be capable, at least sometimes, of upholding the rights of individuals against their community, or their family (Bell, 1993). By defining 'community', as I did above, as consisting of those with whom I enter into negotiation about how we are to live meaningfully together, however, I tie it to both the importance and the meaningfulness of an individual life and to the importance, for the very existence of both the community and of the individual, of meaningful dialogue between the two; thus the identity of persons is seen to be bound up, at least to some extent, by their ability to engage in meaningful relationships with others, having been thrown by birth and circumstance into networks of relationships within which they must negotiate both their identity and the meaningfulness of the world around them. This enables my conceptualization, I believe, to avoid the very real dangers of an over-emphasis on community.

In the previous paragraph I introduced the concept of 'rights' and described some of the problems which arise from too abstract interpretations of rights in contrast to stressing the notion of 'community'. Whilst philosophical discussion of the concept of 'rights' has a relatively short history linguistically, it is true that rights belong to a well-established tradition of ethical reasoning. Their origins can be traced to the recognition by the Stoic philosophers in Ancient Greece of the possibility that the actual laws in a particular community might be seen to be unjust when contrasted with a 'natural law' which is not itself relative to a particular community, and to which everyone has access through individual reflection (Almond, 1991). For this reason the concept of 'universal human rights' which grew out of the 'natural law' tradition has often appealed to those who have felt themselves to be oppressed. It may be argued that it is this appeal to universal human rights transcending any particular community that makes it possible to uphold the rights of individuals against their community, and it must be admitted that in recent years the concept of universal human rights has come to play an important role in the practice of international relations and in the critique of government.

But, whilst the appeal to universal human rights has great power in a pragmatic sense, just how far can one identify 'rights' intelligibly with the concept of an individual over and above her community? To what extent does it make sense to talk of human beings, and consequently their rights, transcending community in this way? I argued earlier that it is not possible to conceive of individuals who are able to step outside of their community. The intelligibility of the concept of universal human rights, insofar as this is understood in terms of the rights of the universal individual, rests ultimately upon the possibility of a similar radical detachment of the individual from human concerns. For it requires an appeal to something like the concept of an 'inner person' independent of social context. The appeal to universal human rights in this individualistic sense is made possible by the contrast between the needs of the community and those of this 'inner person'.

However, as I pointed out earlier, the problem with any approach which demands the radical detachment of the person from his or her community and consequently from all meaningful interaction with others, is that it requires one to lose sight of the fact that human concerns are concerns for us just because of our social embeddedness, because we are human and because our humanity is framed by the fact that we share in ways of life with other people out of which we draw our identity. It is our social embeddedness which makes it possible for us to be individuals. For it is in our social interactions that we negotiate our identity and it is here also that we play our role in the maintenance and transformation of our community. Both individuals and communities appear to

be made possible by their interrelatedness and their interaction.

> ACTIVITY: It seems, on first impression here, that Parker wants to eat his cake and have it too. He wants to have an ethics which values communities and also, at the same time, to have an approach which is based upon respect for individuals. But are these things compatible? Or are the conflicts between the respect for the values which sustain families and communities irreconcilable? Parker believes that they are not. What do you think? Make a list of the tensions between respect for individual children and respect for the values which support families.

In the light of these considerations, it seems that any satisfactory analysis of rights (Almond, 1991) must begin from the recognition that rights are to be located neither in the individual nor in the community, but in the nature of the ethical negotiations between them. Ethical problems arise with respect not simply to individuals or communities in themselves but to the forms of negotiation they undertake, to work out meaningful ways of living together; that is, the ways in which they treat each other. This means that if there is to be a justification of the use of a vocabulary of rights, this can not lie in a commitment to the existence of an abstract 'individual' but must lie instead in a commitment to particular ways of living with others, to particular 'ethical' ways of living. The best expression of this kind of commitment, it seems to me, is Kant's maxim that we should treat each other not solely as 'means' but as 'ends' (Kant, 1909). One can see how such a commitment might lead, in a fruitful way, to a different analysis of rights, in a more socially embedded language, and comprising, on the one hand, a positive right to have an active role in the creation of a meaningful identity for oneself in one's negotiations with others, and on the other hand, a complementary negative right not to be objectified in such negotiations; that is, not to be fixed by it despite oneself.

Such an account could I believe, lead to an enriching of the link between the question of who can be the subject of a right and the question of the duties which such rights imply for others. Consideration of the link between duties and rights in this context must again bring one back to communities, that is, to the idea that both rights and duties are tied in some sense to the nature of our relations to those with whom we have to work out meaningful ways of living together: our community.

This is not necessarily a narrow or restrictive conclusion, for the extended concept of community which I described in the earlier part of this discussion included, deliberately, not only members of a person's immediate family, or their town, culture or nation, but all those with whom it is necessary to work out meaningful ways of living together. Whilst this allows for the notion of degrees of community which most people feel, it is also a reminder of the fact that we do have meaningful relations with a community, whose constituency is diverse and extended, and that these wider relations too bring with them responsibilities and difficulties. This is why, as I argued earlier, homelessness, for example, is a problem for everyone.

For this issue, then, the concepts of the 'social embeddedness of individuals', 'community' and the 'negotiation of meaning' are fundamental, and are to be preferred to a theory of rights framed in individualistic terms; for it leads not to the call for freedom from community but to the call for the right to a voice within one's community. It is for want of a voice, it seems to me, that children run away from home or care in the first place and it is the fear that their voice will not be heard that forces them to remain at risk. It is their community – and the rest of us from that community – which denies them that voice.

ACTIVITY: The pages you have just been reading have introduced some fairly dense philosophical argument into our consideration of how we should work with children and have addressed the concepts of community, ethics, rights, individuals and relationships from a philosophical point of view. This offers us an approach to the child's voice which avoids some of the problems with it which were raised earlier and it also offers the possibility, Parker believes, of a resolution of some of the ethical issues relating to work with young people. In the final part of his paper and of this section Parker goes on to consider the practical implications of his argument. Before you go on to read this section, however, we would like you to go back and read Parker's discussion of the role of philosophy and particularly ethics in work with young people. We ask you to do this because philosophical papers often seem very difficult or impenetrable on first reading and usually need to be read more than once. While you do so, note down any thoughts you have about how this might relate to the practice of working with young people and children. Then read the final section of Parker's paper.

What does this mean for practitioners?

Homelessness enters the lives of most people indirectly, on their television or through the reading of newspapers or perhaps they encounter homeless people in the street. When this happens, homeless children become *de facto* members and victims of our community and hence a problem for us. As participants in such a community, we acquire a duty to do what we can to bring about the empowerment of the children concerned. What our responsibility is depends to some extent upon us, the nature of our lives and our ability to intervene. But, to ignore the issue is to continue to participate in a dialogue of victimization.

Homelessness is also, and primarily, both a personal issue for the children involved and their families and a professional issue for those who come into contact with the homeless through their work (hospital staff, hostel workers, the police, social workers, and others). Some of the problems raised by youth homelessness for those concerned are unique – the combination of working with children, on the edge of the law and often against the wishes of the child's legal guardians gives rise to a range of problems not previously encountered in combination. For many, the idea of third parties becoming involved in the relations between a family and its members or between the social services and a child in its care will be deeply worrying. However, the price we pay if we ignore this possibility (given sufficient safeguards) is a continuing rise in the number of children on the street; itself a deeply worrying prospect. Children, indeed all people, ought to be able to participate, that is to have a voice, in the everyday processes of dialogue which constitute the means by which people work out meaningful ways of living together and out of which they draw their identities. It may be the failure to allow children to take their full part in such processes, and the fact that they feel this so deeply, that causes them to run away in the first place, and if so, it may be the continued denial of this right that encourages them to stay away from those who might otherwise help them.

What is required, it seems to me, is the establishment, at many levels, of fora where children will feel safe and where they will be able to begin to participate in the dialogues which frame their lives. In the UK the Children Act of 1989 has made it possible, subject to stringent supervision, for approved agencies to work for a limited period with children who run away in something like the ways I have indicated. This can only be a good thing. Establishing such refuges would not, of course, stop children running away from home or from care, nor would it stop them ending up on the street, but it would ensure that once there they would very quickly have access to the safety and support they are going to need to re-establish something like a healthy lifestyle.

Youth homelessness itself will continue as long as we fail to reconstruct the nature of family life and life in our community in general in such a way that children feel themselves to be participating in the development of their own and their community's way of life rather than feeling themselves to be its victims. Perhaps the true measure of whether or not one's work with a child, or a parent (or anyone else for that matter), has been ethical is the extent to which they come through

the experience feeling that their story has been heard and that they have been taken seriously.

ACTIVITY: Parker argues that the resolution of ethical dilemmas in practical situations can only happen ethically in a situation where the participants, those with a legitimate interest in the matter at hand, can all participate and have a voice. He is also saying that the real test of whether one's work with children has been ethical is the extent to which they come through the experience feeling that they have been taken seriously and listened to. So it might seem that he is saying that our primary responsibility is our duty to respect the child's voice. But Parker has subtly changed the debate so that an emphasis on listening to children is no longer couched in individualistic terms. The child has to have a voice in balance with the legitimate voices of others. That is, she has to be able to participate in the decision-making process with those who have a legitimate right to be involved. He also suggested that the orientation of such participation ought to be towards the search for agreement about what constitutes the best interest of the child. Finally he has suggested that this can only be achieved by the creation of decision-making fora governed by certain practical ethical principles to guarantee the participation of young people in decision-making.

However, whist this helps to provide us with a theoretical framework for working with young people, it is still quite abstract and in the next section we will develop further the practical ways in which we might work ethically with young people. Before you go on to work your way through the final section of this chapter, we would like you to consider again the question of what principles you think ought to govern decision-making with children and young people. Parker's paper relates specifically to decision-making fora. So, for the purposes of this activity, list the principles which you think ought to govern a meeting between Peter, his parents and the child psychiatrist and perhaps a social worker. After this, we would like you to go on to the next section which is all about making the child's voice a reality.

Section 6: Making 'the child's voice' meaningful

We began this chapter with the statement in Article 12 of the UN Convention on the Rights of the Child that 'the child who is capable of forming his or her own views' should have 'the right to express those views freely'. Article 12 requires that the child's voice should be 'given due weight in accordance with the age and maturity of the child'. In many European countries, Article 12 now has legal force: France, for example, passed legislation in 1993 which requires French law to conform to its prescriptions (Heller, 1997). The British government, too, has formally adopted the Convention. What then does it take to make this notion of 'the child's voice' not just a hollow legal concept, but a meaningful notion in practice?

So far, the chapter has considered some of the following problems in fulfilling the requirements of Article 12:

- A child-centred approach is not universally accepted throughout Europe. It stems from an individualistic discourse of rights which is usually associated with the USA and Northern Europe (although that stereotype didn't seem to fit the Finnish case of Pekka). This may or may not be a realistic model in working with independent children.
- If the child is considered primarily within the family, as tends to be the case in Southern Europe, the 'child's voice' is not necessarily separate from that of the family. But this creates problems for the practitioner who disagrees with the family's opinion of what will benefit the child. Think, for example, of the cases of Peter and Sean.
- In such cases, the child's voice may not be consistently expressed; Peter, for example, changed his mind about the benefit of therapy under pressure from his father. Children's views also change as they develop and mature; at what age does 'the child's voice' represent the child's true wishes?
- Likewise, the family is not always of one voice; in Peter's case, for example, the mother, who had called the police to protect Peter against his father's violence, began by being on Peter's 'side', but in the end she conceded to her husband's opinion about discontinuing psychotherapy. The 'child's voice' may be the voice of either parent, or none. This is even more complicated if we take a psychoanalytic view which problematises what the child really wants, whether the child is expressing rebellion against or identification with one parent or another. Peter's shoplifting, for example, was seen by his psychotherapist as an unconscious rejection of his father's values; it was not an overt expression of his 'voice'.
- Who is the patient? Even if the answer is definitely 'the child', it may not be possible to treat the child independently of the family. If they do not comply with the prescribed treatment regime, they could undermine a decision made according to the child's expressed wishes or the practitioner's opinion of the child's best interests, assuming either of those conflicted with the family's opinion.
- 'Best interests' and 'the child's voice' may be in conflict, however; what the child wants may be inconsistent with what you as a practitioner

thinks would really be best for her. If the decision concerns life-prolonging treatment, involves a once-and-for-all judgement, or entails serious risks of any other sort, is it right to let 'the voice of the child' be the only criterion? Most practitioners would find that seriously irresponsible, a denial of their professional duty of care. The case of the 12-year-old Jehovah's Witness boy with cystic fibrosis illustrated this difficulty.

- 'The child's voice' can only be a reality if it is the child or young person who has the ultimate power to give or withhold consent to treatment. Similarly, the crucial question is not so much 'what treatment is in the child's best interests?' If other agencies also have some power to decide – Social Services, for example – might the child's voice be lost in the welter of conflicting opinions?

- The law typically regards children as 'presumed incompetent' to withhold consent to treatment. Again, this is a serious constraint on making the 'child's voice' a reality. Even competent young people under 18 may be denied the right to refuse a particular treatment regime, as we saw in the case of W.

- Although the rhetoric of 'the child's voice' is widely accepted, in practical terms children's rights often seem to be diminishing rather than increasing. An example of this was the huge increase in involuntary psychiatric treatment for minors in Finland, a country which might be expected to take rights seriously. Legislation which explicitly values the child's opinion is quite strong in Finland; so why is it so difficult to translate new legislation into practice – there and elsewhere? However, once again it is important to remind ourselves at this point that such statistics can easily be misleading and it may be, for example, that the system is now managing to identify correctly and treat patients who were previously slipping through the net in some way.

- Confidentiality may also be an arena of conflict. Does 'the child's voice' extend to 'the child's right to silence'? – for example, in keeping

records of treatment decisions from his or her parents. In the Montjoie affair, we saw that professional norms of confidentiality failed to protect abused children, stifling their 'voices'. This long list of impediments to making the child's voice count could well be discouraging. None the less, the notion of the child's voice is important in practice ethics and law, marking what has been called 'a reconsideration of the child's status, now seen as a subject of rights and not simply an object of protection' (Heller, 1997).

In this final section of the chapter, we want to consider practical ways to resolve the conflicts introduced in the earlier sections, moving beyond the difficulties into conflict resolution in practice.

One crucial issue to resolve is that of *competence*. It is good practice to listen to the child's voice wherever possible, but if the child is incompetent to decide about treatment, he or she is unlikely to have the last word – as, for example, with very young children. We have already seen that in English law, at least, there is a presumption of incompetence in young people under 18. The case of W took this further by denying that even a young person who had been found competent could *refuse* treatment, so long as someone with parental responsibility consented on behalf of the minor. Competence, for someone under 18, is only competence to consent.

Many commentators (e.g. Devereux et al., 1993) argue that this makes a nonsense of consent, and weakens the voice of the child. An alternative position is suggested by Pearce (1996):

Devereux et al. have argued that there should be no difference between giving and withholding consent, because the right to give consent is worthless if it is not accompanied by the right to refuse consent. The logic of this position is clear enough, but it assumes that consent can be conceived in absolute terms and can be considered in isolation from the context in which it is given or refused. If a child declines to give consent for treatment, it might reasonably be assumed that treatment has been refused. However, the refusal could be due to the child's feelings of anxiety and anger, or related to a limited capacity to understand the nature of the request, or perhaps simply a mis-understanding about what is required. The consequences of withholding consent to treatment are usually much more significant and potentially dangerous than simply giving consent – unless one believes that most treatments are either unnecessary or are likely to be more dangerous than the condition for which they were prescribed.

ACTIVITY: Which of these two positions do you agree with? Pearce has given some counter-arguments to the view that meaningful consent is impossible unless the child has the right to refuse. Do you believe these counter-arguments are strong ones? If not, why not?

The focus of this section, as has been noted, is to think about putting the ethical concepts you have encountered into practice, reflecting your own weightings of the importance of 'the child's voice', 'the child's best interests' and 'the unity of the family'.

So, to begin constructing a practical guide to resolving conflicts in working with children, you need to decide how you feel about whether treatment refusal should attract a higher 'tariff' than accepting treatment. If you accept that the two should be distinguished – and in English law, at present, they must be – your guide to practice might begin with this distinction:

• The nature of the decision: consent to treatment or refusal of consent

A practical guide might also want to consider:

• The child's developmental maturity, considered in both emotional and cognitive terms (as required by Lord Scarman's opinion in the Gillick case), and including
• The child's ability to understand the consequences of both treatment and treatment of refusal.

Pearce calls this 'the central issue' in assessing the young person's ability to give or refuse consent. In order to give valid consent, children must have reached the stage of maturity where they have a clear concept of themselves in relation to other people, including an ability to recognize their own needs and the needs of others. Competent children will have an ability to understand the nature of their disorders and know why treatment is deemed to be necessary. They should be able to understand the significance of the risks and benefits of having or not having the treatment. In addition, the competent child will be able to understand these issues in relation to the passage of time and be fully aware of what might happen in the future as a result of having or forgoing the treatment (Pearce, 1996). This ability is usually absent in children under 8, he believes, but almost always present in young people over 14, he believes.

Alderson (1992), on the other hand, has concluded that children younger than 10 years old are able to understand the nature and consequences of treatment quite well.

While noting that these decisions mainly concerned elective surgery, Pearce concedes that 'Alderson highlights the risk of underestimating children's ability to make wise and sensible choices. By excluding young people from the decision-making process, children as young as 4 or 5 years old may feel resentful and angry as they grow older and have to live with the consequences of decisions in which they had no involvement.' This suggests that one item which your practical guide to making decisions should not *necessarily* include is the age of the child. A functional test of competence – being competent to make this particular decision at this particular time – will go further towards making the child's voice count than a rigid age barrier.

ACTIVITY: You've now made a start on a practical checklist of what you would want to consider in deciding how to balance the child's voice, the child's best interests and the unity of the family in making decisions about treating children and young people.

Take some time now to add to your list: What else would you want to know? Then compare it with the 'consent checklist' developed by Pearce in the box below.

A CONSENT CHECKLIST

Factors to be taken into account when assessing competence to give or refuse consent (Pearce, 1996)

(a) The child's stage of cognitive development
     Does the child have a satisfactory under-standing of :
     The nature of the illness?
     Their own needs and the needs of others?
     The risks and benefits of treatment?
     Their own self-concept?
     The significance of time: past, present, future?
(b) The parent–child relationship
     Is it supportive and affectionate?
(c) The doctor–patient relationship
     Is there trust and confidence?
(d) The views of significant others (e.g. other family members and friends)
     Whose opinion influences the child and how?
(e) The risks and benefits of treatment
     What are the risks of treatment or no treatment?
(f) The nature of the illness
     How disabling, chronic or life-threatening?
(g) The need for consensus
     Is more time or information needed?
     Is a second opinion required?

ACTIVITY: **Now apply both Pearce's list and your own version to the following case study (adapted from Alderson, 1992, p. 9. ff.):**

THE CASE OF DANNY

Ten-year-old Danny has neurofibromatosis, which required removal of a major fibroma in his left tibia when he was only two. (His mother had previously died of the disease.) Bone was taken from his right fibula in an attempt to strengthen the left tibia, but after fifteen months in plaster, his lower left leg had to be amputated. His right leg was weakened by the surgery, and he then underwent two attempts at osteostomy to treat a valgus right foot (one that rolls over). Now he is undergoing limb lengthening of the right fibula. As he describes it, 'I'm going to have a bone graft in my right leg. Take a little bit from here (he touches his hip) and put it here (he touches his ankle) to fix it. And get a pin, just put it in and stitch it, then they wait till they heal it.' He smiles and jokes about the forthcoming procedure: 'Then I'll get a wheelchair – be lazy all the time, I like that, better than crutches.'

Danny's parents are less sanguine: they have just learned that another large tumour has to be removed from his left leg stump. They feel that they have little choice but to consent to a further amputation if that proves necessary during the additional surgery, which will be done at the same time as the limb-lengthening. They have not told Danny that his entire leg may have to be amputated. He knows about the new tumour, and has said 'I don't mind them taking the tumour, but I don't want them taking any more of my leg away.' Danny's father says, 'You feel that everyone is doing what they believe to be in his best interest, but they are tending to work a little bit blind.'

ACTIVITY: **Stop at this point in the story and complete your checklist in relation to the limb-lengthening of Danny's right fibula and possible left leg amputation. Has a meaningful consent been obtained? Has the child's voice been heard? What about the parents' position? Then continue reading the case history.**

In the event it proved possible to save the remaining left leg, and the right leg grew well, although Danny suffered a great deal of pain from the limb-lengthening procedure. Now the surgeons want to lengthen the small stump below Danny's left knee. Danny's stepmother explained to the boy that this will give greater leverage to the prosthesis, but Danny said adamantly, 'I don't want them doing that!' He would not explain why; he looked tired and depressed now, with dark circles under his eyes and little of his former chirpy manner. The surgeon gave the family 3 months to think about it, though he hinted that 'it would be interesting to see how the leg responds'. Danny's stepmother was sceptical about the surgeon's motive: 'Is he really thinking about what's for Danny's benefit, or is he just curious?'.

Danny's father replied, 'He genuinely felt that there was some advantage to Danny, But Danny's stepmother argued, 'He's going to senior school soon, he doesn't want another 6 months in a wheelchair. 'In the end, the family refused consent for lengthening the left leg stump.

> **ACTIVITY: Was a decision that respected the child's voice at the expense of his best interests, do you think? Again, compare the factors in this second decision with your own checklist and that used by Pearce.**

There is some uncertainty about what would be in Danny's medical best interests in this second decision. His stepmother also points to the importance of his *social* best interests when she remarks that he is going to senior school soon and doesn't want to begin his time there in a wheelchair. This is an important factor which does not appear on Pearce's otherwise very complete checklist (unless it can be included under Item (d), views of significant others).

Danny showed a great deal of cognitive maturity in the first part of his story: he has clearly grown up early, in the face of long familiarity with his illness. In the second part he may actually seem less mature insofar as he is adamantly unwilling even to consider the additional surgery; is this his pain and fear speaking? Alderton makes the important point that failing to listen to a child's fear, even if it seems irrational, is a form of ignoring the child's voice: 'Children can then be excluded and silenced, perhaps isolated within fears they feel unable to express.' This is a family with intimate and painful knowledge of neurofibromatosis, to which they have already lost one member.

They are perhaps less likely to accede to whatever the doctor says than patients with less experience of long-term illness. So we would say that the family's decision to reject further limb-lengthening appears a reasonable resolution, one which the surgeon has facilitated by giving them plenty of time to think it over.

Limb-lengthening is not a life-or-death decision, but even in terminal illness professional opinion in many countries is beginning to swing round to the view that withholding or withdrawing curative treatment may be an acceptable extension of listening to the child's voice. In 1997, after taking submissions from religious representatives, professional and patient groups, and severely handicapped young adults, the UK's Royal College of Paediatrics and Child Health Ethics Advisory Committee recommended, as we saw in Chapter 1, that withholding or withdrawing curative medical treatment may be considered consistent with the paramount principle of respecting the child's best interests, in these five situations:

(a) *The brain dead child*
   In the older child where criteria of brain-stem death are agreed by two practitioners in the usual way, it may still be technically feasible to provide basic cardio-pulmonary support by means of ventilation and intensive care. It is agreed within the profession that treatment in such circumstances is futile and the withdrawal of current medical treatment is appropriate.

(b) *The permanent vegetative state*
   The child who develops a permanent vegetative state following insults such as trauma or hypoxia is reliant on others for all care and does not react or relate with the outside world. It may be appropriate both to withdraw current therapy and to withhold further curative treatment.

(c) *The 'no chance' situation*
   The child has such severe disease that life-sustaining treatment simply delays death without significant alleviation of suffering. Medical treatment in this situation may thus be deemed inappropriate.

(d) *The 'no purpose' situation*
   Although the patient may be able to survive with treatment, the degree of physical or mental impairment will be so great that it is unreasonable to expect them to bear it. The

child in this situation will never be capable of taking part in decisions regarding treatment or its withdrawal.

(e) *The 'unbearable' situation*
The child and/or family feel that in the face of progressive and irreversible illness, further treatment is more than can be borne. They wish to have a particular treatment withdrawn, or to refuse further treatment irrespective of the medical opinion on its potential benefit. Oncology patients who are offered further aggressive treatment might be included in this category (Royal College of Paediatrics and Child Health, 1997).

ACTIVITY: The Royal College guidelines represent a practical attempt to lay down guidelines for clinical practice in a highly charged area. Do you agree with them? For your final activity, we'd like you to draw up a similar set of guidelines for withholding or withdrawing curative treatment which reflect your own conclusions, after studying this chapter. Try to make them as concrete as possible. Then do the same exercise for some of the other ethically difficult choices which we've covered in earlier parts of the chapter. You might want to include some or all of the following:

- Conflict with one or both parents
- Involuntary treatment
- Knowing when the child is competent to give or withhold consent
- Confidentiality

At the end of this process, you should have your own set of 'protocols', your own personal code of practice, which can be applied to some of the ethically contentious difficulties in working with children and young people.

ACTIVITY: Before moving on to the next chapter take this opportunity to create a summary of key points in this chapter:

Suggestions for further reading

Alderson, P. (1993). *Children's Consent to Surgery.* Buckingham: Open University Press.

Archard, D. (1993). *Children, Rights and Childhood.* London: Routledge.

Franklin, B. (1995). *The Handbook of Children's Rights.* London: Routledge.

Friedman Ross, L. (1999). *Children, Families and Healthcare Decision Making.* Oxford: Oxford University Press.

Murray, T. (1996). *The Worth of a Child.* Berkeley: University of California Press.

Part III

Broader issues in medical ethics

Resource allocation

Introduction

Medical resources are inevitably limited, and decisions will always have to be made between the various ways in which such resources might be used. The amount of money spent on healthcare varies both between countries and within countries over time. Different healthcare systems exist – some more efficient than others. Nevertheless, despite this variation, decisions will always have to be made about the priorities of healthcare spending. This is a profoundly moral matter and raises a wide range of ethical questions: What counts as a just distribution of healthcare resources? How ought we to decide between the provision of different treatments and the treatment of different patients? Given limited resources, what treatment don't we offer? What criteria ought to be used for rationing treatments?

We begin this chapter with an everyday sort of case, about long-term care of the very old. The demographic 'crisis' throughout Europe means that resource questions about the care of older people will become increasingly important; although the elderly are not our sole concern in this chapter, there are several examples concerning them, simply because that is where resource pressures are most likely to come in future. The case of Mr K also highlights conflict over resources between health and social services, between

chronic and acute services, and between families and service providers, with clinicians caught in the middle. In this case individual and social collide. We shall use the case of Mr K as a starting point in trying to work out what guidance can be offered to clinicians and other healthcare professionals over such wider issues of resource allocation.

Section 1: The problem of resource allocation

THE CASE OF MR K

Mr K was a 95-year-old patient in a long-stay ward at Park Prewett Hospital, Basingstoke, North and Mid-Hampshire Health Authority (UK). Like many other hospitals, Park Prewett was under pressure to close long-stay wards and free up resources being used by 'bedblockers'. Legislative changes in the early 1990s meant that there was conflict between health authorities and social services departments over who should foot the bill for long-term care of the elderly. It was in both parties' interests, however, to transfer the responsibility to families, who would pay privately for the care of their elderly members.

At a meeting behind closed doors, the health

authority decided to bring forward the date for closing Mr K's ward by 21 months, to 31 March 1994 instead of 31 December 1995. Although the consultant in charge of Mr K's care had deemed him unfit to be moved, the authority brought in an outside psychiatrist while the consultant was on leave. The psychiatrist conditionally approved the transfer. Along with 23 other elderly patients, Mr K was discharged to a private nursing home – on the very day of the decision. Seventeen days later he died. Four other elderly patients also died within three weeks of discharge from the hospital.

Mr K's son-in-law brought a complaint against the health authority to the Health Service Commissioner, an independent authority established by the Health Commissioners' Act 1993, who has powers to investigate complaints which cannot otherwise be settled in a court of law. In June 1996 the Commissioner condemned the health authority for acting undemocratically. He complained that their decision 'fell far short of the standards of accountability which a public body should display'. Although the health authority had originally claimed that the meeting was 'informal' and therefore private, North and Mid-Hampshire officials now acknowledged that 'the only sense in which it was informal was that it was not held in public'.

The Commissioner declared that his decision should serve as a 'grim warning' to any health authority or hospital trust planning to transfer long-term patients to the private sector. He also expressed 'considerable doubt' that doctors' consent to the patients' discharge had been obtained – let alone that of patients and their families.

The authority's handling of the affair was also censured by a House of Commons Select Committee, which called on ministers to dismiss those responsible. This was a national issue, it was felt, because the authority had flagrantly ignored government guidelines. In December 1997, 8 months after the censure vote by the Commons committee, the authority's chair, Angela Sealey, offered her resignation.

> **ACTIVITY:** Stop here for a moment and make a list of the conflicts you see in Mr K's case. We've mentioned the tensions between the National Health Service and Social Services over who should pay for long-term care of the elderly. What other conflicts are there?

If we use a broad definition of conflicts – to include not only overt conflicts between people but also more abstract conflicts of principle – conflicts between some of the following might have come to your mind:

- The health service and social services
- The family and the public providers (either health or social services)
- Private, for-profit nursing care and state-supported care
- Hospital doctors and hospital managers
- Clinical criteria vs. financial criteria
- Nursing home doctors and hospital doctors – over the issue of Mr K's requirements for hospital-based care
- The best interests of Mr K versus the good of others
- And, of course, the Commissioner vs. the health authority.

How typical is the case of Mr K, do you think? Are cases about resource allocation usually this blatant? In one sense it's very atypical: a particularly flagrant example, clearly an abuse of power by the health authority. And you may also think that the nursing home's professional practices are unusually lax – in accepting the transfer apparently without the clinical sanction of Mr K's consultant hospital physician. But even if Mr K's case is atypically bad practice, the sorts of conflicts which it illustrates occur everyday, even if they're not always this obvious.

In 1999, the British Government introduced changes to the NHS designed to lessen the impact of the internal market on healthcare provision. The biggest changes were those relating to the creation of Primary Care Groups which restore a degree of centralization (at least within a region) and lessen the autonomy of individual general practitioners. Nevertheless, to claim that this has abolished the internal market would be too strong. Hospitals remain trusts, responsible for their own budgets and the purchaser–provider split remains.

Although the immediate background to Mr K's case was community care legislation in the UK, the resource issues it illustrates are by no means unique to British practice. The following commentaries from Greece and Sweden show that resource conflict is a crucial and familiar issue in both Southern and Northern Europe.

Dimitrios Niakas (Niakas, 1997), of the Department of Economics at the National School of Public Health, in Greece, identifies four problems in Mr K's case:

(a) *The problem of accountability for providing services between social and healthcare authorities*
Given the scarcity of resources, and the fact that in many healthcare systems there is a division of these services, battle is joined between these two departments in attempting to save money and transfer responsibility. This conflict over the boundaries of services creates many problems for the elderly and other disadvantaged groups.

(b) *The efficiency problem for policy-makers, who are responsible both for saving money and for improving access to healthcare, reducing waiting lists*
Thus the replacement of long-stay wards in hospitals is necessary, if more patients with acute problems need treatment and care. The transfer of long-stay patients, including the elderly, to other settings (such as nursing homes and home care) seems to be a necessary step for efficiency.

(c) *The ethical problem for the clinician who has to give permission for the transfer, although*

he or she may not know whether the conditions in the new setting will be appropriate to the patient's particular needs
On the other hand, the clinician is under pressure from hospital management, and knows that many acute cases are waiting for admission as well.

(d) *The problem of implementation and social acceptance, even if change were planned and rational*
There will always be losers under any change, but equally, lack of change may be unfair to others. Media coverage may be sensationalistic: for example, in this case Mr K's death was apparently blamed on the transfer, although nobody can provide evidence to prove that.

And Marti Parker (Parker, 1997), of the Department of Social Work at the University of Stockholm in Sweden, confirms that Mr K's case could have happened almost anywhere in Europe:

The case is well chosen in that it is typical of what is happening in many places. Sweden is also closing long-term-stay institutions in an endeavour to decentralize and provide the minimal care necessary. There is also a hope among many politicians that the family will take over more responsibility. Because these decisions are now being made at the local level, with few central directives or standards to go by, and where there is often a lack of competence, there is a greater risk that the 'wrong' decision will be made.

This case could have happened in Sweden. One of the arguments we have heard for decentralizing has been to increase local democracy concerning local decisions. Unfortunately, democracy has actually suffered under decentralization, in my opinion. The case illustrates a similar process in the UK.

There are several issues here. The first is the issue of the decision itself – to move Mr K. A second issue is how the decision was arrived at and implemented – quickly, and without involving the family, or even informing them. A third, related issue is that of consent – of course, a very complicated issue in this age group.

The case, as presented here, does not take into account the fact that moving involves great risk to people in this age group. Any move, even to much better accommodation, increases the probability of death. The fact that 5 out of 24 persons in this age group died within a 3-week period may not be so remarkable, especially after a move. This is regardless of how the decision was made and of whether consent was granted. Even if the decision had been taken under the best, most democratic and humane circumstances, the transfers might still have resulted in the same mortality rate.

Obviously, the circumstances surrounding this decision were scandalous. The families and physicians should have been informed and involved in the decision. The information to the families should have included the risk involved in transfer at this age. The old people themselves should also have been involved to the greatest extent possible. However, the deaths cannot be said to be directly related to the undemocratic process which preceded the decision. We must be careful not to imply a latent causal effect.

The commentaries from Greece and Sweden both remind us not to assume that Mr K's death was directly caused by the authority's decision; but they also emphasize that conflicts over resource allocation extend to other areas than those we have already considered. Three more conflicts are suggested by Niakas and Parker:

• Between saving money and widening access to healthcare
• Between the media and health authorities or hospitals
• Between central and localized decision-making

And we also need to bear in mind the distinction between the *outcome* and the *grounds* of the resource allocation decision and the *process* by which it was made. The Commissioner did not so much criticize the *substance* of the health authority's decision as the *procedure*. He did not lay down an absolute prohibition on discharging long-stay patients, provided that doctors consent, decisions are made publicly, and sufficient notice is given. If the health authority had been willing to wait until the original date projected for the ward's closure, the case of Mr K would probably never have been made public.

After all, as both the Greek and Swedish commentators remind us, even an openly and fairly made decision might have resulted in Mr K's death. So judging by the outcome alone is inappropriate. This is particularly true because, of course, clinicians can't know the outcome of resource allocation decisions in advance. Judging by outcome tends to turn into judging from hindsight.

So what are the criteria by which we should judge the *procedures* behind resource allocation decisions? How do we decide? The second section of this chapter begins to formulate some answers to that crucial question. Before you go on to that section, however, please do this final activity.

> **ACTIVITY: Think of a decision about dividing resources fairly – but this time from outside the healthcare context. You could choose something as trivial as dividing a birthday cake, or something more complicated. How would you decide? What principles of fair distribution lay behind your decision? Make a list of the considerations you would take into account. We will ask you to refer back to this list at the end of the chapter, to see whether your ideas have developed or changed.**

The usual presumption would be that *everyone should get an equal share* of the cake, unless they disclaimed it by saying 'None for me, thanks,' or 'Oh, no, I don't want that much.' So *equality* is one obvious principle to use in decision-making. Some analysts would want to invoke it as what is called a *prima facie* principle. From the Latin for 'at first sight', *prima facie* means that there is a presumption in favour of that principle, in this case 'equality', unless proven otherwise.

However, other principles might also enter the equation: for example, a *medical* criterion that a person with diabetes shouldn't have any cake at all. Or a *first-come-first-served* principle might be relevant for latecomers who complain that they missed out on the division of the cake altogether.

This principle is the rationale for using a waiting list in healthcare resource allocation. What other principles do we use in everyday life to allocate resources fairly?

ACTIVITY: Stop here for a moment and before going on to the next section of this chapter write down a list of the key points raised by this section.

Section 2: Deciding by medical criteria

At the end of the previous section you were asked to think about what principles you would ordinarily use in dividing up scarce resources.

Considering how you would go about distributing things fairly in everyday life may give you some insights into the principles you would use in medical decision-making. But equally, you might well have objected to the exercise on the grounds that making everyday decisions – such as dividing up a birthday cake – is qualitatively different, precisely because they aren't medical decisions. True, medical criteria slipped in through the back door in the cake example, in so far as people with diabetes got no cake, on medical grounds. But, you might feel that this is atypical: most everyday decisions about sharing out scarce goods needn't consider health status.

Medicine also has the advantage over everyday decisions, one could argue, because it represents an objective, frequently quantifiable body of knowledge. In allocating scarce medical resources fairly, isn't the answer just to go by these objective medical criteria? In this view, evidence-based medicine (EBM) can tell us which treatments are the most effective. Those are the treatments to which we should devote maximum resources, EBM advocates might argue. Futile or ineffective interventions don't deserve our scarce resources, and it would actually be unethical to waste money on them.

On the face of it, this looks incontrovertible.

Doing the best we can for patients – perhaps the most basic dictum in medical practice and medical ethics – seems to mean that we should give the most effective treatments to the cases that need them most. Medical criteria are often seen as a value-neutral 'trump card', which puts paid to any further debate about allocation of scarce healthcare resources. On this argument, doctors should stop providing treatment at the point when it becomes medically futile, and that is also the threshold at which the health purchaser – state, insurer or other purchaser – should stop purchasing. So, deciding by medical criteria cuts short any further discussion about allocation of scarce healthcare resources, it is claimed.

This line of argument has a strong common-sense appeal, particularly to doctors who fear that they may be forced otherwise to provide treatment against their clinical consciences (Paris and Reardon, 1992), but we'd like you to think about possible complications in what may seem so obvious an argument.

ACTIVITY: Stop here for a moment and write down three possible arguments against the view that we should decide questions of scarce resources by medical criteria, and medical criteria alone.

There are several sorts of arguments against the apparently attractive option of deciding purely on medical criteria. We chose the following three points.

(a) The terms aren't clear

When advocates of EBM say that no money should be spent on 'futile' or 'ineffective' interventions, they assume that we can all agree on what is 'futile' or 'ineffective'. But, in fact, a range of definitions of 'futile' have been offered by different authors: among them are 'failing to prolong life', 'failing to achieve the patient's wishes', 'failing to achieve a physiological effect on the body', and 'failing to achieve a therapeutic benefit for the patient.' (Halliday, 1997, p. 149). This is not merely a semantic quarrel: it reflects deeper disagreement over both the *utility* or value to be served by treatment, and the *probability* of success. In the long run, of course, we are all dead, and therefore all treatment is futile. In less facile terms, there may be disagreements among practitioners, or between practitioners and patients or their families, about what counts as futile, and things don't always turn out as predicted. Consider the American case below, that of 'baby Ryan' (adapted from Capron, 1995).

THE CASE OF 'BABY RYAN'

Ryan Nguyen was born 6 weeks prematurely, asphyxiated, and with only a weak heartbeat. His clinicians also diagnosed brain damage following seizures, an intestinal blockage, and renal failure which meant that his kidneys failed to clear toxins, although they produced urine. Initially, Ryan was sustained through intravenous feeding and dialysis, but his clinicians doubted that he could be kept alive in this fashion until he was old enough for a kidney transplant, at about 2 years. They wanted to end treatment on the grounds of futility: it was argued that 'long-term dialysis would not only be inappropriate but would be immoral', since it would prolong Ryan's suffering with no chance of improvement.

Ryan's parents refused to accept withdrawal of treatment, despite the hospital's view that imposing 'virtually futile' treatment would be inhumane. The Nguyens sought a second opinion from a neonatologist at another hospital, but that, too, was unfavourable. Finally, they obtained an emergency court order, permitted under the legislation of their home state, directing the hospital to take whatever steps were necessary to maintain Ryan's life, including dialysis. The publicity surrounding the case attracted another hospital's attention, and this third hospital accepted Ryan for transfer. Three days later, surgeons there operated to clear Ryan's blocked intestines. He was shortly able to take nutrition by mouth, and at 3 months he was sent home, not having needed any further dialysis. At 1 year he appeared to be developing normally for his age, free of any permanent neurological deficit; his most recent CAT scan shows no structural problems.

(b) *We can't always get the necessary evidence*

Evidence-based medicine gives a high priority to certain types of evidence, particularly from randomized clinical trials; yet such high-quality evidence isn't always available. This isn't just a matter of the evidence not being available *yet*, because not enough trials have been done – although that, too, is a problem. Drug treatments, for example, are more likely to attract the necessary funding for trials to be carried out – possibly funding from pharmaceutical companies. There might be some alternative treatment which didn't involve the use of drugs – but we would never know about it. 'This could result in some drug treatments being recommended and purchased, not because they are better than alternative, non-drug treatments, but because the *evidence* for effectiveness is better' (Hope, 1995, p. 260).

Outcomes for acute conditions are also easier to measure and test than those for chronic ones, which typically have fuzzier, longer-term parameters. This raises issues about *fairness*. The elderly might be more likely to have chronic conditions, for example; so deciding only to support EBM-approved interventions could inadvertently discriminate in favour of younger people with acute conditions.

Justice

Justice is often seen in terms of fairness (Rawls, 1971), of what principles of fair distribution we could agree to. This is *distributive justice*, the main concern of this chapter, though justice can also be considered in terms of respect for *rights and the law* – crucial in *criminal justice*. What the two branches of justice have in common is that both are concerned with ensuring that individuals receive the treatment that is proper or fitting for them (Miller, 1986). The classic formulation of formal justice is Aristotle's injunction to 'treat equals equally'. This does not mean treating everyone alike: in relation to healthcare, for example, the sick deserve different treatment from the well, and more resources. Indeed, Aristotle also specified that unequals should be treated unequally. It is substantive analysis of what counts as a *relevant inequality* which varies between different philosophical approaches, and, in relation to our concerns in this chapter, between different approaches to resource distribution.

In Section 5 of this chapter we will be going on to explore different approaches to the question of justice. However, it is already clear that we cannot escape ethical debates about *justice* by looking to allegedly scientific and objective medical criteria. Even if in principle it were possible to test every proposed treatment, sometimes it might actually be unethical to run a randomized clinical trial with a particular population, particularly of patients who can't decide for themselves whether to enter a trial: very sick neonates, for example, or elderly people with dementia. This suggests a final point about why it is not sufficient to decide by medical criteria alone.

(c) Even if we had the necessary evidence, we might not want to make it the only criterion for deciding

Patient choice might be another factor to consider, for example. Even if we didn't want to allow patients to choose treatments that were patently and clinically *bad* for them, there might be a certain degree of latitude in letting them choose interventions which suit their particular circumstances, religious or cultural beliefs, or family preferences. In a democracy, shouldn't patient choice also be a value?

Clearly, there are limitations on patient choice, however, when there simply are insufficient resources to satisfy everyone's demands . In the example described below, the UK case of 'Child B', the child patient – or, primarily, her father – 'chose' an expensive treatment with a low probability of success. Evidence-based medicine would probably not have supported the treatment in this child's case. None the less, public feeling

ran high, illustrating the point that evidence-based criteria are often unacceptable for particular classes of patient – notably very sick children. In this case, unlike that of 'Baby Ryan', the decision that treatment was futile turned out to be correct, purely in the sense that the child died. But were other values served by treating the girl? – not least, perhaps, society's sense of solidarity with other parents and children in this tragic situation.

THE CASE OF 'CHILD B'

Child B (later publicly identified as Jaymee Bowen), aged 10, was acutely ill with leukaemia. A bone-marrow transplant had proved unsuccessful. Now both her own doctor and oncologists from London's Royal Marsden Hospital believed she had only a few weeks to live, with further treatment being futile. Although Jaymee's own views in favour of treatment were of uncertain validity – she had not been told how ill she was – her father refused to accept this decision. He located a professor at the Hammersmith Hospital who recommended a further course of chemotherapy followed by an experimental second bone-marrow transplant, which would have to be provided by Jaymee's younger sister. Primarily because the professor had acknowledged that this was experimental, non-standard therapy, and secondarily because Department of Health guidance limited the funding of unproven treatment, Jaymee's Health Authority in Cambridge decided that '*the substantial expenditure on treatment with such a small prospect of success would not be an effective use of resources*' (cited in Montgomery, 1997, p. 65).

Mr Bowen brought a legal action to compel the Health Authority to fund Jaymee's treatment with the experimental procedure. His chances of success looked poor, despite a massive outpouring of public sympathy and extensive media coverage. Normally, English courts are reluctant to intervene in such matters unless it can be shown that the decision was taken in bad faith or was patently unreasonable. Although in a 1987 case (*R. v. Secretary of State for Social Services, ex parte Walker*) the Court of Appeal had stated that courts could strike down decisions about resource allocation, no court had actually done so.

Nevertheless Mr Bowen succeeded, at least at first. In the High Court the Health Authority's decision was quashed, and their powers to refuse treatment on grounds of resource shortage were severely limited. The Health Authority was ordered to reconsider its decision and to spell out its reasoning more clearly, allowing the father a chance to show that the decision had, in fact, been unreasonable. The burden was put on the Health Authority: its duty to recognize Jaymee's fundamental right to life required it to show compelling reasons why other patients should implicitly have priority over her.

However, the Court of Appeal overturned the High Court decision. Whether or not a treatment was life-saving, the Appeal Court held, had no bearing on the general principle that courts could not intervene to determine the merits of the dispute. Courts should not be drawn into resource allocation decisions. Nor should the Health Authority be forced to show where it planned to spend the money that would notionally be saved by not treating Jaymee. The Appeal Court's reasoning was based not primarily on resource shortage, however, but on the weight of medical evidence, suggesting that it was not in Jaymee's best interests to undergo the experimental procedure. So, efficacy of treatment clearly *is* a proper legal consideration.

In the end, a private benefactor came forward, offering to fund Jaymee's experimental treatment. She appeared at first to be doing well after the procedure, but worsened after a few months and died. After her death, Mr Bowen reiterated his satisfaction that everything possible had been done, despite the tragic outcome.

ACTIVITY: Given that there will always be tragic cases, how can practitioners allocate resources fairly? How can we avoid being blown by the media winds into favouring the most emotionally gripping cases? – such as those of Jaymee Bowen. A Norwegian set of guidelines for practical use (from Elgesem, 1996) is instructive, setting out five levels of priorities for healthcare funding. These guidelines were intended to be realistic, reflecting what interest groups and the press would find acceptable – even if that might conflict with consistency of principles. In light of the Jaymee Bowen case, they look even more instructive now than they did when they were first put forward by a government committee in 1987.

We would now like you to read through these guidelines and then undertake the following activity. Firstly, think of two further examples (in addition to those given below, by the Norwegian committee), which you think would fit under each level of priority. Secondly, having thus worked out what are the practical implications of each level of funding, ask yourself whether you agree with these rankings. Would you want to set priorities differently?

Priority level 1
Procedures immediately necessary to save lives in acute physical or mental illness. Examples: emergency surgery; emergency situations in psychiatric care; treatment of severely ill neonates

Priority level 2
Procedures required to avoid longer-term harm to patients or groups of patients, where interventions are well supported by evidence. Examples: diagnosis and treatment of asthma or diabetes

Priority level 3
Procedures with documented effects, but where the consequences of not treating are less serious. Example: treatment of moderately high blood pressure

Priority level 4
Services which are in demand but where there is little or no physiological ill-effect from not treating. Examples: IVF; repeated ultrasound on request during pregnancy

Zero priority
Services which are in demand but which have no documented benefits. Example: special health services for top athletes

Note: Under this scheme, public funding would only be available for levels 1, 2 and 3.

How did you get on with evaluating these levels of priority? We found the zero-level rather puzzling: it seemed to us that the distinction being made was not that the procedures were of no benefit, but that only an elite would benefit from them. And we thought that the refusal to fund IVF might be very unpopular – whereas the committee had said that it was taking public opinion into account. Whether infertility is an illness may be debatable, and whether having children is a right is even more so. But, there is no doubt that good could be done to infertile patients – in patients' own view – by successful IVF. A better justification for not funding IVF, we thought, might be the evidence-based observation that its success rate is rather low (Renard, 1997).

Underlying these five levels of priority in the Norwegian report were five criteria which the commission initially suggested for rationing scarce resources:

- Seriousness of the condition
- Equity in access to health services among all regions and classes
- Length of time patients have to wait for services
- Fairness to disadvantaged groups (defined as single elderly and handicapped people, psychiatric patients and people with learning difficulties)
- The patient's responsibility for the disease, in terms of lifestyle

ACTIVITY: Take a few moments to think about possible conflicts between the criteria.

It seems likely that equity of access to health services for all regions and classes collides with enforcing patients' responsibility for their own condition, in lifestyle terms. Smoking, for example, is typically more heavily distributed among members of the lower social classes than among the better-off. Smoking also illustrates possible conflict between seriousness of the condition and the patient's responsibility for it: should lung cancer and cardiac patients who have smoked be denied resources for their serious condition? An English consultant who refused to perform a heart bypass operation on a cardiac patient who was not willing to give up smoking was, in fact, required to perform the operation, despite his argument that the procedure would have been a waste of resources were the man, as seemed likely, to continue to smoke.

In the end the Norwegian report, in fact, omitted patient responsibility as too contentious a criterion. A more recent version (1997) replaced the five criteria with only three: seriousness of the disease, utility of the procedure, and equity.

ACTIVITY: Do these three criteria cover the appropriate bases for making a decision about rationing resources, do you think?

We wondered if you have noticed the omission of one factor which appears very often in decisions about withholding scarce resources: age. Mr K's case is at the opposite end of the age spectrum from those of Baby Ryan and Child B, but perhaps both sets of cases are really explained by the operation of unexpressed age criteria in rationing. Age considerations, in reverse, explain the special importance society seems to attach to saving children at all costs – as we saw in the public reaction to the Child B case. In Section 3 we will look in more detail on rationing by age, which has raised its controversial head in many countries' practice.

Before moving on to that we just want to emphasize the 'ordinariness' of resource conflicts. Mr K's case was a particularly flagrant example, but hospitals do have to make decisions every day about devoting resources to long-term care of the elderly. This is inescapable, but not necessarily a bad thing. In making judgements practitioners may improve their powers of reasoning, sharpen their skills of analysis and acquire better styles of communication. This is especially true, we would argue, if they can bring ethical analysis to bear in making these judgements. The skill of elaborating judgements about particular cases – what Aristotle termed *phronesis* – is consistent with making better clinical judgements, we think. We have emphasized particular cases in this chapter because we, too, believe in the development of *phronesis*.

The cases of Baby Ryan and Child B were more public and controversial, less common than that of Mr K, and they were also atypical in that they both wound up in court. Legal guidelines were laid down in the Child B case, for British practitioners, which do affect clinical work; but even in the absence of such legal guidelines, ethical analysis can help unravel the reasoning behind the kinds of priorities clinicians have. Some of the ethical values we have encountered so far have included:

- The notion of *distributive justice*, that is, how we can divide up resources fairly
- The concept of *equity* between classes, and of healthcare as a form of reducing social disparity
- The converse notion of desert or responsibility, for example, in the argument about whether people who are responsible for their own conditions deserve fewer resources
and finally,
- The underpinning notion that we cannot escape from social and ethical judgements by taking refuge in medical criteria alone.

We will explore these concepts in greater depth in the remaining sections of this chapter.

ACTIVITY: Before going on to the next section, take a few moments to note down the key points raised by this chapter.

Section 3: Using social criteria to decide on resource allocation

Demographic changes

In Section 2 we asked you to consider a Norwegian model of resource allocation based on the use of priority levels. Whilst doing so, you may have noticed that the priority levels included what might be called 'social criteria' in addition to medical ones. One example of this was the term 'single elderly' in the list of criteria on p. 238. In this section we shall be looking at the use of social criteria as a basis of resource allocation decisions. We shall do so using the example of the elderly.

It is sometimes suggested that the reason for the current debate about the need for the rationing of scarce healthcare resources is demographic change associated with the 'greying' or 'double greying' of the populations of the countries of the European Union and the United States. In November 1991, for example, a Dutch State Commission, chaired by the cardiologist Dr Dunning, published a report called *Choices in healthcare* in which it was argued that choices are necessary for three reasons: firstly, the population is ageing, secondly scientific and technological change is increasingly rapid, attracting funding and publicity, and thirdly, financial resources are limited and cost control is a central goal of Dutch healthcare policy. Earlier on in this chapter we asked you to think about a case of resource allocation which you have encountered in the media or your own experience. To what extent do you think that demographic changes alone can explain the shortage and to what extent was it the result of the other two factors mentioned in the Dutch report? This section takes the form of a reading exercise – based upon an edited version of an article by Ruud ter Meulen on 'Care for the elderly in an era of diminishing resources'.

Care for the elderly in an era of diminishing resources

Ruud ter Meulen

Since the beginning of this century, average life expectancy has risen significantly in the industrialized world. In the early 1900s, the average life expectancy was approximately 50 years. It is currently 76 years for both the United States and for the member states of the European Community.

Life expectancy is higher for women than for men: 73 for men and 79 years for women in the EC. The increase of the average life expectancy is expected to continue: in the year 2025 the average life expectancy will be 80 years, 77 years for men and 82 years for women (Keyfitz and Flieger, 1990).

This increase in average life expectancy, however, cannot be called a success in all respects (Gruenberg, 1977). For whilst individuals do have longer lives they are confronted increasingly with chronic, debilitating diseases which are typical for the later stages of life. The higher one's age, the more one is confronted with chronic diseases such as diseases of the sensory organs, neurological diseases and cardiovascular diseases. In fact, healthy life expectancy, that is the period of life free from diseases and handicaps, has remained the same even as average life expectancy has risen. Consequently, we seem to be living in bad health for an increasing part of our lives (Haan et al., 1991). In view of these figures, what should be the main target of public health policies for the elderly: adding more life or more quality to our (long) lives? (Légaré, 1991).

ACTIVITY: How true do you think it is to say that a greater lifespan will inevitably lead to an increasing period of ill health and dependency? As we read this passage we began to wonder whether changes in lifestyle and particularly in nutrition, as well as medical improvements, will gradually feed through into an increasing healthy lifespan overall. Try to find out what the latest research is on this. Does this support ter Meulen's claim? In his paper Ruud ter Meulen goes on to accept that this might indeed be the case and have some effect, but he argues that:

The gap is too wide to be bridged by these behavioural changes. As for the Netherlands, the Dutch Institute for Preventive Medicine has calculated that the healthy life expectancy for Dutch males is 60 years, while their average life expectancy is 73 years. For Dutch females, the healthy life period ends at age 58, while their average life expectancy is 80 years (Hofman, 1991). Though it might be possible to improve our physical condition (partic-

ularly the capacity of our organs) by healthy behaviour, it will take at least several decades to bridge a gap of 22 years, as is, for example, the case for Dutch women.

He goes on to argue that,

Noting the difference between healthy life expectancy and average life expectancy, we can understand better the increasing demand for long-term care. This is particularly true for the over 80s, the fastest growing age group in the industrialized world: from 16 million in the EC in 1980 to 29 million in 2010 (Taket, 1992). This age group is particularly tortured physically and psychologically by dementia, depression, osteoporosis (including the breaking of hips and arms) and cerebral–vascular accidents. Moreover, 80-year-olds have an increasing chance of smaller, but no less debilitating handicaps, like visual and acoustic impairments, genito-urinary diseases and psychiatric disorders. They are also afflicted by loneliness, social abandonment and poor nutrition (Hamerman and Fox, 1992).

As a result of these handicaps, 80-year-olds are, more than any other age group, dependent on professional care, particularly home care, nursing home care and hospital care. The rapid increase of this age group will result in a sharp rise in the demand for care in the next future.

ACTIVITY: Stop for a moment and consider the likely implications for resource allocation decisions of accepting the claim that the increasing number of sick elderly is responsible for current shortages. What kinds of ethical and practical dilemmas are likely to be a result of this? How do these demographic changes manifest themselves in practice? If demographic changes are indeed the main cause of increasing demand for healthcare resources, one possible response to this might be the use of an age cut-off as a way of deciding who ought to receive treatment. How do you feel about this? Now go on to read the following case study from the Netherlands considering as you do so the ethical questions raised by the idea of age cut-offs.

CASE STUDY: AGE CUT-OFFS

There is in the Netherlands, as in many other countries of western Europe, a chronic shortage of donor organs and because of this there is a waiting list for heart transplant operations. A few years ago it became known publicly that over a period of 5 years, 34 patients had been excluded from this waiting list because they were over 55 years old. Another group were excluded from the list on psychological or social grounds, such as, for example, the fact that they could not speak Dutch. When this happened, there were no medical grounds for such an age cut-off in heart transplant operations. There was known to be some higher risk with increasing age, but nothing which would justify a cut-off as such. During the investigation the cardiologists responsible for managing the list admitted that both the age criteria and the psychological/ social ones were arbitrary but argued that, without such criteria, the number of potential heart transplant patients would rise whilst the number of donors would remain the same. When this selection procedure was made public, it was strongly criticized by a variety of organizations in the Netherlands and, in particular, by the Association of Heart Patients. As a result, the Minister for Welfare, Health and Culture said that he would prohibit the selection of heart transplant patients on the basis of their age. He argued that the selection of patients for medical services should be based upon medical criteria only.

ACTIVITY: In a previous section you looked at some of the problems associated with the allocation of healthcare resources on medical criteria alone. What then are the advantages and disadvantages of the use of age cut-offs as an alternative? You might for example argue along with John Harris (1985) and Michael Lockwood (1988), that the elderly can be said to have had a 'fair innings' or 'fair share' and that younger people ought to get treatment so that they too can share in that which all ought to have. You might, on the other hand, want to argue that all who have need of a transplant ought to be treated equally and treatment ought to be allocated on a first come first served basis. How would you go about resolving such conflicts? How might it be possible to resolve the conflict between the rights of the young and of the elderly? Consider this question as you go on to read the following section of the paper.

Changing attitudes towards the elderly

In his paper Ruud ter Meulen goes on to argue that the association of the scarcity of resources with demographic changes results not simply in limited access for the elderly to healthcare services but also in a growing negative attitude towards the elderly, who are increasingly seen as a burden on society.

The elderly are occupying an increasing number of beds within hospitals, which in some cases results in waiting lists for other, younger patients. The premiums for healthcare insurance are rising in order to pay the increasing costs of the care for the elderly. There is a growing demand for informal care which creates burdens for families and neighbours. These processes might result in a decreasing of the solidarity with the elderly, or at least to a debate about the limits of solidarity between generations.

The attitude to the elderly has never been very positive and may become more negative in times of scarce resources. The phenomenon of elder abuse in nearly all European countries is the writing on the wall (Everaerts et al., 1993). Besides, the elderly already feel that they are discriminated against, covertly or even overtly in the provision of healthcare. Dutch elderly organizations for instance, point to the fact that the majority of waiting lists are for services which are important for the elderly, such as nursing home care, home care, cataract surgery and hip replacements.

Moreover, it should be remembered that demographic change is only partly responsible for the growing demand for healthcare. Much more important is the impact of medicalization and individualization and the decreasing of the solidarity between the generations. The increase of the number and proportion of the elderly is not the main cause of the growing demand for care, but the way the elderly are treated by our society in general and the medical system in particular (Callahan, 1990; Clark, 1989). Such writers claim that the alleged impact of demography on the demand for care is grossly exaggerated: focusing on the demographic process is a way of creating a myth, which hinders an insight into the real causes of the scarcity of resources.

Instead of being blamed, the elderly should be offered new roles and perspectives in our society, by way of retirement policies, voluntary activities and part-time work opportunities. Social values towards the elderly play an important role in the demand for care: a more positive status of the elderly in our society will result in a better health status and a decrease in the demand for care.

This passage suggests that demographic change may be leading to a growing perception of the elderly as a burden and that this will lead to their marginalization and the undermining of the intergenerational solidarity which creates and underpins the sense of duties and responsibilities that together ensure the care of the elderly by the young (on the implicit understanding that their children would do the same for them). It suggests that there is reason to believe that this intergenerational solidarity, like other social structures, is coming under increasing strain because a limited number of the young have to provide for an ever-increasing number of dependent elderly. When we were reading this, we found ourselves wondering whether intergenerational solidarity has really declined or whether the young are simply less able to care for their elderly relatives because of the other demands of contemporary life. In the next section Ruud ter Meulen takes up this question.

One of the main issues of an ageing society is the solidarity between the generations and the obligations between the young and the old. In former times, these obligations were firmly established. The young had a duty to support their elderly parents with financial and other material means. The old in turn, supported the young, for example, with education and care for children while the parents were at work. These obligations were based on the principle of reciprocity: the young supported the old, while the old supported the young (Callahan, 1987).

Besides the mutual support between young and old in the family, there was, from the beginning of this century, a sense of solidarity between the generations. On the basis of the principle of solidarity the old were increasingly supported financially in their access to medical and social services. This solidarity is expressed in the payment of health-care insurance premiums, premiums for pension schemes and taxes which are used for services for the old.

Both forms of intergenerational solidarity are coming increasingly under strain. First, there is a continuous change in the dependency ratio between the young and the old. A decreasing number of young people have to support financially an increasing number of older people. This a general problem for an ageing society, which poses not only a problem for healthcare, but also for other services for the elderly, like pension schemes. A solution for this problem might be to allow (or to force) the elderly to work longer than the retirement age at this time. This strategy is complicated by a shortage of jobs, which in the future will continue to be the case because of the ongoing entrance of women into the labour force. The change in the dependency ratio results in an increase of premiums for pensioning and healthcare insurance. The young will have less to spend for themselves and for the care for their children. The tension between the young and the old will continue to rise (De Jouvenel, 1990).

Solidarity between the generations is also strained by another process. In former times, this solidarity was supported by traditional living arrangements, like the family and the neighbourhood. Recently, these arrangements and structures have been subject to profound change. Instead of the traditional family with two parents, other forms of living together or of child-rearing have developed. Children are not living in the same neighbourhood as their parents, but are moving to other cities or parts of the country. Traditional values such as altruism and solidarity have to be adjusted to these new living arrangements. As a result, there is a vagueness about the obligations of the young to the old.

One must not forget, however, that we are talking here about general processes. Sociological studies show, that on the micro-level families still play a dominant role in the care for the elderly (Johnson, 1993). Solidarity between the generations is a multidimensional concept: family members who are living at a geographical distance may still feel a strong sense of solidarity, while family members living close to each other may have grown apart in a social sense (Johnson, 1993).

The relations and obligations between generations are of extreme importance for every society. For the future, the values of reciprocity and solidarity must be underlined. None the less, we have to rethink these values and adapt them to a changing society.

ACTIVITY: To what extent, after reading this passage, do you feel that the decline in social solidarity is a real phenomenon? If it is, one solution to this divide and to the fracture of social solidarity would be to argue that the allocation of healthcare resources ought to be determined according to principles with more of a community-based, or 'communitarian' focus. That is, the criterion upon which decisions ought to be made is the extent to which a certain pattern of allocation would tend to support and increase social solidarity and community well-being.

It might be argued that this would tend to lead to decisions opposed to those which would have been made on the basis of an age cut-off. The implication of such an argument would be that we would spend *more* money on the elderly than on the young, the resulting increase in social solidarity being argued to lead to a decrease in demand for healthcare and to an easing of the scarcity of healthcare resources. But such claims are inevitably based upon empirical projections about the likely effects of such actions and it is open to opponents to claim the opposite. Indeed, Daniel Callahan, for example, is a well-known communitarian who does argue for age cut-offs. List the advantages and disadvantages of such an argument and approach.

The goals of medicine

Daniel Callahan has argued that one of the reasons for the shortage of resources is the distorted aims and goals of modern medicine, and this is reflected also in the Dunning report's emphasis on technology as a causal factor. Callahan argues that emphasis on life-extending treatments both costs a great deal and leads to an increased period of dependency rather than of health. Now read the following passage from Ruud ter Meulen's paper and consider the extent to which the emphasis of modern medicine on technology and on life-extending treatment is responsible for the shortage of resources.

The increase in average life expectancy in this century is partly due to the successes of medicine, particularly preventive and acute care medicine. Especially in the last two decades, medicine has succeeded in the extending of life. In view of the increasing chance of chronic, debilitating diseases at the later stages of life, we have to consider whether a further increase of life expectancy is desirable.

One of the main priorities of scientific research in medicine is to find the causes of ageing, in order to increase the maximal life expectancy. Though a fundamental breakthrough is not to be expected soon, researchers are already talking openly about a maximal life expectancy of 130 or even 140 years. Ageing is considered as a disease and not as something we have to accept as part of our human condition. Some years ago, Leon Kass stated that healthcare is more oriented towards fighting diseases which are the main causes of death, than focusing on the main causes of poor health (Kass, 1981). One fatal condition is exchanged for another. Human immortality, Kass says, seems to be the main goal of medicine. Medical progress is measured in terms of life years that have been won. Differences in level of health between countries are measured in average life expectancy.

The total elimination of the main killer diseases in old age, such as cancer and heart disease, would not have much effect on the average life expectancy. If these fatal diseases are fully eliminated, the average life expectancy at birth would rise by 6 or 7 years, while the average life expectancy at 65 years of age would only rise by 1 or 1.5 years. Instead of focusing on an unattainable ideal, the physician might do better to recognise the finiteness of human existence.

The dominant orientation of medicine towards the quantity of life, instead of quality of life, also manifests itself in the increased use of life-extending care for very aged persons. In particular, cardiosurgical treatment (e.g. bypass grafting and percutaneous transluminal coronary angioplasty) is increasingly used for persons above 80 years old. A leading Dutch cardiologist said recently that age is not an indication against such treatments, in cases where they are used for people in a good condition (Koster, 1990).

We must be careful, however, not to accuse medicine of having only a one-sided approach. We are ourselves very willing to reap the fruits of the progress of medical technology (Callahan, 1990). In its attempt to prolong our lives, medicine is acting on a desire that has been governing our culture for several centuries. From the beginning of the Modern Age, that is around 1600, we have been fascinated by the idea that human life is something which can be extended and that death can be postponed (Achterhuis, 1988). The scarcity of resources is, for a large part, determined by a cultural process, in which the extension of life is made an absolute ideal. One forgets, however, that we are all going to die some time, in spite of all efforts to extend life. Life cannot be extended into eternity (Callahan, 1990). This is not possible, but it is

also not desirable. A longer life will result in worsening health. Moreover, the meaning of life is closely connected to the finiteness of life. The Dutch philosopher van Tongeren states in this respect, that the quality of our life is mainly determined by our attitude towards death (Van Tongeren, 1990).

ACTIVITY: If it is true to say that modern medicine's emphasis on life-extending treatment is at least partly to blame for lack of resources, what are the implications of this for how we view old age? Is it true, as Daniel Callahan claims, that the attempt to extend the life of the elderly is somehow to demean it and to deny the value of old age as a distinct period? If we continue to consider active, future-oriented life as the only valuable life, this might indeed lead us to overlook the distinct values and features of old age. But need it necessarily be the case that we have to reject such treatments in order to respect this period of life? What does this have to say about our attitude to death and the end of life? What does the idea of 'stages of life' mean to you? Stop for a moment and attempt to describe in your own words just what it is that makes the end of life a distinct period. How difficult was this? Do you now feel that the valuing of this period of life is made more difficult by life-extending treatments or more easy? If so, how?

The desire for a long life goes together with a devaluation of old age as a distinct and meaningful period of life. In a society which values health and long life in a dominant way, old age can only be seen as a deviation or even as a disease which must be fought or suppressed (Cole, 1988, 1992). Old age is no more than a prolonging of middle age, without a meaning of its own. Considering the fast maturation of the young, on the one hand, and the pursuit of a long and active life, on the other hand, we are moving, as Bernice Neugarten styled it, towards an 'age-irrelevant' society in which 'eternal youth' is the universal norm (Moody, 1991a).

The increasing medicalization of old age is linked to the absence of a view on the meaning of old age (Callahan, 1987). The medicalization of old age, and therewith the over-utilization of healthcare services may be stopped when we recognize ourselves as fragile and mortal beings. According to Callahan (1987), fragility and mortality will only be accepted, when we know how to give meaning to the last stages of our life.

The growing need for care, particularly long-term care for chronic diseases, poses an important problem for the allocation of healthcare resources. As long as the healthcare budget is not allowed to increase (that is, as part of the GNP), there will continue to be an increasing scarcity of resources for long-term care facilities, like nursing homes, home care and homes for the elderly.

One possibility might be a reallocation of resources from acute care to long-term care. According to Callahan (1987) the increasing scarcity of long-term care must be addressed by the introduction of an age limit for expensive life-extending treatment, paid from collective funds. After reaching a 'natural lifespan' (which is not a biological, but a biographical measure), elderly patients should not receive life-extending therapies. In exchange, the elderly should have an increased access to long-term care facilities.

Callahan's proposal has been strongly criticized as a kind of 'ageist' discrimination (Barry and Bradley, 1991; Binstock and Post, 1991). Gerontologists and liberal ethicists have argued that every age has its own aims and that no one can determine for another whether this life is completed or this 'natural lifespan' has been reached. There is no reason to believe, they argue, that an old person would value his life less than a younger one. When one considers only years of life instead of life only, one shows no respect for the unique value of the human person, which is the moral basis for our society.

On the other hand, there is some truth in the argument that people who are 75 years old have had a 'fair share' of life, or 'fair innings' (Harris, 1987). We all have the moral intuition that to die young is a sorrow and a tragedy, but that to die at an old age is a sorrow, but no tragedy. In a situation in which treatment possibilities are limited,

and a choice must be made between a person who had a fair share and one who had not, it would be reasonable to choose for the latter.

When we read this section we wondered how true it is that the costs of caring for the elderly are in fact due to high-tech life-extending treatments. There is some reason to doubt Callahan's claim about the financial savings to be made by cutting life-extending treatments. Increases in healthcare expenditure as a result of old age tend not to be the result of the use of life-extending treatments, but are, in fact, largely due to the cost of visits to general practitioners and of hospitalization. The majority of admissions for the elderly are for life-enhancing care, that is care designed to improve those physical functions which are needed for normal daily activities and not for life extension. The operations most commonly carried out on the elderly in Dutch hospitals, for example, are cataract surgery, prostate surgery, hip replacement and treatment for inguinal ruptures. The most common form of life-extending treatment (coronary bypass grafting) appears only at number 14 in this list.

Only a negligible proportion of the patients in nursing homes are treated with life-extending technologies, like artificial ventilation, resuscitation and artificial feeding. It is true to say that, for each person, the majority of their healthcare costs are incurred at the end of life, particularly in the last 12 months of life. These are, however, mainly costs for nursing and caring and only for a negligible part for aggressive, intensive treatment for patients who are moribund. Professor ter Meulen agrees:

Limiting acute, life-extending care to the elderly will, at this moment, not solve the allocation problem. Though there may be an ethical argument in favour of setting limits to the elderly, there will be no financial gain. Moreover, the introduction of age criteria will reinforce the discrimination against the elderly and the process of scapegoating of the elderly for the scarcity of healthcare resources. Besides, there will be strong resistance with the medical profession toward age limits: every physician will try to get the best treatments for their patient.

However, there is an increasing tendency, particularly in the United States, to put very old people on life-extending therapies. The number of people above 80 years old who are getting organ transplants, open heart surgery or are put on renal dialysis is increasing. A study by Hosking et al. (1989) revealed that there has been a large improvement in post-operative survival after surgery among patients 90 years of age and older in the past two decades. While in 1972 Denney and Denson found a 30-day surgical mortality rate of 29 per cent for patients 90 years of age and older, Hosking found a 30-day case fatality rate of 8.4 per cent. Although a direct comparison between both studies was not possible, the outcomes of Hoskings' study suggests that elderly persons at a high age are tolerating better the stress of surgical procedures. This could have been the result of better surgical and anaesthetic advances, as well as of the improvement of medical care (Hosking et al., 1989). However, there was no clear sign of improvement in survival over years in the study period.

Callahan's proposal of setting limits is, in fact, an attempt to prepare for a future where expensive life-extending therapies have become normal procedures for people over eighty or even ninety years of age (Callahan, 1994). We should be careful indeed, not to try to increase the average life span by expensive technological devices, but instead focus our efforts on an improvement of long-term care facilities. However, this process of re-orientation and re-allocation should not be done by way of direct and overt age limits for clinical procedures on the micro-level. It is politically more feasible to reallocate resources for the elderly by indirect means, for example, by the setting of research priorities (more money for research for chronic diseases) and the allocation of resources on the macro-level (more nursing homes instead of Intensive Care Units) (Moody, 1991b).

Finding extra resources in the family

We hinted earlier that much of the strain of underfunded health services inevitably has greatest impact upon families. The strain is taken by them. And this points to the fact that as health-care resources become more limited, pressure will build for health services to find resources externally in the form of informal care and by requiring patients and their families to contribute to the costs of their treatment or care in the form of 'co-payments' (see Glossary). Now continue your reading of the paper by ter Meulen.

There is a fundamental belief in most industrialized countries that national governments have an obligation to supply resources for the care of the elderly and, in particular, for long-term care. Because of the increasing number and proportion of the elderly, however, and the growing demand for care, families, relatives and neighbours will inevitably get involved in the care for chronically ill and even debilitated elderly family members (or neighbours). Daughters in particular are coming under an increasing pressure to care for their elderly parents (Abel, 1991). Family care imposes considerable strain on the caregiver. It may be a heavy physical and psychological burden for the individuals, who may fall ill themselves. Moreover, caregivers have to invest time and money in the care of their parents, which may impede their own contributions to pension schemes (Evers and Olk, 1991).

Informal caregivers not only have obligations towards their parents, but also towards their own children. Moreover, they want to realize their own life plans by way of professional career or by private activities. These plans and obligations are threatened when they have to care for their dependent parents. Though most individuals feel an obligation to care for those who cared for them in their childhood, there is an increasing vagueness about the way these obligations are to be balanced against other obligations. This vagueness results in feelings of uneasiness and feelings of guilt.

The gap between the demand for care and the supply of care is too high to be bridged by efficiency measures. Rationing or prioritizing of services will be inevitable. However, national governments are not prepared to make such hard choices. Instead of removing entire services from the basic package, the Dutch Government, for example, is removing parts of these services and expecting them to be paid out-of-pocket by individuals, who are allowed to take a private additional insurance for these (parts of) services. In particular, non-medical services, like housecleaning for dependent elderly people, are to be paid by the individuals out of their own pockets. Furthermore, the Government is introducing an increasing number of deductibles and co-payments, particularly for long-term care. Co-payments are already existent for services reimbursed by the Exceptional Medical Expenses Act, like psychotherapy and nursing home care. Co-payments for home care, already existent for some time, have been increased in the past years, though they are bound to a fixed maximum amount each month.

Co-payments, compulsory deductibles and private additional insurance, are in fact the policy of the Dutch Government to cope with the scarcity of resources. This policy of increased financial contributions by individuals will have a significant impact on the solidarity of the higher with the lower income groups as well as on the solidarity of the high risks with the low risks. Both 'income' and 'risk' solidarity are the pillars of the social

healthcare insurance. Such financial contributions are a greater burden for lower income groups than for higher income earners, even if these contributions are income dependent and fixed to a maximum level. The same applies for the premiums for a private additional insurance, which are easier for the better-off. This additional insurance will endanger risk solidarity as well. Such an insurance is a private legal insurance against health damages. Acceptance of persons with high risk (for example, persons with chronic disease) is not obligatory for such a private insurance.

The increase of financial responsibility upon the individuals in healthcare insurance is, in fact, part of a change within the entire system of social security of the Welfare State. For example, in 1993 there was a dramatic cut in the benefits (and the eligibility criteria) for the industrial disability insurance. Individuals were allowed to negotiate privately or collectively for a private additional insurance to bridge the gap between the new benefits and the old ones, in case of enduring disability for work. This policy is meant to decrease the part of the collective expenditures in the Gross National Product. The Government has no objections against private expenditures for healthcare or other forms of social insurance, even if they raise the total amount of expenditures. By keeping down the collective part, the compulsory premiums for healthcare and other social insurance are kept low and incomes (before tax) will not have to be increased.

The shift from public expenditure towards private will inevitably result in a greater gap between the well-off and the lower income groups. This divide is reinforced by the introduction of market forces and nominal premiums in the national healthcare insurance. Individuals are free to insure themselves for services not included in the basic package by an additional premium. This additional premium allows individuals to insure themselves for a better quality of care as well, for example, in the up-and-coming private clinics. These clinics do not have waiting lists and ensure the client of a quick and comfortable service for their complaints. An increasing number of business corporations are making contracts with these clinics. Part of the costs of sickness payments made by the employers are costs of time waiting for a treatment in a hospital. By a quick service in private clinics these costs can be reduced.

The elderly are affected most by this policy, because they have low incomes and are more dependent on healthcare services, particularly home care and long-term care (where co-payments will be dominant). However, instead of rationing by objective criteria, most nations will address the scarcity problem by rationing by income, and thus by age. The gap between the haves and the have-nots will be further increased by liberalism, individualism and economic competition (market mechanisms).

The elderly as a political force

The elderly are set to form an increasingly large proportion of the electorate and thus have the potential for an increased political influence. This might be one way in which the elderly might be able to enhance respect for this period of life, changing the perception of them as a burden.

Though the ethical issues described above, are common for most industrialized countries, there are national and regional differences in the way these issues are addressed. For example, the very low prestige of the elderly in the post-communist countries of Central and Eastern Europe contrasts sharply with the relatively well-off position of the elderly in the Western world. Remarkable also are the large differences in the way the elderly are organized in Western Europe and the United States. In the US the elderly are a powerful lobby

group with strong political influence. In Europe on the contrary, the elderly are hardly organized and have (thus far) little political influence. This situation might change in the near future: in the Netherlands political parties for the elderly have entered Parliament in the past national elections and are pulling away votes from the traditional parties.

Though the ethical issues manifest themselves in various ways, national governments of the developed countries have taken hardly any measures in this respect. Most of these governments are well aware of the changing demographic situation, and some have taken some measures to improve the medical, social and economical situation of the elderly. However, long-range planning is absent almost everywhere. This is particularly true for care for the elderly, where acute care is still dominant in respect with long-term care and social care. The need for long-term care will raise serious moral problems in the institutions as well as in families caring for their elderly parents. However, the greatest victims of this lack of planning will be the elderly themselves.

ACTIVITY: Are there any organizations for the elderly in your country or your local area which have entered into this debate? What are they arguing about and what has been their contribution to the debate? Make a note of the key points raised by this section.

Section 4: Health economics, markets and healthcare rationing

In Section 3 we asked you to undertake a guided reading exercise about allocating scarce medical resources by age criteria. Rationing by age appears at first to coincide with rationing by evidence-based medical criteria – discussed in Section 2 – in the very rough sense that older people are likely to have less favourable outcomes. However, this is a very rough guide indeed, and, in fact, a genuinely evidence-based analysis would reveal that age is by no means a reliable indicator of treatment success. For this reason, and others suggested in the paper by Ruud ter Meulen on which the reading exercise was based, rationing healthcare by age alone turns out to be an unjustified form of discrimination which contradicts both the principle of justice – treating equals equally – and good clinical practice. In justice, conceived as treating equals equally and unequals unequally, age of itself does not constitute one of the substantive relevant inequalities which justify a smaller share of the 'cake'. We shall be returning to a discussion of this question in Section 5 when we look at the work of Norman Daniels.

THE CASE OF MARGARET DAVIS

If anyone is a testament to the benefits of high-tech medicine can offer the elderly, 98-year-old Margaret Davis is that person.

Davis, who turns 99 this month, is doing well after undergoing open heart surgery at Emory University Hospital in Atlanta for replacement of her aortic valve and double coronary artery bypass surgery – the oldest patient ever to undergo the procedure at the hospital.

'I feel great', says Davis, 'and I can breathe again'.

Even her own doctor, however, concedes that performing such complex, costly procedures on people of advanced age raises ethical issues, especially as the nation begins to talk about 'setting limits' on care as a way to conserve medical resources.

Joe Craver, M M, the Emory cardiothoracic surgeon who operated on Davis, says his patient was physically capable of undergoing surgery and was leading an active life until her illness slowed her down. She was living independently, and pursuing hobbies such as fishing and playing bridge. She had had coronary artery disease for some time, but felt fine until last spring, when she began experiencing shortness of breath.

'Except for her heart problems,' Craver says,

'she was in good shape. Physically, she was better equipped to withstand surgery than most people in their 70s.'

While there was some risk involved, Craver says, surgery was the only alternative doctors could offer Davis. Without it, he says, she probably would not have lived longer than 6 months (*Medical Ethics Advisor*, 1993).

You may be wondering by now, however, whether we will ever come to a definite agreement about what the substantive relevant inequalities really are. If not – and agreement does seem unlikely – then why not bypass the entire attempt to find a philosophically satisfying set of criteria for rationing scarce healthcare resources? Why not let an impersonal mechanism such as the market determine the allocation of scarce healthcare resources? Perhaps letting the market decide would be actually fairer *and* more efficient than trying to intervene with principles of justice on which no ultimate agreement can be reached. By being the most efficient means of allocation, it would also be the fairest insofar as there would be minimum waste. By lessening waste, and allowing national health services to concentrate on the neediest cases, markets have even been argued to increase social solidarity – although solidarity is generally seen as a socialist value and markets as associated with liberal individualism, on opposite sides of the political spectrum. The Dutch Secretary of State for Health, for example, stated early in the 1990s that, by introducing a market in healthcare, the costs of care could be reduced and that this would result in either a lower price for healthcare insurance or at least a slower rate of increase in premiums. Markets have become a dominant concept in healthcare throughout Europe, and few practitioners have escaped the effects of injecting market mechanisms into health services.

This proposition – that markets in healthcare are both the fairest and the most efficient means of allocating scarce resources – is the proposition which we will examine critically in Section 4. You will undertake two more guided reading exercises: the first on the *use of economic evaluation in healthcare allocation*, and the second on *markets, community and healthcare rationing*. Whereas Section 2 mainly dealt with *medical* criteria for resource allocation, and Section 3 the *social* question of age cut-offs and solidarity with older people, Section 4 concerns *economic* criteria, and we will also examine some concrete cases about cost and benefit. Thus economic models of resource allocation will be our concern here, in contrast to Section 5, which will consider philosophical models.

We will conclude that an economic analysis, in fact, has much the same effect as an explicit decision to ration by age: it discriminates, although not intentionally, against older people. More generally, economic analysis is *not* value-free, and the market ideology rests on a shaky construction of unexamined philosophical views. So we cannot just bypass ethical debates about resource allocation by letting the market decide.

To put it another way, so far our discussion has assumed that governments, health authorities, or other purchasers must intervene to allocate actively resources between competing recipients. We have conceived this as a problem in distributive justice, treating equals equally and unequals unequally. But, according to proponents of markets in healthcare, such active intervention is neither politically desirable nor economically efficient. Can we avoid value choices about whom to favour by letting the impersonal mechanism of the market decide?

ACTIVITY: Stop for a moment and think about 'markets in healthcare'. What does the term mean to you?

The term 'market' may seem out of place in healthcare. To many people, a market is a physical location in which goods are exchanged between individuals: what can this possibly have to do with medicine?

One economist has written, 'Originally a market was a public place in a town where provisions and other objects were exposed for sale; but the word has been generalized, so as to mean any body of

persons who are in intimate business relations and carry on extensive transactions in any commodity' (Jevons, quoted in Marshall 1936, p. 270). This takes us a little further, by making it plain that a market need not occupy one physical space. But its discussion of 'intimate business relations' and 'extensive transactions in any commodity' still jars somewhat, when applied to healthcare. A more helpful definition emphasizes the co-ordinating role of the market in transactions of all kinds, not necessarily in business or commodities: 'The crucial feature of the market as a co-ordination device is that it involves voluntary exchange of goods and services between two parties at a known price. Through a complex set of such exchanges the economic activities of people who are widely dispersed and who are entirely unaware of each other's existence can be co-ordinated' (Levacic, 1991).

Now read this selection by the Belgian economists Diana de Graeve and Ines Adriaenssen, of the University of Antwerp: 'Use of economic evaluation in healthcare allocation.' (You will find that unfamiliar terms are highlighted in bold; please look in the Glossary at the end of this chapter for a definition.)

The use of economic evaluation in healthcare allocation

Diana de Graeve and Ines Adriaenssen

Resources, such as people, time, equipment and knowledge, are scarce. This is the main reason why choices must be made concerning their allocation. For the majority of goods and services, this allocation decision is left to the market. In the medical sector, however, market imperfections such as uncertainty, **external effects** and information asymmetry hamper an **efficient** allocation via the market. Allocation decisions with respect to medical care, are often made by government or health authorities. Economic evaluation becomes an aid to these decision-makers when deciding among different uses for scarce resources.

Two features characterize economic evaluation. Firstly, it deals with both the costs (C) and consequences or effects (E) of activities. Secondly, economic analysis involves the comparison between two or more alternatives. These two characteristics lead us to define economic evaluation as the comparative analysis of alternative courses of action in terms of both their costs and consequences. Economic evaluation thus calculates the additional cost that is needed to obtain an additional benefit. . . . In the case of comparing two alternatives, this can be written mathematically as $(C2-C1)/(E2-E1)$. This ratio is called a cost–effectiveness ratio.

Measurement of costs

The costs of a medical intervention consist of all additional resources used in the intervention. Two concepts are important when measuring the use of resources: opportunity cost and marginal cost.

The costs of using resources for some purpose should be measured as their *opportunity cost*. In perfect markets, the market price is a good approximation of opportunity cost. However, the healthcare market is not a perfect market. Prices are often 'negotiated tariffs' (e.g. negotiated fees for services). In other instances healthcare services may be provided free (e.g. by the voluntary sector). Economic evaluations also use *marginal* or incremental costs, the additional costs needed to introduce or expand the healthcare programme.

We can further distinguish direct, indirect and intangible costs. Direct costs are associated directly with the medical intervention. This does not mean that only medical costs can be included, however: direct costs include both medical expenses (e.g. drugs, physician care, nursing treatment) or non-medical expenses (e.g. travel costs to and from treatment centres, special equipment purchased for the home). Indirect medical costs include cost of medical treatment in the additional life-years obtained through the treatment, which would not otherwise have been expected, while indirect non-medical costs refer to costs asso-

ciated with reduced productivity due to illness, disability or premature death. Intangible costs cover pain, anger and suffering occurring as a result of the intervention.

ACTIVITY: Stop for a moment and try to apply these categories of cost to a treatment decision which you recently had to make for yourself or in discussion with a patient. How many of these categories did you take into account?

We found many of the categories quite unexpected and difficult to apply, particularly indirect medical costs – which seemed an odd way to consider what to us is a benefit, added life-years. We felt more comfortable with intangible costs, which are close to the more familiar idea of iatrogenic harm, from the Greek for 'harm arising from the doctor'. That is, these are costs arising from treatment which has gone wrong, or from side effects even from treatment which proceeds as expected.

Measurement of benefits

There are four basic types of economic evaluation:
(a) Cost–minimization analysis
(b) Cost–effectiveness analysis
(c) Cost–benefit analysis
(d) Cost–utility analysis

ACTIVITY: Note the possibilities of differentiation here. To many practitioners, all economic analysis is the same; no doubt you've heard the complaint that 'all that counts these days is money'. One purpose of reading this article by two economists is to gain a more sophisticated view.

The identification and measurement of the costs is similar in the four types of economic evaluations. The measurement of the consequences, that is, the health improvement, differs, however. Let us first discuss how benefits can be measured.

When alternatives accomplish the same desired outcome, the economic evaluation is essentially a search for the least expensive alternative. An analysis such as this is called a cost–minimization analysis. Such an analysis is only justified, however, when there is good evidence of the equality of outcomes – a condition which is often lacking.

ACTIVITY: Try to think of an example from health-care provision. One that comes to mind is generic v. name-brand drugs: the justification for limiting pre-scribing to a generic list, at least, is that the generic drug is usually as effective.

Usually, the health improvement gained through various interventions differs in one or more dimensions. The easiest case is when the health improvement which we wish to compare is limited to one dimension: for example, lives saved, years of life gained, or number of days without pain. In this case we would not automatically lean towards the least expensive programme. Rather, we would compare the cost per unit of beneficial outcome (i.e. cost per year of life gained). Such an analysis, in which costs are related to a single common effect that may differ in magnitude between alter-native interventions, is usually referred to as a cost-effectiveness analysis.

More realistically, the desired outcome usually differs in several aspects between the alternatives (e.g. physical, emotional and social quality of health, as well as quantity of life-years). In order to come up with a single summary score, we can translate all the effects into monetary terms. An analysis that measures both the costs and the con-sequences of alternatives in terms of money is called a cost–benefit analysis. . . . Willingness to pay, established through survey methods, is a theoretically sound monetary valuation of health improvement, although the methodology to measure this valuation is only just developing. Another method is the 'human capital' approach, which limits measurement of benefits to increased (market) productivity and values the productivity on the basis of market earnings. In this way it dis-criminates against the elderly, housewives, and people with severe disabilities because these groups are less likely to be employed.

ACTIVITY: Can all effects be translated into mone-tary terms, do you think? Note that the authors recog-nize the problems in doing so without using indicators that favour certain groups: either those who can pay for health improvements, or those with human capital that can be translated into market earnings. (The two groups overlap.) Already we are beginning to see how the attempt to create value-neutral, quantifiable indicators does not avoid difficult ethical questions about justice and fairness.

Finally, the fourth method of economic analysis is the cost-utility calculation. The best-known type of cost–utility analysis involves Quality-Adjusted Life-Years (QALYs), which combines duration and quality of life in so-called utility-adjusted life-years. Instead of simply comparing how many life-years can be saved through various interventions, QALY analysis weights in how much value or utility people attach to a year in a particular status: complete freedom from pain, moderate pain, minor disability, major disability and so forth. The weights used reflect individual prefer-ences, standardised between 0 and 1. The value of zero corresponds to death, whereas one equals perfect health. The results of such a cost-utility analysis are expressed in terms of the cost per QALY.

Type of analysis	Unit of measurement of benefits
Cost–minimization analysis	No measure (assumed equal)
Cost–effectiveness analysis	Unidimensional 'natural' units (e.g. life-years)
Cost–benefit analysis	Monetary units
Cost–utility analysis	Utility units (e.g. QALYs)

Imagine, for example, that the patient's state of health after a certain treatment receives a utility of 0.75. This means that the patient is indifferent between 12 months in health state X and 9 months in perfect health. Thus comparisons between treatments can be undertaken without having to translate them into monetary values.

ACTIVITY: Think about the ethical as well as the economic advantages and disadvantages of QALYs. On the face of it, they appear to give a voice to patients' individual preferences, which can be weighted into an economic analysis. And they don't translate everything into monetary terms. On the other hand, when QALYs are used as the basis of health policy decisions, all preferences must be aggregated, and this leads to ethical problems. The medical ethicist John Harris (Harris, 1987) has attacked QALYs because they require an unsupported leap from what I would prefer for myself to what I would prefer for you.

To put this argument another way, **utilitarians** – who seek to maximize total **welfare**, as does cost–utility analysis – are sometimes accused of overriding minority preferences. The utilitarian philosopher John Stuart Mill claimed 'that happiness is a good: that each person's happiness is a good to that person; and the general happiness, therefore, is a good to the aggregate of all persons.' (Mill, cited in Haydock, 1992, p. 185). It is the jump from the second premise to the conclusion that is faulty. In the extreme, it might increase the general happiness of a fascist society for a particular race to be exterminated, and in Mill's view it would therefore be a good to the aggregate of all persons in that society, including the members of that race.

To apply this to healthcare, try to think of a specific example in which the preferences of the majority and those of minorities may collide. One that comes to my mind is the rationalization of services in London, which, it was felt, was receiving a disproportionate share of resources because of the concentration of major teaching hospitals there, while its primary care services were often poorer than the average because of the large number of single-practitioner inner-city services. The Tomlinson report recommended closure of some hospitals in favour of improving primary care; but although all Londoners might arguably benefit from better primary care – which everyone uses – the minorities served by the closed hospitals will not.

It is not clear how we are supposed to benefit from a system which maximizes aggregate utility if we are denied treatment in the name of aggregated preferences throughout society as a whole. But politicians and health purchasers must make decisions for aggregates, not individuals. This takes us back to the difficult questions about distributive justice with which we have been wrestling throughout this chapter. 'The utilitarian principle is concerned with the interests of the majority, but justice is concerned with the interests of each person equally' (Downie, cited in Dickenson, 1995, p. 230).

Before concluding our discussion of benefits, we should note that costs and benefits frequently occur at different times. For example, vaccination against pneumococcus pneumonia occurs in Year 1, when the costs are incurred; but illness will be prevented for 5 years, not just for Year 1. People are not indifferent with respect to timing: they prefer benefits now and costs in the future.

ACTIVITY: This is one constraint on using a cost–benefit ratio in economic analysis. What other similar constraints might there be?

Costs and benefits are also incurred by different parties: for example, GPs would be responsible for costs in the vaccination example, but hospitals would be the gainers insofar as they would not have to treat people who would otherwise develop severe pneumonias. Similarly, the costs of providing national health services fall on taxpayers, but the benefits accrue disproportionately to older people simply because they are more likely to be ill. In a pay-as-you-go system such as the UK's, the current generation of taxpayers is financing the care of the elderly. This is what makes the allocation of scarce healthcare resources a contentious political issue.

Economic evaluation and allocation of resources for the elderly

Economic evaluation itself is indifferent to age. It only looks at costs and benefits that will be generated through a healthcare intervention, aiming to maximise health benefits within a given budget. Take the example of two proposed interventions:

(a) a vaccination campaign against hepatitis B for babies
(b) a vaccination programme against pneumococcus in the elderly

Suppose that the costs of the two campaigns are the same, and that benefits are measured in QALYs. Then the cost–utility style of analysis will favour the programme which generates the most QALYs.

ACTIVITY: Which programme will this be?

The 'winner' will be programme (a), because more potential life-years with good quality of life can be gained for babies. Older people have a shorter life expectation, and a greater likelihood of chronic disease in the remaining years, so that their quality-weighted life-years will be fewer.

Age may influence costs as well as benefits generated by an intervention, however. Older patients, in general, generate higher treatment costs than younger individuals, with the exception of children. They often have higher risks for complications, poorer initial health, and longer time requirements for recovery. For example, it has been found that hospital treatment costs for pneumococcal pneumonia in Belgium were about twice as high for the over-65s as for younger adults. In addition the probability of hospitalization is, respectively, 10 per cent for younger adults as against 30 per cent for the over-65s (Lombaert et al., 1997). A similar positive correlation between age and treatment costs was found for HIV-related disease and AIDS (de Graeve et al., 1997).

Indirect non-medical costs are also clearly related to age, reflecting as they do reduced productivity due to illness. They are most often measured as the market wage rate which the individual would have received during days of absence, in the human capital approach. In principle pensioners do not have market productivity or indirect non-medical costs. Thus a medical intervention which shortens illness duration and saves on indirect costs will put non-economically active people at a great disadvantage.

Cost and effectiveness are not independent. The increased cost generated in treating older people arises because older people tend to respond less well to treatment and because their capacity for rehabilitation is less. For example, whereas 80 per cent of patients under 60 who have suffered a hip fracture are able to walk at 1 year, only 6 per cent of those older than 90 make such a recovery. Another example is that of influenza vaccine, which is approximately 60 per cent effective in younger adults but only 50 per cent effective in the elderly.

It is clear that age will have an impact on the costs and benefits generated by a medical intervention, although the overall effect on net benefit, cost–effectiveness or cost–utility ratio is not always evident. A review of six studies found evidence for an increase in the cost–utility ratio with age (Baltussen et al., 1996). Another study comparing administration of simvastatine and cholestyramine vs. no intervention in reducing cholesterol levels also showed an increase (Tormans et al., 1990). (These results were subsequently used in a proposal to exclude older people from reimbursement for simvastatine on their national medical insurance – a measure which was heavily debated and eventually scrapped.) But the opposite correlation is also possible, as the results of vaccination against influenza virus or pneumococcus bacteria show.

ACTIVITY: So far the economists' discussion has focused on the implications for older people of applying economic analysis, demonstrating the political and ethical implications – the implications for distributive justice – of applying what appear at first to be neutral forms of cost–benefit analysis. Increasingly, we can see that this leads to discrimination against the elderly, unless we consider age to be one of the categories which we will actually want to compensate for under a system of justice which considers it to be one of the substantive inequalities that demands compensation.

Does cost–benefit analysis sometimes inadvertently 'discriminate' against any other groups in society? Think about this question for a moment before going on to the next paragraph.

Our own answer is yes: against women and the disabled for example, as women outlive men by an average of 6 to 7 years; but few cost–benefit analyses take this into account. If, for example, age cut-offs were implemented, they would deprive women of more life-years than they would do for men, because women live longer. The counter-argument might be that QALYs actually discriminate against men; because treatments are cheaper for women in terms of life-years gained per intervention. Women, however, have a higher morbidity and lower quality of life in their final years, with more chronic illness and, since QALYs would also have to take this into account, the overall effect might well be to penalize women.

This leads into the second possible example, disability. One might also argue that disabled people are penalized in QALY analysis for having a 'lower quality of life'. Because QALYs require us to rank different states of health and disability, and then allocate resources according to these rankings, they enshrine in policy judgements value judgements about disability which many disabled rights groups would reject.

In both cases, certain groups are penalized in cost–benefit analysis but whether or not this counts as 'discrimination', although the discrimination is not overt, the consequences for women and the disabled may be unjust. We would need a more comprehensive theory of justice to give a formal answer to this question, but our intention here was simply to show that what purports to be a value-free and fair system may have consequences which harm vulnerable groups.

Conclusion

In an economic evaluation of alternative medical interventions, costs and outcomes are compared with the aim of maximizing beneficial health outcomes within a given budget. Interventions are thus prioritized according to cost–effectiveness, cost–utility ratio, or net benefit (efficiency). This information, however, is only one element upon which decisions about allocating healthcare

resources should be based. Equity considerations are also important, and could equally well be put into practice in order to promote equality consciously. Clearly, a trade-off between equity and efficiency may be necessary.

Moreover, economic evaluation only looks at the efficiency problem in allocating resources; it does not look at social acceptability or political feasibility. It can never become the sole instrument upon which to decide resource allocation. It is only one input factor. As Drummond et al. state (1987), economic evaluation is not intended to be a magic formula for removal of judgement, responsibility and risk from decision-making . . . though it is capable of improving the quality and consistency of decision-making. At root, it is a method of critical thinking . . . placing difficult choices out in the open for discussion.

In their conclusion De Graeve and Adriannesen emphasize that 'economic evaluation only looks at the efficiency problem in the allocation of resources . . . [not] social acceptability or political feasibility'. We have already suggested that economic evaluation is not value free; it results in outcomes, such as fewer resources for older people in a QALY analysis, which raise issues about fairness between generations and which generate political 'heat'. But when such outcomes appear to be the result of market forces rather than deliberate political decisions, they may well appear to remove 'judgement, responsibility and risk from decision-making'. It is worth looking in somewhat more detail at the concept of efficiency, which has become something of a Holy Grail in the politics of healthcare throughout Europe, even in nations with the most strongly socialist, non-market modes of provision. As Mats Thorslund, Åke Bergmark and Marti Parker write (1997b):

What generally characterizes so-called political first-order decisions is an increasing emphasis on 'efficiency' aspects. Measures to increase efficiency may, at least at a rhetorical level, offer temporary respite from the sometimes unpleasant task of prioritizing. When there is doubt about the efficiency of a field or sector, a cutback in resources may serve two different purposes. Firstly, it can be regarded as an incentive to improve overall efficiency and to develop better methods. Secondly, decisions on cutbacks may rest upon the presumption that the resources in the margin of an area can be reduced without any damage to what is considered to be its central task or 'core function'.

In Sweden, as in many other countries, the 1980s saw a substantial improvement in efficiency. There was an emphasis on home-based services which made it possible to decrease the number of institutional beds in many municipalities. During the 1970s and much of the 1980s, care services were actually in need of trimming. Through reorganization and better co-ordination of professional groups, the need for institutional beds was decreased. However, much of the slack in the system has now been removed, and . . . it is doubtful whether further substantial savings can be made.

Sometimes efficiency savings are not controversial, as the Swedish example partly illustrates. It is generally accepted that efficiency advances the interests of both individuals and society; but is this always so? Even anti-marketeers have generally accepted the proposition that allocative efficiency – rewarding the most efficient producers by allocating them a larger share of resources – promotes distributive justice by minimizing scarcity of resources. In addition, there is sometimes claimed to be an element of merit or desert in giving the most resources to, say, hospitals which most successfully reduce their waiting lists or which provide maximal care at minimal cost. At least, this is so in political rhetoric, although it may not seem so fair to, for example, inner-city hospitals with more than their 'fair' share of social problems, hampering them from easily meeting targets for maximizing patient episodes.

ACTIVITY: **Think back again to the case of Mr K. Would you say that the decision to discharge him was taken on efficiency grounds?**

Our own answer is that the decision could actually be seen as inefficient. The Swedish social work professor, Mats Thorslund, points out that so-called 'bedblockers' cost a hospital less than acute cases, and continue to decrease to the level of the hospital's 'hotel' costs of care. We must avoid the trap of assuming that decisions ostensibly taken on economic grounds are necessarily efficient!

It is now time to move on to the final exercise in Section 4, in which we will ask you to read 'Markets, community and healthcare rationing', by Donna Dickenson. The purpose of reading this article is to illustrate how some general principles of economic analysis – which you read about in de Graeve and Adriannesen – have been put into political practice in one national healthcare system, that of the United Kingdom – and why. Again, suggested activity breaks in the reading will highlight particularly relevant, controversial or difficult concepts and arguments. Dickenson's paper analyses the reality of the 'internal market'; although this market approach has been somewhat de-emphasized in the most recent White Paper on the NHS (1998), there is still substantial talk of the reliance on markets and contracts.

Markets, community and healthcare rationing

Donna Dickenson

The United Kingdom's National Health Service appears to be evolving towards an ideologically mixed system. Officially, markets and individual choice are the new orthodoxy, replacing earlier norms of communal solidarity. More privately, it is acknowledged that markets in healthcare exclude a sort of *lumpenproletariat*, or perhaps lumpenpatienten – and that this group is likely to be disproportionately made up of elderly people. The so-called 'demographic time bomb' is accepted uncritically as entailing higher and higher health-care costs as the population 'greys' – even though studies in the US and Canada have found no association between ageing of the population and higher health expenditure, and even though Japan and other countries have a far higher proportion of elderly citizens than does the UK. There is more open talk of a two-tier model of healthcare services delivery and rationing, whatever the original commitment of the NHS to providing a universal service. Not only is there a two-tier system in relation to waiting times for patients of fundholding and non-fundholding general practitioners; there is also open acknowledgement of the likelihood that the NHS may well become a provider of core services only, for a less fortunate core of the population (Hamm, 1996).

This hybrid is intellectually and morally unsatisfactory to pure pro- and anti-marketeers alike. It provides neither a pure 'free market' nor a socialist engine of community solidarity in healthcare. For those who see freedom from fear over healthcare bills as a basic duty which society owes the elderly, it is ethically wrong and practically worrisome to let state-financed healthcare degenerate this way. From the pro-market viewpoint, the optimal distribution of resources should occur naturally in a free market, according to Coase's theorem. There is no need for state intervention, which is construed as interference with free choice.

In the already-established state medical service, markets cannot occur naturally, but they can be created artificially – contradictory though this may appear. An internal market has been set up within the NHS to separate the funding of healthcare from its provision, following principles set out in the 1989 UK government White Paper Working for Patients (DOH, 1989). Purchasing is the province of health authorities, such as that in the case of Mr K, and fundholding general practitioners; providing is done by general practitioners as gatekeepers into the service, and by hospitals, themselves reorganized into independent trusts competing with other providers on free-market principles.

ACTIVITY: If you live in the UK, think of some examples of how these market changes have affected the NHS. If you are not a UK resident, think of any parallels in your own country. Market provision is less common in the Scandinavian countries; for example, in Sweden services for the elderly are still provided primarily within the public sector (Thorslund et al., 1997a, b).

But can markets in healthcare ever be 'free'? Since market mechanisms were introduced into the NHS in 1991, a number of modifications of 'free' principles have occurred. The thrust of these 'reforms' has not necessarily been socialist or communitarian, however. Rather, the managed market notion has replaced the hope of a purely 'free' market, I would argue. The political issue, then, is who does the 'managing', and whether those decisions benefit particular groups disproportionately – or harm others, such as the elderly.

Even in healthcare systems which were never overtly socialist, such as that of the United States, a managed market is the reality, a free market largely rhetorical. Who gets treatment is effectively decided by health-insurance plan managers, directors of Health Maintenance Organizations, and officials of companies providing insurance plans or HMO membership to their employee: by the phenomenon of 'managed care'. The decision about whom not to treat is made in the first instance on the basis of who is covered by one of these categories, or who is not a player in the market; the rest form the 43 million Americans with no healthcare insurance. (A 1996 statute now limits the discretion of insurance firms to refuse coverage to bad risks, further limiting the perfect freedom of the market.)

In the second instance, decisions about how extensively to treat those who do qualify for care are increasingly made not by clinicians, but by administrative policy within HMOs and insurance firms. These bodies are market creations and players, true, private rather than public; but they operate in a very different fashion to what an unreconstructed advocate of markets as enhancing free choice might imagine. For example, a US psychiatrist who requested a brain scan for a patient with depression and chronic headaches, Donna Encheff, was denied the request by the patient's HMO on the grounds that the patient's condition had already been classified as psychological, not physiological. After litigation was threatened, the health plan finally agreed to a scan and surgery for what turned out to be a venous angioma which might have threatened paralysis or death. The 'iron hand of bureaucracy' which Weber so detested lies more heavily, arguably, in private bureaucracies than in public ones.

ACTIVITY: Would it be possible for such limitations on clinical freedom and judgement to occur in your own healthcare system? Consider whether the injection of market mechanisms affects doctor–patient relationships, more broadly. If so, how? One example from the UK concerns cervical screening targets for GPs. The percentage of women to be screened has been set very high in these targets, putting pressure on GPs to screen more women or lose their entitlement for this work. But, elderly women and women from some ethnic minority groups are often unwilling to come forward for screening. Particularly given the unreliability of some cervical cytology results, as publicized extensively in recent cases of large numbers of women having to be recalled, GPs face a difficult ethical and professional dilemma.

In the UK universal entitlement remains the rationale; but whereas Americans who can afford specialist treatment are free to engage the consultant of their choice, if their insurance provider agrees, the British healthcare 'consumer' must still go through her general practitioner for access to more specialized treatment. In advocating an internal market, the Conservative government stressed that patients would, in fact, be free to 'shop around', but this was misleading. The term 'internal market' as first popularized (by Enthoven, 1985) did envision something like that, but this was not the model eventually adopted (see also Mullen, 1991). In many ways, patients are less free to choose than they were under more centralized mechanisms of allocation. If a district health

authority or fundholding GP does not have a contract with a particular hospital, patients can no longer ask to be referred there, as they could have done before the 1991 market mechanisms. Allowing patients to 'shop around' would require their home authorities to reimburse them retrospectively, as in Continental insurance systems, but successive UK governments, both Conservative and Labour, have not chosen to grasp that particular nettle.

A further limitation on both market efficiency and equity for disadvantaged groups is the deliberate preference given to private providers. Once again, this is not a pure market, but a managed one, which deliberately sets out to benefit private nursing homes and private insurance schemes for long-term care. This was certainly a factor in the case of Mr K. A case in Leeds, however, seemed to establish that hospitals could not discharge patients at will to private care, regardless of the ability of their families or of their local services to pay. The Conservative government under John Major gave great prominence to a 'partnership' scheme to provide private insurance cover for long-term care, a measure which was intended to defuse controversy about the displacement of elderly people from long-stay wards and other forms of public provision. But it refused to provide costings, and many commentators suspected that private insurance firms would be unable to provide as much cover as would be required (Walker, 1997).

I have sought to establish that the NHS internal market is neither a pure free market nor an expression of socialist solidarity. The values which inform allocation of the community's healthcare resources in the internal market are expressed surreptitiously, only emerging in publicity surrounding 'hard cases' such as that of Mr K. There is a hidden ideology masquerading behind the surface objectivity of letting the market decide.

How then can we reassert a more communitarian ideology of healthcare distribution? The usual answer is that we should revert to the older, more socialist values of the NHS, but that land of lost content seems more real now that it is lost than it did then, perhaps. Consensus within the entire community on the fundamental values of the health service was less the order of the day in 1948 than we now think, in hindsight (Webster, 1994; Seedhouse, 1994). In addition, other changes outside the realm of healthcare lessen rather than increase communal solidarity: for example, the progressive diminution of the value of the state pension and the necessity for personal pensions based on an individual's contribution record and her pension fund's luck in judging the stock markets (Walker, 1996).

A different sort of communitarianism might argue that how we conduct the resource debate itself creates the values behind the health service: that they are not immutable principles waiting to be discovered, but values created by the process of decision-making itself (Edgar, 1999). From this perspective, healthcare is not only instrumental to individuals, but also to the well-being of community solidarity. It can be seen as a public forum in which notions of health and appropriate use of healthcare resources are negotiated. Neither the fixed model of healthcare delivery as a market system, nor the metaphor of healthcare as the engine of socialist solidarity can capture this view, although it is closer to the second insofar as the socialist image does at least recognize that there is a debate about values going on.

I find this an attractive and innovative notion, but I am not sure where it leaves those who most urgently need the debate to be resolved: the elderly in long-term care. It will take a conscious and considerable effort to mobilize their views in the communal forum. Without the political will to do that, the idea that our healthcare system reflects a communal discourse and creates communal values could easily become a form of justification for discrimination against vulnerable groups such as the elderly. If older people are receiving a smaller proportion of resources, that argument might run, it must be the will of the community. Although the public outcry about cases such as that of Mr K suggest that this may not, in fact, be the will of the people. In the meantime, if the inadequacy of market provision is forced onto the political agenda, however, by

shocking cases such as that of Mr K, then perhaps we do stand a chance of recreating communal solidarity.

Even in Sweden, where solidarity is still the official value, there is a need for more open discussion of these issues. Indeed, because decisions are typically made administratively rather than democratically, 'often the basis for these decisions is not stated openly; sometimes it is obscure, even to the decision-makers themselves. For example, the general trend in care services has been that younger and relatively healthier pensioners are receiving less help, that less money is being spent on home help services, and that institutional care is receiving more financial support. The strategy that seems to be implicit in these decisions (although not stated openly) is *focusing*, that is, to concentrate resources to those individuals with the greatest needs' (Thorslund et al., 1997a).

Need is actually a philosophical criterion for resource allocation, often set against *merit*. Both in market systems and in more centralized decision-making, values and philosophical concepts cannot be avoided. It is now time for you to move on to Section 5, which summarizes philosophical models.

ACTIVITY: Take a few moments here to make a note of the key points raised by this section.

Section 5: Philosophical models of resource allocation

In this chapter we have been addressing the question of *distributive justice* in relation to the allocation of scarce healthcare resources. We have explored some possible explanations for the existence of such scarcity and whether or not it is, in fact, a growing problem in relation to healthcare. In the previous section you saw that there are those who argue that the demographic time bomb is something of a myth. However, whether or not we are in fact witnessing a phenomenon of this kind, the fact is that resource allocation and questions of distributive justice are inevitable in any healthcare system, no matter how well funded. Decisions will have always to be made about how to distribute healthcare: how much ought we to allocate to each region, to each kind of treatment, to primary, secondary or tertiary care and so on. We would want to argue that such distribution inevitably raises important ethical questions for those who have to make these choices. We have, throughout this chapter, looked at a variety of other ways in which healthcare allocation decisions could be made, whether on grounds of medical criteria, age, or economics, but in every case it has proven impossible to side-step ethical considerations. In this section we want to address such considerations in relation to distributive justice more directly.

ACTIVITY: Think back for a moment to the example with which we started this chapter, that of distributing pieces of a cake. What did you decide would be the ethical way in which to divide it? On first reflection we might be tempted to allocate the cake equally among those who want it. However as we suggested earlier, following Aristotle, whilst justice requires that we treat equal cases equally, he also reminds us that it is unjust to treat different cases as if they were the same, and this suggests that a commitment to 'equality' cannot mean that we treat all people the same. We might, for example, decide to allocate the pieces of cake on the grounds of need. If a starving man comes into my house I may decide to forego my share of the cake and give it all to him, even though this might go against the principle of equality. On the other hand, I might decide to give a larger portion to my brother and take a smaller piece myself because he has been working hard all day to collect the ingredients which go into my cake-making and he deserves to be rewarded. Desert, equality and need (see Glossary) are three possible guiding concepts for the ethical distribution of the cake or of healthcare resources. Can you think of any more? List them here and we will return to them at the end of this section.

John Rawls – justice as fairness

John Rawls has argued in his book *A Theory of Justice* for a procedural model of justice. What this means is that he attempts to create a method or procedure which, if followed, will lead to a just outcome. He suggests that, in order to allocate what he called primary social goods (such as money and healthcare) in a way which is just, we ought to imagine ourselves making the decision in a hypothetical situation which is characterized by two features. The first feature is that we, as the decision-makers, have to imagine that we have perfect knowledge about the society about which we are making the decision. We would, for example, know all the statistics which were relevant to the decision; we would know the likelihood of success of various treatments, and we would know which age groups are more likely to require certain treatments, etc. In fact, we would have to be capable of knowing all there is to know about the society in question which is of relevance to our decision. The second feature of this imaginary situation would be that we would have absolutely no knowledge at all of our own position in this society. So, for example, we would not know whether we were male or female, a child or elderly, sick or healthy, rich or poor. Rawls calls this imaginary situation the 'veil of ignorance' and suggests that, from behind this veil, it is possible to make an ethical and just decision about the allocation of primary social goods such as healthcare resources.

ACTIVITY: Our first response to this is to ask what would the likely outcome of such a process be and would it be an outcome that we would find ethical? Try this for yourself. Using Rawls' model how would you go about allocating healthcare resources? How would this help us to resolve difficult choices like the one involving Mr K?

Rawls argues persuasively that, in such a position, the rational and just thing to do would be to argue for the equal distribution of resource, except if by distributing resources unequally one could improve upon the situation that would be achieved by the worst-off member of the society in the case of an equal distribution. He calls this the *difference principle*.

What would be the implication of this principle for the distribution of healthcare resources in the cases we have already seen? How would it bear upon the use of age cut-offs in resource allocation?

Norman Daniels – Equality of opportunity

Let's go on now to see how Rawls's model of procedural justice is applied to healthcare by one theorist, Norman Daniels, by reading an extract from a paper by Masja van den Burg and Ruud ter Meulen on 'Age as a criterion for distributing scarce healthcare resources'.

Age as a criterion for distributing scarce healthcare resources

Masja van den Burg and Ruud ter Meulen

Another proposal for age cut-offs has been made by Norman Daniels in his book *Am I My Parents' Keeper?* (1988). According to Daniels the much-discussed competition for resources between the young and the old is misleading in so far as it suggests a conflict between different groups of persons. The issue of distribution should be considered from a diachronic perspective. In fact, it is a matter of individual, prudential decision-making how to distribute resources over the different stage of one's own life. The criterion of age does not differentiate between persons, but between life stages within a person's life. At any particular stage of life, all persons will be treated the same. In this respect the age criterion is different from other criteria such as race, sex or religion.

The starting point for Daniels's theory of distributive justice is the clearly perceived self interest of the individual. According to Daniels an age-based allocation of scarce healthcare may be justified. However, it should never be put into practice until we have a society in which general principles of justice are realised. A just distribution of social goods requires a 'fair equality of opportunity' for all, not only in regard to healthcare, but also to income and education.

Within Daniels's theory of just healthcare a fair share of healthcare is determined by *what is necessary to maintain a fair equality of opportunity over a lifetime*. The allocation of available healthcare services will then be determined by what a prudent individual would choose. Prudential planning requires neutrality toward the different life stages. For this, Daniels uses the hypothetical contract theory of Rawls and his idea of the 'veil of ignorance'. Behind the veil of ignorance prudential planners do not know their age, health condition and other personal circumstances. In this 'original position' Daniels suggests, it would be prudent for individuals to secure a roughly equal opportunity at each life stage to carry out their plans of life, whatever they may be. It is rational to maximize the chances of living a normal lifespan. Because their fair share of healthcare will not provide all possible beneficial care for all their health needs, the allocation between the different life stages will be affected by age-related differences in needs (Daniels, 1988).

Like Rawls, Daniels creates a hypothetical situation in which prudential planners are confronted with a scarcity of resources. To simplify the situation they can choose between two distribution schemes. In the first scheme no one over 75 years is offered any high-cost life-extending technology. Persons younger than 75 years will have access to all life-extending treatments. Under this scheme everybody reaches the age of 75 years, and then immediately dies. In the second scheme resources are strictly allocated according to medical need. Only one of the high-cost technologies can be developed and made available to all who need it. This scheme offers an 0.5 probability of living to age 50 and a 0.5 probability of reaching age 100. Life expectancy is identical to the first scheme of distribution.

Prudential planners would prefer the first scheme of distribution. Daniels offers two reasons.

Firstly, prudential planners know that the inci-dence of disease and disability is greater between ages 75 and 100, and so the quality of life is com-monly greater under the first scheme than under the second. Secondly, the most important life plans will be completed by the age of 75 years. This makes the 50-75 period more important than the 75–100 period. Daniels underlines that age cri-teria are only justified if the savings are used for long-term care for the elderly.

ACTIVITY: How does Daniels' use of Rawls's model of justice as fair equality of opportunity compare with your own? What are the implications of the model when assessed using the three concepts we intro-duced earlier of *equality, need and desert*?

Daniel Callahan – Setting limits

Earlier in Section 3 of the chapter we encountered the work of Daniel Callahan in our discussion of age cut-offs. Callahan offers a philosophical per-spective which is sometimes seen as opposed to that of Rawls in that it is **communitarian** rather than individualistic. Rather than using a principle of equality and rights as the basis of decision-making, communitarians suggest we should base our ethical consideration of questions such as these on the concepts of the natural lifespan, the good society or community, and on the notion of a balance between rights and responsibilities. Read the following section from van den Burg and ter Meulen's paper and try to identify the ways in which this approach differs from the one outlined earlier.

In view of the increasing scarcity of healthcare services, there has been a widely discussed debate about the allocation of these services, first in the US, but now also in many European coun-tries. Distributing scarce healthcare resources involves many ethical issues. It requires that the goals of medicine are defined and the choices made should reflect major values in society. Besides this, these choices will have considerable

consequences for the accessibility to healthcare services.

Since the 1980s, several proposals have been made to re-allocate these services. One of these proposals is to set limits to the elderly in their use of expensive life-extending care. The most debated proposal for such age-based rationing is made by Daniel Callahan in his book *Setting Limit*s (1987).

Callahan proposes to set limits on life-extending care for the elderly in exchange for better access to long-term care facilities. According to Callahan, we should set limits to the use of expensive medical technology which extends the lives of elderly people only for a few weeks or months. Instead, this technology should be allocated to the young, in order to increase their chances to reach old age.

Callahan's proposal should be seen from a com-munitarian point of view. For communitarians the source of norms and values should be found in society. Criteria for justice are rooted in a moral tradition. In this view modernism and individual-ism are obstacles to the development of a shared meaning of old age. Our pluralistic society embraces individual liberty and is opposed to a shared notion of the good life which is considered coercive. There are no shared values or even dis-cussion of these values which could give meaning to suffering and decline in life, and the concept of a whole life is absent. Both of these are required, Callahan suggests, in order to give meaning to old age and death.

In Callahan's opinion we need a community-based notion of the meaning of old age. The life cycle and the concept of a whole life are of con-siderable importance for ageing, dying and death. The meaning and significance of old age have much to do with the role of the elderly in society. In his view, old age is a period of consideration, reflection, disengagement and preparation for death. The elderly are the conservators of the moral tradition, they are able to integrate the past with the present and the future. They have insight in the way in which the generations are connected with each other. In these roles and functions, the elderly have obligations toward the young. The young need the old to develop a meaningful perspective on their lives, as a coherent whole.

The goals of medicine should be defined in this normative framework. The goal of medicine is not the extension of life as such, but the avoidance of premature death and the achievement of a full and natural lifespan. After that point Callahan speaks of a tolerable death: the event of death at that stage in lifespan when one's possibilities and life goals have on the whole been accomplished and one's moral obligations to those for whom one has responsibility have been discharged. At that point death is understood as a sad but none the less acceptable event. The natural lifespan and tolerable death are thus defined in terms of the fulfilment of a biographic life. When the natural life span has been achieved, medicine should be directed at improving the quality of life and the relief of suffering. This means the control of pain and the active effort to promote physical functioning, mental alertness and emotional stability.

This understanding of old age and death justifies limitations on some forms of medical care for the elderly. Our social obligation to the elderly, he suggests, is to help them live out a natural lifespan. After that point it is legitimate to set limits to life-extending treatments, in favour of life-enhancing care, that is care which tries to improve those physical functions which are needed for normal daily activities. In Callahan's opinion age criteria should be used as part of a national healthcare policy. They should not be considered as medical, but person-centred or biographic criteria.

Callahan's proposal requires a full-scale change in thinking and attitudes. Therefore, he argues that it is time to start a public debate. When consensus on the use of age criteria has been reached, it must be implemented in public policy. Callahan underlines that a policy of age-based rationing can only be morally acceptable within a society that recognizes the positive values of all ages (Callahan, 1987).

ACTIVITY: Communitarians have sometimes been criticized for emphasizing tradition and community at the expense of the rights of individuals. And this can be seen to be expressed most clearly in the concept of the 'good life' or the 'good community', for they leave open the question of who is to decide what would *count* as the good life. This is particularly important in relation to the question of age cut-offs, for what counts as the good life might be said to vary both with age and between people. It is open to us to reject Callahan's particular conception of the good old age. Stop for a moment and list some of the advantages and disadvantages of the communitarian approach compared to Rawls and Daniels, before going on to read the next excerpt from the paper.

Now, finally, bearing in mind these different theoretical approaches based on fairness, equality of opportunity and the good life and also the three concepts of need, desert and equality, we would like you to finish this chapter by reading the following report of some empirical research in the Netherlands which involved carrying out interviews with doctors about how they go about making resource allocation decisions. In the light of your consideration of the various perspectives and the issues raised by this chapter, we would like you to use this reading as an exercise. Try to identify the arguments the doctors are using and note them down. When you reach the end of the reading, address each of these arguments in turn and identify their weaknesses and strengths using the arguments and counter-arguments you have explored as you have worked your way through this chapter.

Age as a criterion for distributing scarce healthcare resources *(cont.)*

Masja van den Burgh and Ruud ter Meulen

It is healthcare practitioners who decide upon the distribution of medical care. In a recent study we interviewed 11 Dutch physicians. The main goal of the interviews was to find out how physicians deal with tough choices. Which criteria and arguments influence the process of selection? Special attention was paid to the role of age and the position of the elderly. In the analysis of the interviews, a distinction will be made between the indication and the selection.

Scarcity of resources

First of all, physicians find it difficult to imagine that there will be a scarcity of healthcare resources in the future. If there is a scarcity, they believe that it is created because of budgetary constraints by the government. Many physicians argue that there are enough financial resources in the Netherlands and that the government should enlarge the healthcare budget.

If it is true that as a consequence of a limitation of resources we cannot do our work any more, we cannot justify this situation towards our patients. And I think that the patients should know that it is not the physician who is responsible for the lack of care, but the politicians.(. . .) However, if the politicians are going to tell me which patient I have to refer to the Intensive Care Unit, I will leave the hospital and start working for a pharmaceutical company.

However, other physicians argue that the decision-making would be much easier were the government to make explicit choices and set limits:

If in a situation of scarcity, you have to make a choice between different persons, the government should set the rules for such decisions. The government should make it clear to the voters, that this government has decided that everybody above 90 years does not get a hip replacement. In my opinion I should not have to explain this decision in the treatment room.

In cases where the scarcity is caused by political decisions, the politicians should set the limits for who will get what kind of treatment. As long as the government does not make such choices, most of the physicians will do their best to give every patient the treatment he or she needs. However, this does not apply to heart transplantation, where the scarcity is not the result of political decisions, but of a lack of supply of donor organs.

Age and indication for treatment

On a clinical level, physicians sometimes have to decide between patients. In such situations, age is an important factor for determining the medical appropriateness of medical treatments. In the opinion of the physicians, age is related to the medical condition of the patient and the expected medical benefit. From a medical point of view, the elderly are in a less favourable position. Growing old involves fewer chances of success and more chance of complications. But physicians agree that age alone is not decisive for the medical appropriateness of a treatment. They think it is better to look at the biological age, instead of the chronological age. This is illustrated by the following quotations:

Age does play an important role, but not as an absolute fact. We cannot use a formula: this man has a biological age of 86 years. However, it may be true that an elderly person can't stand a certain treatment any more. So, certain treatments will not be given to older persons. As an example: a 90-year-old person who needs resuscitation, will not get it, because from experience we know that he or she will not survive.

Another physician said about age:

When a colleague proposes to treat an 85-year-old, there will be an intensive discussion, until a consensus is reached. The result can be that the treatment will not be given. Age is an easy and objective substitute for supplementary problems. An 85-year-old with heart problems, nearly always has other problems too, which complicates the treatment. So, you talk about age, but in fact you mean the whole physical condition of the patient.

Quality of life considerations are taken into account. They are determined by the medical, social, psychological and mental condition of a person. Important aspects are vitality, co-morbidity, the social context and the future perspective of patients. These factors are negatively related to age. In general, elderly patients will not be treated as aggressively as younger patients.

Age and selection for treatment

The principle of beneficence is difficult to realize in a situation of scarcity. Physicians are expected to provide optimal care to patients. Beneficence obliges them to act in accordance with their interests. Scarcity in healthcare may force them to withhold an appropriate treatment, which may cause medical and/or social harm for the patient involved. The reluctance to accept scarcity and the selection of patients is illustrated by the following quotation:

It is important to be clear about the indication and that has nothing to do with scarcity. As a doctor you cannot accept it when a politician or a hospital director says that some kind of appropriate care will not be provided. These people don't know what they are talking about.

Scarcity, due to a lack of money is not accepted. In practice, physicians try to find solutions, or, if that is not possible, create one.

When the shortages in healthcare are due to, for example, a lack of organs, it is hard to steer clear of scarcity. This kind of scarcity is considered to be absolute. Physicians are forced to select patients. Different arguments and values are relevant for the selection procedure. The position of the elderly in the process of selection depends on the weight physicians attach to these values. It is not always clear which selection criteria are acceptable. Is it justified to use utilitarian criteria in order to maximize the medical benefit? Can it be justified to base the decisions with regard to selecting patients on the notion of the natural lifespan? Below, the arguments of the physicians are grouped under the headings equality, efficiency and the natural lifespan.

Equality

From the legal point of view, equity and equality are leading principles. Persons who are equal from a medical viewpoint, should be treated equally. The question is whether age can be considered as a medically relevant criterion. Several authors argue that chronological age cannot be considered as a medical criterion (Jahnigen and Binstock, 1991). Therefore, the principle of equality is being violated when physicians distinguish between patients on grounds of their differences in age.

In the interviews with the physicians it appeared that the principle of equality is taken into account. However, this barely influences the medical decision-making with regard to the selection of patients. Physicians think that people who are equal in a relevant sense, must be treated the same. However, in their view age is a medically relevant criterion. Therefore, for them it is justified to distinguish between people of different ages.

I have learned that it is unethical to say that 5 years of life for a 25-year-old has more importance than 5 years for a 75-year old. In general, for the 75-year-old, it is as much important to see his grandchild as it is for the 25-year-old to see his child. But this argument does not take into account that age might be an indicator for concomitant diseases.

Some physicians stated it more explicitly:

You cannot say that when you take age into account in your decision-making, that is a kind of discrimination. There are medical and social arguments that lead you to start a different treatment for a 90-year-old than for a 46-year-old. In that sense, age is not a discriminatory criterion. Age is a medical criterion.

Even when the chance for success is equal for a 25-year-old and for a 75-year-old, the 25-year-old gets priority on the basis of the duration of the benefit:

It is not age, but the situation of the patient, his rate of success, the time that is left. So, the proportion of the investment compared to the benefit. An operation at the age of 75 that results in hospitalization of many months and a benefit of 1 year longer life at best, is different compared to an operation on a person of 25, because the benefit is much greater in the latter case.

Efficiency

Efficiency is promoted by utilitarian arguments. The principle on which utilitarian arguments are based is 'the greatest good for the greatest number'. The objective is to realize maximal health benefits with minimal costs. Potential candidates for a medical treatment are compared to each other; priority will be given to patients who are expected to have the greatest medical benefits.

Patients who statistically have lower chances of success will be excluded. This is illustrated by the following quotation:

I think that you have to choose for the patient who is expected to have the best results. You ought to use such a scarce resource as efficiently as possible.

In most cases, priority will be given to younger patients. The elderly are in a less favourable condition with regard to utilitarian criteria. In general, the rate of success of medical treatments are lower for elderly people. Risk of co-morbidity increases with age and elderly patients normally have diminished physiological reserves. Furthermore, the benefits of life after extensive treatments are lower for the elderly, because of limited life expectancy. Most physicians argue that it is reasonable to apply age criteria for heart transplantation. Some are in favour of flexible age criteria, others believe in strict age criteria. The following quotations are illustrative:

The whole situation is determined by the scarcity, you have to do something. And I believe that doctors use the following principle: how long can a patient profit from a medical treatment? And a younger person has a longer profit than an older person. (. . .) In 90 per cent of the cases age is decisive.

In situations of absolute scarcity, physicians favour the patients with the best chances:

It is a matter of supply and demand. So, in case of absolute scarcity, those persons (. . .) with the best possible medical outcome will be treated first.

Imagine that two people need at the same time a complex treatment, then you will favour the patient with the fewest supplementary problems, and with the best prognosis after treatment. When I have two ruptured aortic aneurysms, one of 40 years old and one of 70 years old, then the 40-year-old will probably be treated first.

Under normal circumstances physicians do their very best for the individual patient. Beneficence is the leading principle. However, under conditions of absolute scarcity utilitarian arguments are used in medical decision-making. Physicians weigh lives and compare patients. Priority will be given to patients with the best rates of success. The objective is to maximise the medical benefit.

The natural lifespan

The notion of the natural lifespan seemed reasonable to some physicians. For them it is important not to forget that, at a certain point, life comes to an end. In their opinion, it is fair to give everybody the chance to grow old. They do not think it is a matter of discrimination if it is decided on non-medical grounds that a 25-year-old person gets a treatment and a 75-year-old person does not get it. One physician argued that a different treatment on the basis of age is acceptable:

This is not bad, because discrimination always takes place. I mean you have to distribute the scarce treatments. You can close your eyes and start a lottery, but that does not solve the problem. In such cases I would give priority to a 25-year-old. That looks reasonable to me. If you let people participate in a lottery, you walk away from your responsibility.

This physician thinks that it is more reasonable to give everybody a fair chance to become old than to treat everybody equally. However, this moral notion cannot easily be framed into a rule. Another physician who was in favour of the philosophical argument about 'natural lifespan' argued:

This is reasonable: the glass may be half empty or the glass may be half full. Of course, for the one person life has just started, for the other there is just a little left. The further you are on the road, the more you are looking back and the less you can look forward. That is all true, but you cannot turn it into a general rule.(. . .) We do not need rules, but we need an ethics which guides our decision-making.

Most of the physicians in this study stuck to their own rule that only medically relevant facts may influence clinical decision-making.

At the end of their article, Masja van den Burg and Ruud ter Meulen comment that:
Using utilitarian criteria in the selection procedure conflicts with the principles of dignity and equality. Using utilitarian criteria involves a comparison between human lives and implicates that

some (longer) lives have more value than other (shorter) lives. Dignity and equality do not allow lives to be weighed against each other. Finally, when utilitarian criteria become the leading principle in the selection procedure, access to healthcare services for some groups of patients may be threatened, especially the elderly. When scarcity increases in future, it can be expected that utilitarian criteria will be used more often and that elderly people will get into an increasingly less favourable position.

The objections to the application of utilitarian criteria need to be taken seriously. Physicians, who continue to be confronted with scarcity in future, have to be aware of the ethical implications of their choices and decisions. In medical education attention should be paid to the ethical dimensions and aspects of clinical practice. This may contribute to the prevention of being discriminatory against the elderly.

When resource allocation decisions are being made we need to be wary of making the vulnerable worse off than they already are. What the case studies and other materials in this chapter show is that, whilst medical, economic and legal consid-

erations are central to any decision-making process, it is not possible to avoid the pressing ethical and moral questions with which we are confronted as practitioners in an era of limited resources.

ACTIVITY: At this point, before you go on to the next chapter, make a list of the key points raised by this section and add them to your other lists to make a summary of the key points raised by this chapter.

Summary of key points from this chapter:

Suggestions for further reading

Callahan, D. (1987). *Setting Limits: Medical Goals in an Ageing Society*. New York: Simon and Schuster.

Daniels, N. (1988). *Am I my Parents' Keeper? An Essay on Justice between the Young and the Old*. New York: Oxford University Press.

McKie, J., Singer, P., Kuhse, H., and Richardson, J. (1998). *The Allocation of Healthcare Resources*. Brookfield, VT: Dartmouth Publishing Co.

Rawls, J. (1971). *A Theory of Justice*. Cambridge MA.: Harvard University Press.

Thinking about ethics: autonomy and patient choice

Section 1: The importance of autonomy in medical ethics   Section 2: What is autonomy?   Section 3: Autonomy: alternative models in European law   Section 4: Medical ethics: alternative models

Introduction

Human rights and the associated emphasis on liberty or freedom belong to a well-established tradition of ethical reasoning. Their origins can perhaps be traced to the recognition by the Stoic philosophers in Ancient Greece of the possibility that the actual laws and conventional practices in a particular community might be seen to be unjust when contrasted with a 'natural law' (Almond, 1993). For this reason the concept of 'universal human rights' which grew out of the 'natural law' tradition has often appealed to those who have felt themselves to be vulnerable or to be oppressed by the powerful. For the appeal to a concept of universal human rights transcending any particular community and its laws makes it possible to call for the upholding of the rights of individuals against their community and against such laws, and in recent years the concept of universal human rights has come to play an important role. It helps us to recognize and express the importance of the protection of the weak and vulnerable.

In medicine this has tended to be expressed as the belief that the protection of vulnerable patients and the practice of ethical medicine can best be guaranteed in a context of patient-centred medicine, that is in medicine which places a very high value on respect for autonomy and patient choice. An emphasis on patient-centredness means that, in cases where practitioners wish to

override the expressed wishes of a patient, the burden of justification lies with the practitioner.

The demand for this kind of respect for autonomy and patient choice in healthcare practice has increasingly been recognized officially. Below are three examples of this. Although there are a very large number of other such expressions, the ones we have chosen here as examples are the Italian Deontological Code (Codice di Deontologia Medica (25 Giugno 1995)), the Declaration of Helsinki 1964 (as amended by the 41st World Medical Assembly in Hong Kong 1989) and the Finnish Act on the Status and Rights of Patients, 1992.

Italian Deontological Code (Codice di Deontologia Medica), Article 31

- Doctors should not undertake any diagnostic or therapeutic activity without the informed consent of the patient.
- Consent, in written form in those cases where specific diagnostic and therapeutic procedures or possible consequences for the patient's physical integrity make necessary an unequivocal expression of the patient's will, is an integral part of, not a substitute for, the informed consent mentioned in Article 29.
- Diagnostic procedures and therapeutic treatment entailing serious risk for the patient's safety must be undertaken only when absolutely necessary and after adequate information

on possible consequences is given. Proper evidence of consent must follow.

- Furthermore, when a patient who is able to understand and decide explicitly rejects intervention, doctors must refrain from any diagnostic or therapeutic procedure, because no action is allowed against the patient's will, save only in cases mentioned in Article 33 below (Translated by Dr Carlo Calzone, Calzone, 1996).

Declaration of Helsinki

- In any research on human beings, each potential subject must be adequately informed of the aims, methods, anticipated benefits and potential hazards of the study and the discomfort it may entail. He or she should be informed that he or she is at liberty to abstain from participation in the study and that he or she is free to withdraw his or her consent to participation at any time. The physician should then obtain the subject's freely given informed consent, preferably in writing. (Declaration of Helsinki, Basic principle 9, 1989)

Finnish Act on the Status and Rights of Patients

- The patient has to be cared for in mutual understanding. If the patient refuses a certain treatment or measure, he/she has to be cared for according to the possibilities available in another medically acceptable way in mutual understanding (part of Section 6 of the Finnish Act on the Status and Rights of Patients, Statute No 785, 1992 – enacted 1993).

Few today would dispute the importance of autonomy and of an emphasis on the value of the patient's voice and informed choice to ethical medicine. Recently however, the call for more patient autonomy has come under challenge from some of the quarters where it might previously have been expected to find a powerful resonance. For example, some of those arguing for the need to protect minority ethnic and cultural rights have asked whether the call for individual rights is compatible with the recognition of a diversity of cultures and of cultural identities and have argued that a more sophisticated concept is required. In this final chapter of the workbook we look more closely at the methods of medical ethics itself and investigate the extent to which the concepts of 'autonomy' and of 'patient choice' are capable of resolving the types of ethical question we have been exploring throughout this workbook and the extent to which they need to be either supplemented or perhaps replaced by other approaches. We start with a short critique of autonomy by Dolores Dooley from the National University of Ireland at Cork.

Section 1: The importance of autonomy in medical ethics

Autonomy, feminism and vulnerable patients

Dolores Dooley

Moral and political philosophy [and medical ethics] is under challenge to look again at some of its fundamental concepts and commitments. This challenge within the disciplines is not simply about theoretical considerations but coincides with cultural and demographic changes throughout the western world; such changes are bringing pressure to bear on societies to re-examine their respect for and treatment of multicultural and marginalised groups in their cultures, examples of which are diverse religious groups, women, minority racial groups and homosexuals. A familiar liberal traditional position affording a plethora of rights to citizens needs revision, it is argued, because it has made the fundamental mistake of universalizing its key concepts. It has assumed that all citizens can be understood as homogeneous: having the same expectations, values, political beliefs and aspirations for the good life. But citizens are, in reality, much more diverse than universal concepts reflect. The 'fit' between theory and reality is loosening

(Young, 1989). Against this background of cultural and ideological changes, ethnic, religious and gender subgroups within societies are increasingly looking for what Amy Gutmann describes as the 'recognition of every individual's uniqueness and humanity [which] lies at the core of liberal democracy, understood as a way of political and personal life' (Gutmann, 1994).

Is a democratic pursuit of equality and liberty rights for diverse and morally pluralist groups of human beings compatible with social harmony? Is the pursuit of liberty for diverse moral views problematic for the conscience of others who may disagree with how some individuals choose to use their liberties? Finally, are certain political accommodations necessary if a people within a state are to live constructively with ethnic, sexual and religious diversity? If so, what are these accommodations?

In this chapter we will be going on to look more closely at the concepts of 'autonomy' and of 'patient choice' in medicine and healthcare more widely. Just what does it mean to be autonomous? What are the conflicts between autonomy and other values? How ought such conflicts to be resolved?

We would like you to begin by reading the following account of the case of Peter Noll from Switzerland.

THE CASE OF PETER NOLL (this case is based on Peter Noll's own account)

When he was 56 years old, the Swiss law professor and author Peter Noll discovered that he had advanced cancer of the bladder. He was advised to have surgery but chose not to. In his book *In the Face of Death* he explained why he chose to refuse treatment.

Survival chances in bladder cancer are relatively good, especially if the surgery is combined with radiation treatment. How favourable the odds were was a matter of statistics – about 50 per cent. In response to my questions, [the urologist] says

that sexual intercourse would no longer be possible since there could be no erection; but there was no other essential limitation – biking, sports in moderate measure, even skiing. Patients who survived the critical first 5 years all grew accustomed to the curtailed life. When I explained that I would never consent to such an operation under any conditions, he said that he had great respect for such a decision but that I should really get as much information as possible from other doctors as well. Did I want to take the X-rays with me? I said no; the case seemed quite clear to me.

What bothers me is the loss of freedom; having others in charge of you, to be drawn into a medical machine which controls a person and which one cannot fight. Naturally, intolerable pain will disturb me too. In order to escape it, one enters the machine that takes away pain and at the same time freedom. And it's precisely this enslavement that I don't want.

I don't want to get sucked into the surgical–urological–radiological machinery because I would lose my liberty bit by bit. With hopes getting more and more reduced, my will would be broken and in the end I will end up in the well-known dying chamber, which everybody tends to give a wide berth – the outer office of the cemetery.

Peter Noll died nearly a year after his diagnosis during which he had lived alone and administered his own pain relief. However he had continued to write, to work and to meet his friends until the last few days of his life.

As a part of his preparation for death, Peter Noll planned his own funeral.

ACTIVITY: Peter Noll argues forcefully for patient autonomy. Take a few minutes to consider how far you think the emphasis on autonomy and patient choice should be pursued? What do we do if patients make choices about their treatment about which we feel uneasy or which appear to be at odds with our assessment of their best interests? What if the patient's choices conflict with the other demands we feel upon us as part of our commitment to the practice of ethical medicine? Can you think of any other ethical features of ethical medicine with which patient choice might conflict? Make a list of what you consider to be the key 'principles' of ethical medicine. Start the list with something like 'Place a particular emphasis on the value of the patient's autonomy and choices'. We would like you to keep this list close at hand as you progress through the chapter, adding to it when possible. Once you have completed your list, spend a few minutes going through it, identifying ways and circumstances in which each of the principles might conflict with 'autonomy and patient choice'.

We would now like you to read the following commentary on the Peter Noll case by Christian Hick who is a doctor from Germany.

The right to refuse treatment

Christian Hick

Treatment refusal as the realization of a 'free death'

For Aristotle, things in medicine seemed to be clear.

We deliberate not about ends but about means. For a doctor does not deliberate whether he shall heal, nor an orator whether he shall persuade, nor a statesman whether he shall produce law and order, nor does anyone else deliberate about his end. They assume the end and consider how and by what means it is to be attained (Aristotle, Nichomachian Ethics III,3).

But today, on the contrary, we must deliberate not only about means but also about the ends of medicine. The very meaning of health, as the end of medicine, is submitted to our power, as becomes evident in predictive genetic testing. It is questionable, and this is where our consideration of the right to refuse treatment starts, whether medical treatment provides the patient with the health he is expecting, with the experience of personal health, of health adapted to his conception of existence and of a human life.

In his autobiographical book, which takes the form of a diary, Peter Noll records his thoughts

from the moment of his being diagnosed with bladder cancer until immediately before his death. The relevance of this day-to-day description of the progression of an incurable disease for the discussion of the 'right to refuse treatment' lies in the motives Peter Noll had for his refusal. In fact, the whole book can be seen to some extent as a long, written, argumentative meditation explaining his refusal, a refusal which might *prima facie* seem unreasonable.

ACTIVITY: Take a moment at this point to re-read Peter Noll's account of his reasons for refusing treatment. While you do so, try to pick out and note down Noll's own arguments for asserting his right to refuse treatment and any comments you might like to make about these arguments. Then go on with your reading of Hick's commentary below.

Taking the quotations above, together with the arguments Noll presents in the rest of his book, the following reasons are those he gives for his refusal of the treatment offered.

Negative reasons
- After the treatment he will need an artificial urine collection device
- Sexual intercourse will no longer be possible
- There is a 50–50 chance of a relapse

Positive reason
- To have certainty about one's death instead of a mere statistical possibility of death or survival.

This 'positive' reason is, for him, the most important one and seems to be, at the same time, the one most easily overlooked by medical professionals who have difficulty imagining themselves in the role of such a patient. The certitude of death, even if it should occur earlier is in general easier to deal with than the incertitude which lies in the statistical possibility of healing. Certitude permits planning, active coping and the shaping of one's life, incertitude breeds passivity and might very well spoil the rest of one's lifetime. Noll refuses treatment because he wants to master his own death. This presupposes that dying is not merely an objective, biological process but, as life, a personal affair. In this way Noll discriminates between three different ways of dying:

- Sudden death by accident
- Prolonged dying controlled by the 'medical machinery'
- 'Self-controlled' dying – 'to see death as it comes'

The positive reason Noll gives for refusing medical treatment lies in the possibilities he sees in a 'self-controlled' dying, which permits the integration of death into the biographical life of an individual:

It is a real chance to see death as it comes. Firstly, there is nothing left to be taken into consideration; nobody can take from you more than your life. Secondly, one can prepare oneself and bring everything to a close.

As a way of clarifying his view on the relation between personal freedom and death, Noll quotes some famous passages from Montaigne's Essays, especially Chapter XVII of the first book entitled, 'That to study philosophy is to learn to die'.

The premeditation of death is the premeditation of liberty; he who has learned to die, has unlearned to serve. There is nothing of evil in life, for him who rightly comprehends that the privation of life is no evil: to know how to die, delivers us from all subjection and constraint.

And how should one premeditate death in an intensive care unit, how should one find any link from death in a 'machine' with the preceding part of a free and personal life story? To refuse to be treated seems by this view to be the only way to safeguard a person's liberty and biographical integrity. And in the second book of his essays Montaigne continues, as does Peter Noll in quoting him, as if he had foreseen the problems of modern medicine and the pitfalls of 'healing' – when there is nothing left to heal.

The common way of healing goes at the expense of life: one is incised, one is cauterized, our members are cut off, food and blood are taken away. One step further and we are definitively healed.

> **ACTIVITY: What do you think are the strengths and weaknesses of Noll's arguments? Are some of them stronger than others?**

When we read through the case, we felt that some of the arguments were quite weak. The idea that he was any more certain that he was going to die because he didn't get treatment for his cancer just isn't true. Clearly, there is an obvious sense in which we are all certain to die from the moment we are born. What Noll is perhaps reasonably sure about now is that, without treatment, he is going to die 'sooner' than he would with treatment, but even this is not certain. Noll might perhaps have replied that, at least by refusing treatment, he has kept control of his death, for he has made the decision. But even here, it would have been him who made the decision had he decided to accept treatment.

His argument that he now has certainty about the form of death rather than statistical possibility is again wrong. If he continues to live a 'normal' life for a year (as he did) then during that year there was as much chance as before that he would be killed by a 'sudden accident' or by a heart attack, for example. So certainty is not gained by his choice, nor are statistics avoided. Moreover, the idea of having a self-controlled death and of 'seeing death as it comes' could as easily be re-interpreted as a reason to go on living and to accept the treatment. Certainly, the quotations from Montaigne could, and perhaps should, be interpreted as calls for us to use the awareness of the certainty of the finite nature of our lives as a motivation to enhanced living not as a reason to choose death now. If life is indeed enhanced by the anticipation of death, then one ought perhaps to attempt to have more of it rather than less. The most certain way to take control over death and to make it certain would be for Noll to kill himself and he does not suggest this.

What Noll may, in fact, have been attempting to avoid was the 'unnatural' death and the unnatural life (one with a colostomy bag and one without sex). For he suggests that medicine and the 'medical machine' are inevitably the enemies of autonomy and that being 'treated' necessarily involves a loss of self, especially at the end of life. What do you think about these claims?

Noll argues that personal autonomy and patient choice ought to be the guiding principles in medical ethics. There is a sense in which the case itself might be seen as extreme but it usefully brings the concept of autonomy and patient-centred choice into question. For, how can we have patient-centred care if the patient doesn't want care?

THE CASE OF PETER NOLL *(cont.)*

Peter Noll's friends varied in their responses to his decision to refuse treatment. He wrote,

The expression of respect seems, to a certain extent, to be a standard response, for I heard it several times afterward. Naturally, it is appropriate to show a patient who chooses metastasis instead of the technological prolongation of death a certain admiration, even though, strictly speaking, he hardly deserves it, for he really has only a choice between two evils, and it is almost purely a question of taste as to which he prefers.

But, his friend Ruth informed him that his decision was found to be difficult to accept by several of his friends.

You see, you're upsetting people with your decision. If someone has cancer, he goes to hospital and has surgery – that's what's normal. But if someone has cancer and goes around cheerfully like you, it gives people the creeps. They are all of a sudden challenged to confront dying and death as a part of life, and that they don't want. Nor are they able to do it as long as they are not in your situation. That is why it is irritating and confusing that you sit here and say 'I have cancer' while refusing to go to the hospital. If you went to the hospital, everything would be all right. Then everything would be fine again; people could visit you, bring flowers, and after a certain time say, 'Thank God, he's been released' and again after a certain time, 'Now he's back in', and they'll come again with flowers, but always for shorter periods. But, at least they would know where to find you. They would know that you hadn't been run over by a car but have cancer and that you were going to the hospital to have things cut out, all as it is supposed to be. You scandalize them (this isn't the way she expressed it) – you are showing them that death is in our midst and you are acting it out before their very eyes; they suddenly are forced to think of what they have always suppressed. And, of course, they think only of themselves. Which makes it all the worse. They cannot help imagining what their own fate will be at some future time.

Whilst there is obvious irony in Ruth's comments, it does seem to be important to recognize that decisions like that taken by Peter Noll are always inevitably going to affect people other than the patient him or herself. How would we feel about Peter Noll's decision if he was the single parent father of dependent children, for example? Should factors such as these make a difference? If not, why not?

We would like you to return now to the conflicts between autonomy and other principles of ethical medicine which you listed at the start of this chapter. In their groundbreaking book *Principles of Biomedical Ethics*, Tom Beauchamp and James Childress identified what have come to be known as the 'four principles of biomedical ethics'. They suggested in that book that ethical problems in medical ethics are best analysed using a framework provided by the principles of 'autonomy', 'beneficence', 'non-maleficence' and 'justice' and this has come to be known as the principlist approach.

Four *prima facie* moral principles [can be identified] which seem defensible from a variety of theoretical moral perspectives and can, I believe, help us to bring more order, consistency and understanding to our medico-moral judgements. These principles – respect for autonomy, beneficence, non-maleficence and justice – plus attention to the scope of each of them – may not give us the answer to a particular medico-moral problem. But they can and do give us a widely acceptable basis for trying to work out our answers more rigorously. If, when confronted with a medico-moral problem, we consider the possible relevance of each of these principles to the particular circumstances then it seems to me that we are at least unlikely to omit any relevant moral concerns (Gillon, 1985, p. viii).

ACTIVITY: Below is a very brief account, using extracts from Beauchamp and Childress (1994), of each of these terms. As you read through their account of the four principles, we would like you to compare them with the list you made earlier and see how they compare. Do you think that it would be possible to regroup your principles so that they fit easily gathered together under these four headings? If not, what are the problem areas which make this difficult?

The four principles of biomedical ethics

Respect for autonomy

. . . we start with what we take to be essential to personal autonomy, as distinguished from political self-rule: personal rule of the self that is free from both controlling influences by others and from personal limitations that prevent meaningful choice, such as inadequate understanding. The autonomous individual freely acts in accordance with a self-chosen plan. . . . A person of diminished autonomy, by contrast, is in at least some respect controlled by others or incapable of deliberating or acting on the basis of his or her desires or plans (Beauchamp and Childress, 1994, p. 121).

Non-maleficence

The principle of non-maleficence asserts an obligation not to inflict harm intentionally. It has been closely associated in medical ethics with the maxim 'primum non nocere': 'Above all [or first] do no harm'. . . . An obligation of non-maleficence and an obligation of beneficence are both expressed in the Hippocratic oath: 'I will use treatment to help the sick according to my ability and judgement, but I will never use it to injure or wrong them (Beauchamp and Childress, 1994, p. 189).

Beneficence

. . . In ordinary English the term 'beneficence' connotes acts of mercy, kindness and charity. Altruism, love and humanity are also sometimes considered forms of beneficence. We will understand beneficent action even more broadly, so that it includes all forms of action intended to benefit other persons. 'Beneficence' refers to an action done for the benefit of others; 'benevolence' refers to the character trait or virtue of being disposed to act for the benefit of others; and the 'principle of beneficence' refers to a moral obligation to act for the benefit of others. Many acts of beneficence are not obligatory, but a principle of beneficence, in our usage, asserts an obligation to help others further their important and legitimate interests (Beauchamp and Childress, 1994, p. 260).

Justice

It is more difficult to isolate an explanation of justice in either Beauchamp and Childress or Gillon as their discussion of this concept is both extended and subtle. However, for the purposes of this chapter it is sufficient to say that both Beauchamp and Childress and Gillon present an essentially Aristotelian account of justice. For example, Beauchamp and Childress claim that,

Common to all theories of justice is a minimal requirement traditionally attributed to Aristotle: Equals must be treated equally, unequals must be treated unequally. This principle of formal justice sometimes called the 'principle of formal equality' is 'formal' because it states no particular respects in which equals ought to be treated equally and provides no criteria for determining whether two or more individuals are in fact equals. It merely asserts that whatever respects are under consideration as relevant, persons equal in those respects should be treated equally' (Beauchamp and Childress, 1994, p. 328).

It seems inevitable, as both Beauchamp and Childress and Gillon accept, that there will always, in real cases, be conflicts between these principles which will need to be resolved in order to make an ethical decision. We would now like you to go on to read a paper by Juhani Pietarinen from the University of Turku in Finland in which he explores such conflicts. Pietarinen argues that, whilst several 'principles' are often claimed to be central to ethical medicine (he lists five examples), in actual fact the overriding moral consideration ought to be that of 'justice'.

As you read his paper through, consider whether or not you think his attempt to resolve the conflicts between these principles in favour of justice is successful. If not, can you think of other ways in which, in real cases, practitioners might go about balancing the demands made upon them by conflicting ethical considerations such as these?

Conflicting ethical principles in intensive care

Juhani Pietarinen

Suppose a mentally competent person suffers from a serious illness causing her severe and occasionally intolerable pain. Let us suppose also that her prognosis is not good and that her condition is likely to deteriorate quickly both mentally and physically. She is not expected to live for very long. To keep such a patient alive would usually involve certain special and often quite expensive medical treatment (tube feeding, oxygen and resuscitation equipment, surgical interventions, antibiotics, etc.).

What would the ethical care of this person require? Would it mean keeping her alive by all means possible? Or could it also mean under certain circumstances limiting intervention to minimal pain-controlling measures? Could it also under certain circumstances mean the withholding of treatment altogether?

There are several intuitively plausible ethical principles upon which it is sometimes claimed decisions concerning intensive care such as this might be based. However, as we shall see, these

principles tend to conflict with one another, and this means that we have to find a method for solving such conflicts.

Some of the most commonly cited ethical principles in healthcare are as follows:

- *The principle of self-determination*
A competent person has the right to make and carry out decisions concerning her state of health.

- *The principle of care*
The healthcare professionals have the moral obligation to benefit their patients and not to harm them.

- *The principle of respect for human life*
The healthcare professionals have the moral obligation to preserve and promote the life of their patients.

- *The principle of justice*
The patients should be treated in accordance with the requirements of fairness.

- *The principle of cost-effectiveness*
Healthcare decisions should aim at the greatest net balance of expected utility.

ACTIVITY: How does Pietarinen's list of principles compare with your own? Do you have more or less than him? Is it possible to fit your principles under his headings? If not, why not?

One way in which conflict between principles might be resolved would be if it were possible to identify a hierarchy of principles. That is, if some of the principles always overrode the others. Do you think it would be possible to put your principles into an order of this kind? What kind of problems do you face in the attempt?

Now go on to read Pietarinen's analysis of the relationships between the various principles. His aim in this paper is to emphasize the importance of justice in decisions concerning intensive care. Do you think he succeeds in this?

If there are no serious defects in either the patient's ability to control her desires and actions, or in reasoning which might vitiate the important decisions and choices she has to make, or in the information upon which the decisions at hand are based, then the patient can be called competent (or autonomous; see Harris, 1985, pp. 196–201). The principle of self-determination should have a prominent role in the case of competent patients. When patients are fully informed of their situation and there are no obvious defects in their ability to control their desires, or to reason and make decisions, then they are very good authorities in deciding on the nature of their care, i.e. withholding intensive life-prolonging measures and their decision should be respected.

Perhaps the most common way to support the principle of self-determination is to appeal to Immanuel Kant's requirement of respect for persons or to John Stuart Mill's requirement of the freedom of individuals. My argument is that the right to self-determination belongs to the basic rights (or 'liberties' in the Rawlsian sense) of a just society. Equal right to self-determination is therefore an essential part of justice.

Under what circumstances does this principle of self-determination come into conflict with the other principles I have listed?

The principle of care might be said to conflict with the principle of self-determination in cases of patients who have a fatal disease but who don't want intensive life-prolonging measures. One of the most important ethical guides for doctors and nurses has long been the dictum *'primum non nocere'* or 'above all do no harm'. If this is accepted, then the obligation not to harm people is more stringent than the obligation to benefit them. When the case of refraining from using certain medical treatment is considered from this point of view, a serious problem arises: the decision not to treat someone as efficiently as possible will have as a consequence a more rapid deterioration of the condition of the patient than there would have been under the non-minimal treatment. The decision seems to conflict with the principle of non-maleficence that is included in the principle of care.

However, the principle of care also demands a commitment to beneficence. Why should avoiding

harm always have priority over doing good? Preventing illnesses and disease is an important objective of healthcare, but so is recovering from illness and injury as well as the relief of pain. Indeed, in some form or other the beneficence of human beings must be the main aim of medical care and healthcare in general (see Gillon, 1985, ch.13). Looking from the point of beneficence, the principle of care can be made compatible with the minimal treatment decisions in the care for the dying person. There are good grounds for thinking that they will be more beneficial to patients than intensive life-prolonging procedures. What is more essential here, however, is the fact that medical paternalism of the kind above is against justice. It denies the status of an autonomous individual as the ultimate authority in matters of her concern.

ACTIVITY: Pietarinen argues that, whilst there may appear to be a conflict between the 'principle of care' and that of 'self-determination', they are in this case at least in fact compatible if it can be shown that intensive life-prolonging procedures are less 'beneficial' than minimal treatment. Under what conditions do you think that this might be the case? And under what conditions do you think it would be right to override the patient's self-determination in their best interests or in the principle of care?

Take a few moments to look back at the chapter on 'ethical decisions at the end of life' where we tested the hypothesis that the goal of medicine at the end of life ought to be that of 'relieving suffering'.

We would now like you to continue with your reading of Pietarinen's paper and, while you do so, to see if you can pick out and write down the various stages in his argument.

Perhaps the most serious argument against minimal treatment or non-treatment decisions can be developed from the viewpoint of the principle of respect for human life. According to this principle the life of human persons is intrinsically valuable, and it is therefore our moral duty to promote the life of persons and to refrain from destroying it. As John Harris puts it, 'an irreplaceable part of what it is to value life must be a belief that it is better that people live rather than die, and die later rather than earlier' (Harris, 1985, p. 53). In medical ethics, this means that healthcare professionals, doctors and nurses who adhere to the principle of 'respect for human life', have an obligation to prolong life by taking medical measures to do so.

But how fundamental is this obligation? Is it an absolute requirement in the sense that it overrides all other moral and non-moral considerations? Another difficult issue is the notion of 'life' here. Should we give 'life' in this context the same meaning as in the biosciences, or give it a meaning that reflects certain important social conditions and experiences characteristic of human beings? It does not seem plausible to think that to prolong the biological life of persons would be an absolute obligation of doctors and other healthcare professionals. It is a typical *prima facie* obligation, valid to the extent that there are no other obligations or other moral considerations of comparable importance at stake, prima facie obligations can by definition be overridden under certain circumstances.

Firstly, respect for a person's self-determination requires that, if a patient sincerely and clearly wants to avoid protracted care, this should count as an overriding reason for not attempting anything more than minimal treatment. Sometimes, for example, continued treatment may involve conflict with values that are of the utmost importance to the patient, as in the paradigmatic example, blood transfusions for Jehovah's Witnesses who refuse them. Secondly, protracted intensive care may, in fact, mean a gross violation of both the requirement of beneficence and that of non-maleficence, when it is so painful that it would be inhumane to submit anyone to it. And, thirdly, providing intensive care for one person seems to be unjust when the resources it requires might be used for the care of other and perhaps greater numbers of persons (cf. Harris, 1985, pp. 57–58).

Are these considerations compelling enough to override the requirement of preserving the patient's life to the very end, at any cost? It seems to me that the answer must be affirmative. It is very difficult to see why we should give greater importance to unqualified biological life than to something that might properly be called human life, i.e. life worth living for human persons. The reading of the principle of respect for life will depend very much upon how we understand the value of life, whether we judge it to be 'primarily a value to the person whose life it is or of some independent importance' (Harris, 1985, p. 58). The moral considerations above strongly recommend the former.

How did you get on with this task? Sometimes it can be incredibly difficult to pick out the claims being made in a text in bioethics. We have picked out the following structure up until this point.

(a) According to the principle of respect for life, it is our duty to promote life and refrain from destroying it.

(b) In medicine this means that practitioners have to take medical measures to do so.

(c) Biological life is less valuable than 'human life'. By this he means 'life worth living for human beings'.

(d) It is not plausible for the preservation of merely biological life to be an absolute obligation of practitioners. It is only a *prima facie* obligation. Which only stands unless it conflicts with other obligations of comparable importance.

(e) Self-determination is an overriding principle and obligation. Especially when to go against self-determination means overriding the patient's values.

(f) The principle of care (beneficence and non-maleficence) are also overriding when the intervention causes intolerable pain.

(g) The principle of justice may also be overriding if it uses resources which should be allocated to others.

(h) These three considerations mean that the principle of respect for life should sometimes be overridden.

My final remarks concern the two remaining principles, the principle of justice and the principle of cost-effectiveness. It seems obvious that they do not cause any serious problems in the case of patients insisting on minimal care only. It is neither unjust nor against utility calculations to choose a minimal care for persons who seriously want it. The situation is different, however, when the patient has not indicated their will or if they expressly want protracted intensive care.

According to the Roman Catholic doctrine of ordinary and extraordinary means, 'one is held to use only . . . means that do not involve any grave burden for oneself or another' (Pope Pious XII, 1957). In other words, saving life is morally obligatory only if its pursuit is not excessively burdensome or disproportionate in relation to the expected benefits (Gillon, 1985, p. 141). This means, in effect, that a solution to the very serious moral problem of how much doctors should strive to keep their patients alive would be found in calculations of cost-effectiveness.

I think it is not morally acceptable to make such a strong appeal to cost-effectiveness in intensive care decisions. If the patient wants to live, then the withholding of even extraordinary means seems unjustified. It would be against the patient's right to self-determination, against the requirements of care and against the principle of respect for human life. We cannot justify such violations simply by appealing to high costs. Even when we cannot judge whether it is in the patient's interests to live, but her staying alive does not seem to be a burden to her, it is questionable to stop life-prolonging care by appealing to high costs. We should rather appeal to justice. The capacity of intensive care units is limited, and a patient receiving expensive intensive care is doing so at the expense of other patients who need similar care but must be excluded from it. Moreover, the funds used to provide intensive care could often be used in a more effective way to provide different types of care for others (Brody, 1988, p. 35).

Justice requires that the intensive care system is fair for all citizens. This means firstly, that everyone ought to have an equal right to it, and, secondly, that the allocation of resources among the various fields of healthcare should be fair and, thirdly, that all individuals should have an equal opportunity to get intensive care.

The crucial question in allocating resources is not what would be a sufficient share of intensive care but what would be a just or fair share. But what kind of distribution of healthcare resources would be fair? And what kind of procedure would guarantee an equal opportunity for people to life-prolonging services (e.g. a 'first-come-first-served' or a triage approach?). These are very difficult questions and cannot be answered without a full-scale theory of justice.

My argument has been that the most important moral problems of intensive care tend to come back to the question of justice. This means that solutions to the kinds of problems I have described will be as acceptable as the theory of justice upon which they are based.

We end this section having begun the process of investigating the importance of autonomy to ethical medicine and having problematized to some extent, the claim that respecting autonomy and patient choice is a simple matter of doing what the patient asks. We have also looked at the conflicts between respect for autonomy and other important values in medical practice. We shall be returning to these questions again throughout this chapter. In the next section we will be going on to look at just what is meant by 'autonomy'.

Section 2: What is autonomy?

In Section 1 we looked at the conflicts between respect for autonomy and other principles and values in ethical medicine. Bearing this in mind, we are now going to look more closely at the concept of autonomy itself. This is a theme which has emerged in several places throughout this workbook as a whole, most notably in the chapter on 'long-term care', and it seems to lie at the heart of the question of what counts as ethical medicine. What do we mean by autonomy and how do the various interpretations of autonomy relate to medical practice?

This section will go on to take the form of a reading exercise using a paper by Veikko Launis from Finland, but we would like to start off by asking you to read the following case study in the light of your work in the previous section.

THE CASE OF CARL

Carl suffers from dementia and for this reason lives in a residential nursing home. During the day, Carl seems fine. He functions well but towards the evening, and in particular when it is time for him to go to bed, Carl becomes very distressed, irritable and nervous. This manifests itself in a desire to wake up the people in the beds and rooms around him. The staff have tried their best to help Carl to relax and to find ways of avoiding his feelings of nervousness. They have tried letting him stay up for longer and they have tried talking to him and trying to soothe him. But as soon as the 'coast is clear' he leaves his bed and starts waking the others. Recently, the staff have used some sedatives but these too have failed to solve the problem. The night staff find it very difficult to manage and the other residents are clearly suffering. What ought to be done?

At a staff meeting several suggestions have been made. One of these was to set up a 'gate' around Carl's bed and another was to 'lure' Carl into taking a sleeping pill.

ACTIVITY: The case of Carl is a much more everyday kind of case than that of Peter Noll. Even so, the problem with which the staff at Carl's home are faced might in some ways be said to be more complex and challenging. What would it mean to 'respect autonomy' in this case? Clearly, there are conflicts here between Carl's autonomy and the interests of others. Nevertheless, having made the decision that Carl's behaviour is unacceptable in a residential setting such as this, how can the staff act in such a way as to respect his autonomy? What would be your decision? Give reasons.

In order to get a sense of the variety of different approaches to the concept of autonomy, we would now like you to go on to read a paper by Veikko Launis of the University of Turku which introduces three different ways of describing autonomy: what he calls the 'Kantian', the 'Humean' and the 'Millian-Frankfurtian'. As you read the paper, consider the case of Carl under each of these descriptions. What would this conception of autonomy mean both in the case of Carl and in that of Peter Noll?

The concept of personal autonomy

Veikko Launis

While the general notion of an autonomous person as a self-determining and self-governing agent is familiar to everyone, philosophers differ remarkably in their interpretation of it as well as in the value, or 'normative weight' they place on it. Some philosophers and ethicists regard personal autonomy as the main principle (or starting point) for their theory, whereas others (the ethical pluralists) take it to be simply one morally important notion among others. There is a wide disagreement in the philosophical literature even on whether it makes sense to attempt to explicate a single meaning of 'personal autonomy' at all (Christman, 1988).

In what follows, I shall not try to provide a new interpretation or definition of 'personal autonomy' nor to attempt to answer the question of whether or not the concept of personal autonomy has a central or single meaning (of which everyone who masters the language is supposed to be aware). What I wish to do, however, is to discuss three rival conceptions of personal autonomy that have been prominent in the philosophical literature. I believe, although I do not have the space to argue the point here, that the choice between these conceptions is relevant to the normative question of how the medical treatment of vulnerable patients, especially children and the mentally ill, should be carried out.

If we leave aside the significantly different question of autonomy (of the will) as a basic condition of moral agency (Lindley, 1986), there are at least three different ways in which the meaning of 'autonomy' can be understood. In these conceptions, autonomy is not regarded as a condition of moral agency but as an ideal feature of persons who are in some meaningful sense independent, rational and capable of self-control. Following Richard Lindley's terminology we can call these conceptions 'Kantian', 'Humean' and 'Millian–Frankfurtian'. I shall consider each in turn.

The Kantian conception of autonomy

According to the Kantian conception of autonomy, an individual is autonomous if she is guided not by contingent inclinations and desires but by reason (or morality) alone. Insofar as a person's behaviour is determined by passions and desires, she is not acting fully autonomously. In this account, to be fully autonomous is to be a fully rational agent – a person motivated by purely rational principles. The rationality requirement is thus included in the conception of autonomy itself.

It should be noticed that the Kantian conception of autonomy is a *substantive* conception and not simply 'formal', since it implies that there are certain decisions or choices (the content of) which cannot qualify as autonomous, no matter how they are made. According to some defenders of this view, such decisions include, for example, the decision to commit suicide and the decision to use addictive drugs such as heroin (because no rational agent would make such a choice).

Many philosophers have argued that the Kantian conception is far too restrictive. For instance, in his famous essay 'Two concepts of liberty' Isaiah Berlin criticizes a view relevantly similar to the Kantian conception (he calls it positive liberty) as follows:

Once I take this view, I am in the position to ignore the actual wishes of men or societies, to bully, to oppress, torture them in the name, and on the behalf, of the 'real' selves, in the secure knowledge that whatever is the true goal of man (happiness, performance of duty, wisdom, a just society, self-fulfilment) must be identical with his freedom – the free choice of his 'true', all be it often submerged and inarticulate, self (Berlin, 1969).

While Berlin's criticism is by no means conclusive, there appear to be many other good reasons to oppose the substantial (or non-formal) interpretation of autonomy. To provide just one, anyone defending such an account will face the overwhelming difficulty of distinguishing those decisions that can qualify as autonomous from those that cannot.

The Humean conception of autonomy

The Humean conception of autonomy is, in several respects, contrary to the Kantian conception. According to the Humean view, actions and decisions are autonomous in so far as they are the result of proper deliberation, that is, in so far as they are not based on false or irrational beliefs or faulty reasoning. In this view, a person's behaviour may well be – and actually is – determined by her inclinations and desires without this being detrimental to her autonomy (Lindley, 1986, pp. 28–43). The account underlines the fact that reason alone can never be a motive of any action or decision. As Hume himself puts it, 'it can never oppose passion in the direction of the will'.

The Humean conception of autonomy is a purely formal conception, since it implies that any given decision or choice, regardless of its content, can qualify as autonomous, as long as it is made in the appropriate way (Husak, 1992, pp. 83–84).

It is not contrary to autonomy (or reason), Hume states, 'to prefer even my own acknowleg'd lesser good to my greater, and have a more ardent affection for the former than the latter'. To be autonomous is simply to act on those (rationally permissible) inclinations and desires one happens to have, and, according to the defenders of this view, there is no reason to believe that those decisions and choices that are somehow unusual or 'odd' must always result from improper deliberation.

According to the critics of this view, the Humean conception of autonomy is, in contrast to the Kantian, far too permissive and minimalist. As Richard Lindley notes, it 'gives insufficient weight to the role of the agent as a deliberator, who can stand back from pushes and pulls, and decide how much weight to give to his various inclinations' (Lindley, 1986, p. 33). Those who advocate the Kantian conception seem to be right, critics of the Humean approach claim, in that autonomy requires from a person the ability to act contrary to (at least sometimes) existing desires and inclinations.

The Millian–Frankfurtian conception of autonomy

The Millian–Frankfurtian conception of autonomy combines in many respects what is best in the Kantian and the Humean conceptions. Where the Kantian conception holds that autonomy requires a person to be totally free from the slavery of her contingent desires and inclinations, the Millian–Frankfurtian conception requires merely that the person's desires and inclinations (on which she acts) be genuinely her own. As Mill himself remarks, they must be 'the expression of his own nature', and not merely the products of external influences. The Millian–Frankfurtian conception thus acknowledges the Humean claim that acting on strong urges and inclinations is not inconsistent with autonomy. However, the conception takes from the Kantian critics of the Humean approach the recognition that human beings are not just the passive victims of whatever inclinations and desires they have (as the Humean con-

ception of autonomy seems to assume). An autonomous person does not automatically act on her desires and inclinations, but subjects them to rational scrutiny (Lindley, 1986, pp. 44–70). Lindley puts the matter as follows:

We all have desires, often conflicting desires, of various strengths. Because we have a will we are able to deliberate about our desires. Autonomy requires that our will is as we want it to be. In other words, the desires which actually motivate us should be the desires we want, after all deliberation has taken place, to motivate us. Someone of whom this is not true, is not in control of his own conduct (Lindley, 1986, p. 66).

To make the Millian–Frankfurtian conception still clearer, it is helpful to make use of a distinction drawn by Henry Frankfurt in his influential paper, 'Freedom of the will and the concept of a person'. According to Frankfurt's account, there are different levels of desires and preferences. In addition to what he calls 'first-order desires', there are 'second-order' (and perhaps even higher-order) desires, that is, desires about the kinds of lower-order desires we want (Frankfurt, 1971). Personal autonomy requires that an agent's decisions and actions be in accordance with her (authentic, self-selected) highest-order desires and preferences. That is to say, they must be in accordance with what the agent judges to be in her best interests.

Concluding remarks

According to the Millian–Frankfurtian conception of autonomy, there are no substantive ends or lifestyles that would be required by autonomy alone. People's values and goals differ considerably, and there is no objective way to prefer one to another. Like the Humean account, the Millian–Frankfurtian conception is thus based on a purely formal (and value-neutral) interpretation of personal autonomy.

Despite its advantages, the Millian–Frankfurtian conception of autonomy cannot of course specify necessary and sufficient conditions for being an autonomous person. At best, it can give us a hint of what is necessarily required for an adequate analysis of this practically important and in many ways ambiguous concept, 'autonomy'.

In the next section we will be going on to explore the various ways in which autonomy and patient choice have been expressed in European law. Then, in Section 4, we shall return to the question of concepts of autonomy by looking at some alternative, contemporary, conceptions of medical ethics which place less emphasis on autonomy.

Section 3: Autonomy: alternative models in European law

In the previous two sections of this chapter, you've seen some case examples testing the limits of autonomy. In this section, we will be looking at its limitations in law, and conversely at new initiatives to give it greater weight.

Before we do that, however, we need to point out that autonomy is actually a concept from ethics, not law. Autonomy doesn't appear in the index of major texts on healthcare law (e.g. Montgomery, 1997) whereas it notches up more references than any other entry in the index for a classic text in ethics, Beauchamp and Childress's *Principles of Biomedical Ethics*. Perhaps that seems a trivial observation; but the differences go deeper than that. Autonomy may, or may not, be the ethical value which legal systems are most concerned to protect.

Although Beauchamp and Childress argue that 'rules requiring consent in medicine and research are rooted in concerns about protecting and enabling autonomous choice by patients and subjects' (Beauchamp and Childress, 1989, p. 67), this is not universally true, even if it holds for the United States. In English law, for example, the legal requirement of consent has quite a different basis, and if we had to name one value which the English law of consent is concerned to protect, we would say that it is trust between doctor and patient.

This difference is consistent with the fact that, in English law, there is no right to *informed* consent, as there is in the United States. In the common law which underpins both systems, treatment without consent is regarded as a civil wrong (the tort of battery). Whereas a doctrine of informed consent has grown up in the United States, particularly since the Second World War, the original requirement for consent, which persists in England, is primarily required as a defence to an alleged tort of battery. The older underlying reasoning has less to do with enabling autonomous choice than with preserving the patient's bodily integrity and the physician's professional integrity, with keeping alive the value of trust in the fiduciary relationship between doctor and patient.

To put it another way, the basis for consent in English law is not the patient's autonomy, but the doctor's duty to provide the patient with the information needed (Trew, 1998, p. 280). It is a doctor-centred standard, arguably even a paternalistic one. By contrast, the standard for consent in American law is what the reasonable patient would want to know, not what the reasonable doctor would want to reveal.

One might argue that this is much the same thing, because in both legal systems we are talking about the information needed to make an autonomous choice. But, whereas Beauchamp and Childress identify their primary concern as autonomous choices and *actions* – 'Consents and refusals are actions, not persons' (Beauchamp and Childress 1989, p. 68) – English law's concern is with the bodily integrity of the *person*: 'Every person's body is inviolate' (*Re F*, 1990). And whereas American law, from which Beauchamp and Childress appear to be generalizing, is rooted in constitutional rights to privacy and property, English law lacks any such constitutional rights. To sum up, 'fully informed consent . . . is not the law in England' (*Sidaway*, 1985); it is an American doctrine. To argue backwards from the right to fully informed consent to patient autonomy won't work in England because there is no right to fully informed consent.

More generally, European models concerning autonomy and consent are likely to be different from the dominant American literature on autonomy. The overall theme of this section, then, is that autonomy is not the sole value of any European legal system. Although the bioethics literature, particularly in the USA, was dominated by the concept of autonomy until recently (with a few long-standing exceptions, such as the work of Daniel Callahan), the legal codes under which European practitioners work are not.

But within Europe we can distinguish different levels of emphasis on autonomy. We will now ask you to read an article by Donna Dickenson which suggests that there are at least three principal models in European healthcare law, each with its own dominant ethical values. Rather than a unitary 'Western' cultural and legal framework in which the rights of the individual are paramount and autonomy is the core value, there are at least three 'different voices' (following Gilligan, 1982). In one of these systems patient autonomy is much more important than in the other two, but even there it is not the sole value.

ACTIVITY: Now read the article, 'Three different models in European medical law and ethics' (based on Dickenson, 1998). As you read, make entries in the following table, whose meaning will become clear as you read; we will compare notes at the end.

	Southern Europe	Western Europe	Nordic Europe
Dominant concept			
Dispute solution			
Legal examples			

Three different models in European medical law and ethics

Donna Dickenson

European medical law and biomedical ethics can be contrasted to dominant American autonomy-based approaches, even though they are all frequently conflated as 'Western'. But at least three 'different voices' within European law and bioethics can also be identified:

- The deontological codes of southern Europe (and Ireland), in which the patient has a positive duty to maximize his or her own health and to follow the doctor's instructions, whilst the physician is constrained more by professional norms than by patient rights

- The liberal, rights-based models of Western Europe, in which the patient retains the negative right to override medical opinion, even if his or her mental capacity is in doubt
- The social welfarist models of the Nordic countries, which concentrate on positive rights and entitlements to universal healthcare provision and entrust dispute resolution to non-elected administrative officials.

Law in general, and medical law in particular, is about conflict resolution: for example, what to do when patients and their doctors disagree about what treatment is best, or whether treatment has been adequately carried out, and at what expense. Essentially I shall argue that the three models' solutions to such disputes are as follows:

- The patient has a positive duty to follow the doctor's instructions and to maximize his or her own health and well-being, a requirement which is often enshrined in constitutional provisions (Southern Europe)
- The patient has a negative right to override medical opinion and to pursue his or her own notion of individual well-being, by resort to the courts if necessary (Western Europe)
- Disputes are unlikely to arise in the first place if a proper social welfare system is in place; if they do come up, they should be resolved in an administrative manner by appointed officials, not by favouring either doctors' duties or patients' rights (Nordic countries). Another way of conceptualizing this third way, however, is in terms of positive rights and entitlements.

Of course, these three models are caricatures of much more complex realities, but like all models, they have their analytical uses. It is particularly interesting, I think, to disentangle the Western European rights-orientated models from the Nordic administrative one, since the two are often confused. There are anomalies, of course: Ireland, though not part of southern Europe, rejects the liberal rights-orientated model of the person, enshrining a positive duty of seeking to promote

one's own health in its constitution in the Italian fashion. Here, the influence of the Catholic Church is clearly important; yet that does not explain why the Netherlands, with a very substantial Catholic population, has embraced the individualist non-Catholic model so wholeheartedly. In the case of Ireland, the discourse of choosing one's own moral principles is comparatively new; yet the Irish do not entirely reject the Kantian notion of self-enacted moral principles. The Church is now coming under fire for failing to educate children in ethical skills, in the ability to stand back and reflect on one's own values. But, although Ireland has never experienced Fascist rule – unlike the countries of southern Europe – there is a long-standing absence of pluralism at official levels (though not in the population), according to at least one Irish writer (Dooley, 1997).

'Medical deontology' is the term which the professional codes of southern Europe typically use to describe their approach. (This includes France, for example, Decret no. 95–1000 du 6 septembre 1995 portant la code de deontologie medicale, a formal legislative act rather than a professional code.) Adapted in 1845 as the term 'deontologie medicale', the phrase really denotes what Americans and northern Europeans would probably term 'professional ethics'. In one article on the Italian code, medical deontology is defined as 'the discipline for the study of norms as well as those pertaining more strictly to professional performance' (Fineschi et al., 1997). This is actually rather close to the vocational model of medical ethics which prevailed in America and Western Europe until recently, in which 'medical ethics [is seen as] a matter of right attitude and certain proscriptions of behaviour' (Ashcroft, 1998).

This is the doctor's side of the bargain; the corresponding virtue in patients is to obey the virtuous doctor. In Italy, for example, where codes of medical ethics date back to the Fascist period, there is a positive duty in the name of the collectivity to maximise one's own health and to allow the doctor free rein in the exercise of his or her beneficence. To the extent that this duty is positively enjoined on doctors, for example, by Article

28 of the Deontological Code, it would actually be morally wrong and legally dubious to stand in the doctors' way. Thus if relatives of a handicapped person or a child refuse consent to treatment, the doctor has a duty of beneficence to proceed regardless. Although the same article deals extensively with the patient's right to informed consent, 'in actual clinical practice doctors are given substantive discretion to resolve potential conflicts between the right of patients to be informed and the need to ensure their compliance' (Calzone, 1996). Despite formal guarantees against enforced treatment in Article 32 of the Italian constitution, physicians tend to rely on implicit consent except in surgery, when formal written consent will normally be obtained. Overall, the aim of the 1995 code is to promote compliance with medical advice rather than patients' rights.

Nevertheless the 1995 code also represents a partial evolution away from paternalism, towards a more equal form of doctor-patient relationship. Article 4, for example, specifically calls on the physician to 'respect the rights of the individual'. This sounds much more like the discourse of autonomy rather than that of medical paternalism. In specific areas such as medical confidentiality, the 1995 code also represents an advance towards the liberal model on its 1989 predecessor: the old practice of informing next of kin of a terminal diagnosis but withholding the information from the dying person is specifically prohibited. On many other vital questions, however, the code is silent, e.g. in relation to advance directives. Here, the professional's duty of beneficence is presumed to fill in the gaps. Where assisted reproduction is concerned, the Code is quite explicit, particularly in proscribing commercial contract motherhood. The neo-liberal model emphasizing freedom of contract is specifically rejected. Overall, the paramount values in the deontological codes are the professionalism of physicians and the dignity (rather than the rights) of patients (Lebeer, 1998).

It has been said, however, that dignity is what is allotted to those who are not in charge. The second model in European law, of which I take the Netherlands as a strong example and the UK as a weak one, is much more concerned with patients' rights. Of the three European models, this is the closest to the dominant emphasis in American biomedical literature on autonomy (e.g. Engelhardt, 1986), but it is still crucially different from US law and practice, particularly in its British variant.

Whereas the Italian code of professional conduct is intended to be 'as free as possible from the strict confines of the law' (Barni, 1991), the rights-orientated approaches of Western Europe rely on the law to enforce patients' rights. And whilst it has been said that in Greece the patient is in some sense defined as a defective person, not fully competent (Peonidis, 1996), Western European practice more typically refers to patients as 'service users' and upholds the assumption of competence (at least for adults) even in very extreme circumstances. In the 1993 English case of *Re C*, for example, a 68-year-old paranoid schizophrenic whose delusions included the belief that he was himself a world-famous vascular surgeon was judged competent to reject the preferred management plan of the real vascular surgeon who was treating him for a gangrenous leg. On the other hand, the standard for consent in UK law remains what a reasonable doctor would disclose rather than what a reasonable patient would want to know; in this and other aspects of the law, the British model represents at best a weak form of the patients' rights approach, arguably closer to the professional duties model of southern Europe. A strong version of the patients' rights model is to be found in the Netherlands, particularly in regard to mental health legislation.

As in the UK, the assumption of patient autonomy is not vitiated in Dutch legislation by a finding of mental incapacity. Where the Netherlands goes further, however, is in affording even compulsorily detained patients the right to refuse treatment for psychiatric disorders. In the Mental Health Act for England and Wales, a distinction is made between refusal of physical treatments, which is allowed, and refusal of treatment for mental illness, which is not (s63). Dutch legislation dating from 1994, however, gives the compulsorily detained mental patient the right to accept or refuse the treatment plan which the psychiatrist draws up. The law thus makes no distinction between the rights and treatment decisions of a competent patient and an incompetent patient, which some Dutch commentators find an extreme version of the patients' rights position (Berghmans, 1997b; Verkerk, 1998). A series of consultation rounds between physician and patient gives even the compulsorily detained patient the upper hand in cases of conflict, unless he or she is a serious danger to himself or herself, or to others. Consent from family members cannot override the patient's own refusal, whereas in most Southern European systems, familial proxy consent is important. In English law, too, a family member cannot decide on another's behalf; indeed, too close influence from a relative counts as duress, which makes consent to treatment invalid (*Re T*, 1992).

Dutch legislation is also scrupulous about requiring consent to admission, even from autistic, learning-disabled or senile patients, where English law and practice allow for informal admission (R v Bournewood, 1998; Shah and Dickenson, 1998; Livingston et al., 1998; Eastman and Peay 1998). Unless the patient actively consents, formal mechanisms for treatment must be invoked; in contrast, English practice relies heavily on informal admission in the absence of active resistance. In the Netherlands, where the 1994 legislation was strongly influenced by the patients' rights movement, the decision regarding compulsory admission must be a formal one, and it is entirely separate from the decision regarding compulsory treatment. Thus the onus is on the medical professional in both cases to prove that compulsion is necessary.

Of all the European jurisdictions, then, the Netherlands seems the closest to the dominant American model; but even there practice must be seen in the context of a national insurance-based system of healthcare provision, a very different set of structures from that in the United States. The existence of universal health services there, and in the UK, demonstrates that patient choice and autonomy are not the only values; solidarity with less advantaged members of society is also crucial.

If we look particularly at structures and delivery mechanisms, we begin to move into the territory of the third model. Giving rights to patients is only one side of the coin; they also need to be given the structure and facilities to actuate these rights, many Dutch commentators argue – particularly where vulnerable groups are concerned (e.g. Ter Meulen, 1996). The 1994 legislation also provides for patient advocates, a kind of ombudsman, in all hospitals; but the most complete version of the administrative model of conflict resolution is found not in the Netherlands but in the Nordic nations.

Here the paradigm I shall examine is the Finnish Act on the Status and Rights of the Patient (Statute no. 785, 1992, which came into force on 1st March, 1993), and the earlier Patient Injury Act (1986). Although one strand in the 1992 Finnish statute is strengthening legal guarantees of patient autonomy, the patient's rights are still primarily conceived in the social context, against the background of the mature Nordic welfare state (Lahti, 1996). To put it another way, social justice is the pre-existing value, to which autonomy is being added now that a certain level of general welfare has been attained – the opposite of the American model, in which universal provision has still to be attained but awareness of patients' rights is high.

> . . . [I]n public debate the human rights, the legal protection of an individual as well as the rights of consumers and, accordingly, the rights of clients/patients were emphasised to a greater extent than before. This has to do with the advancement of the general level of well-being and knowledge in a welfare state. People were no longer content with the realisation of the fundamental rights of the individual. Instead, they demanded further improvements in social security and increased possibilities for individuals to take actively [*sic*] part in the decision-making that concern [*sic*] them, as well. In addition, certain changes in the structure of the health and medical care system have increased the pressure to enhance the rights of patients (Lahti, 1996).

However, patients' civil and social rights may come into conflict:

So two main emphases can be recognized in the development of Finnish health law during [the] last few decades, and some tension may occur between them: on the one hand, the strengthening of the patient's freedom rights (in particular, the right to self-determination) and the procedural guarantees of her legal protection and, on the other hand, the enhancement of the individual's social rights (e.g. by increasing health services and the possibilities for access to medical treatment (Lahti, 1994, pp. 208–9).

In the classic Nordic model, resources and social structures to support the rhetoric of rights, to transform them from negative liberties to positive entitlements are part of statutory provision; dispute resolution is primarily through non-elective administrative channels, rather than through civil litigation or criminal prosecution, as in the United States.

In Finland the control over the healthcare and medical personnel has for a long time focused on the administrative sanctions and ethical self-regulation of the personnel. Criminal trials brought against medical personnel have remained very rare. . . . The interests of the patient as well as of the health and medical care personnel would be better served if the disagreements arising from the patient's care and treatment could be settled as flexible [*sic*] as possible in each unit of health and medical care (Lahti, 1994, p. 210).

Indeed, the source of the greater concern for patient autonomy in Finland was a government official, not a grass-roots demand, a professional organization or a court decision: in 1973 the Parliamentary Ombudsman stated that Article 6 of the Constitution Act, which protects personal liberty, extended to patient self-determination and bodily integrity. Following this announcement and a lengthy consultation, a no-fault system of injury compensation was enacted in 1986, in line with the Finnish preference for flexible resolution of disputes and their distaste for litigation. One ramification of this is that failure to obtain consent is not actually grounds for compensation; only worsening of the patient's condition as a result of that failure. For example, Lahti cites the case of a dentist who failed to obtain the patient's consent before removing four teeth which could

have been filled. The Supreme Court ruled that there was no action in law for failure to obtain consent, but that damages could be paid because there were no acceptable medical grounds for removing the teeth. 'It should be noticed that a therapeutic measure performed in the absence of the patient's consent is not considered — exceptional cases excluded — punishable as an offence encroaching on life, liberty or bodily integrity, i.e. as a crime in the nature of assault and battery. . . . In this respect a patient's right to self-determination is not protected . . .' (Lahti, 1994, p. 213). Although this example predates the Patient Injury Act, positive effects of treatment still would not count as injury in Finland. By contrast, in the American case of Mohr v Williams a woman had consented to an operation on her right ear, but the surgeon had erred: it was the left ear which required surgery. He operated on the left ear without her consent, and was held liable for battery despite the actual benefit to the patient. This comparison illustrates the far greater value which the American system sets on patient choice and self-determination as such, rather than on benefit to the patient.

Similarly, in the 1992 Act the provisions on competence and right to refuse treatment for children and young people are left very open, with the rather vague provision that a competent minor has to be treated 'in mutual understanding'; the model for resolving any conflicts does not involve recourse to the courts in adversarial fashion, but administrative intervention. There is no formal definition of competence or of informed consent. Instead, it seems to be assumed that conflicts can be resolved in the public healthcare system precisely because it is a public healthcare system, with the virtues of universality and solidarity built in. The act's principal drafter has described it as a 'soft law' aiming to avoid sanctions, concentrating instead on influencing practitioner attitudes (Lahti, 1996). In contrast, representatives of the nascent Finnish patients' rights association describe the idea of the rights-aware patient as a foreign import, and look to the Netherlands for their model

(Södergård, 1996). This movement criticises the ombudsmen as mere officers of the 'system'; unless the liberal notion of separation of powers is preserved, patients' rights advocates argue, there can be no real accountability. But this view, typical of the second model, appears to remain a minority one.

Clearly, there is some movement in each of the three models towards increasing the weight given to autonomy; equally clearly, autonomy is not the sole value in any of them. This movement is two-way: the concept of autonomy is likely to be changed by its encounter with other, pre-existing values in these three legal systems. Autonomy is not simply being imported unaltered into previously 'primitive' systems; what emerges from these new developments will be something very different from the standard model of instrumental, rational individualism.

ACTIVITY: How did you get on with this exercise? To what extent do you think Dickenson's analysis of the European legal situation is an accurate reflection of differences of emphasis on ethical values? As Dickenson herself emphasizes strongly, whilst a model of this kind has analytical uses there is sure to be significant variation 'on the ground'. Can you think of any examples of cases/ judgements or situations which do not fit this model?

Before moving on to the next section make a list of the key issues raised by this chapter.

Section 4: Medical ethics: alternative models

In Section 3 we saw that no European legal system is as autonomy-conscious as American law. Autonomy is working its way into systems based on other core values – such as the Finnish one – but it will be incorporated in a very different way, building onto the prior value of universal provi-

sion in the Nordic example. These new initiatives in law will produce a new sort of hybrid, a different kind of autonomy, perhaps.

Similarly, new initiatives in theory have also challenged the dominance of standard notions of autonomy in medical ethics. There is increasing dissatisfaction with 'the notion, which nowadays is almost obsessive, of respect for the patient's autonomy' (Silva, 1997). But this opposition is not rooted in medical paternalism; it does not seek a return to the 'bad old days' of 'doctor knows best'. Indeed, it can be seen as a logical progression in the notion of autonomy, an extension of it to groups previously excluded – particularly when we look at feminist ethics. These new models seek to refine the notion of autonomy rather than replace it altogether. (In passing, the second theory we shall present, virtue ethics, is actually not new at all, in the sense that it consciously evokes classical Greek philosophy, particularly Aristotle; but we will not pursue this point further.) In this section we will look at three such models and ask what lessons they offer for practice, where a narrow model of autonomy may well be insufficient. They are as follows:

- Narrative/feminist ethics
- Virtue ethics
- Deliberative ethics

Our way of proceeding in this section will be through guided readings of three articles, one for each of the three models. We begin with narrative/feminist ethics, in an article by the British philosopher Susan Mendus, 'Out of the doll's house.'

You will see that Mendus uses Ibsen's play *A Doll's House* as an extended metaphor and explanatory device. We think this use of literature is important in teaching medical ethics, enriching our responses and moving beyond the exclusively scientific training which most doctors and medical students have had since early adolescence. But, it will take a little more unravelling than you may be used to, so we suggest that you read it actively, using the grid below. As you read, please begin filling in this table, a similar activity to what you did for the three different legal systems in Section 3. What we want you to concentrate on is, firstly, what criticisms the new model offers of the standard autonomy-centred model in principlist medical ethics; secondly, what alternative concepts it stresses as equally or more important; and, thirdly, what concepts it retains from the standard model.

	Narrative ethics	Virtue ethics	Deliberative ethics
Critique of autonomy model			
Alternative concepts to model			
Retained concepts from model			

Out of the doll's house

Susan Mendus

Autonomy is, without doubt, one of the most important concepts (maybe the most important concept) in modern moral and political philosophy. John Rawls (1971), Ronald Dworkin (1977) and Joseph Raz (1986) (three of the most influential political philosophers of the late twentieth century) all accord a central place to autonomy, and all agree that political arrangements are to be judged in large part by their ability to create the conditions in which people may lead autonomous lives. Autonomy is crucial [in this view] for individual flourishing and, by extension, for a good society. But what exactly is autonomy? Here agreement runs out:

. . . [T]he term is used in an exceedingly broad fashion. It is used sometimes as an equivalent of liberty, sometimes as equivalent to self-rule or sovereignty, sometimes as identical with freedom of the will. It is equated with dignity, integrity, individuality, independence, responsibility and self-knowledge. It is identified with qualities of self-assertion, with critical reflection, with freedom from obligation, with absence of external causation, with knowledge of one's own interests. It is related to actions, to beliefs, to reasons for acting, to rules, to the will of other persons, to thoughts and to principles. About the only features held constant from one author to another are that autonomy is a feature of persons and that it is a desirable quality to have (Gerald Dworkin, in Christman, pp. 54–5).

Autonomy, it seems, is a 'catch-all' term, lacking clear definition and deployed primarily for the purposes of evincing approval. Cynically, we might say that nobody knows what it is, but that whatever it is, it is a good thing for individuals to have and for society to promote.

My aim is to question that conclusion. I want to argue that the assumption that autonomy is a desirable quality to have, and the concomitant assumption that political arrangements are to be judged (in some part) by their ability to foster autonomy, overlooks an important set of prior considerations. When those considerations are taken into account, autonomy will be seen to be less important to individuals than is usually supposed, and, by extension, to be less central to the construction of social and political policies. In brief, I shall suggest that we should worry less about autonomy than most moral and political philosophers are inclined to do.

First, however, I must say something about what I take autonomy to be. As has already been emphasized, the philosophical literature is replete with diverse and often contradictory accounts. However, one prominent claim, and the one I shall concentrate on here, is that autonomy is a personal ideal according to which individuals are authors of their own lives. To be autonomous is to be able to live out one's plans, projects and aspirations and, in that sense, to 'write the story' of one's own life. Thus Joseph Raz, subscribing to this conception, defines autonomy as follows:

The ruling idea behind an ideal of personal autonomy is that people should make their own lives. The autonomous person is a (part) author of his own life. The ideal of personal autonomy is the vision of people controlling, to some degree, their own destiny, fashioning it through successive decisions throughout their lives (Raz, 1986, p. 369).

ACTIVITY: Does this definition of autonomy fit the case of Peter Noll? Consider this entry in his diary after he learned the diagnosis of bladder cancer:

What bothers me is the loss of freedom: having others in charge of you, to be drawn into a medical machine which controls a person and which one cannot fight. Naturally, intolerable pain will disturb me too. In order to escape it, one enters the machine that takes away pain and at the same time freedom. And it's precisely the enslavement that I don't want.

We think it probably does: what Peter Noll most feared was that the narrative of his life (and death) would be written not by himself but by what he called 'the medical machine'. Once he consented to the surgery and radiation for his bladder cancer, he felt, the script would be out of his authorship: things would take their own course, and he would be sucked into one procedure after another.

The notion of exercising autonomy as writing one's own script also entails possible conflict with the approved roles, the conventional script, and this aspect of Peter Noll's case can be seen in a comment from his friend Ruth after his decision to refuse treatment:

You see, you're upsetting people with your decision. If someone has cancer, he goes to the hospital and has surgery – that's what's normal. That's why it's irritating and confusing that you sit here and say 'I have cancer' while refusing to go to hospital. If you went to the hospital everything would be all right: people could visit you, bring flowers, and after a certain time say, 'Thank God, he's been released', and again after a certain time, 'Now he's back in' . . . but at least they would know where to find you (Noll, 1989).

By exercising his autonomy in the sense of refusing to read from the socially acceptable script for cancer sufferers, but insisting instead on writing his own narrative, Noll placed himself outside the bounds: people no longer knew where to locate him in the usual story – not just literally.

Now continue with your reading of Susan Mendus:

On this understanding, then, my life is a story and what matters is that I should, so far as possible,

write that story myself. Of course, and as Raz is at pains to point out, such authorship can never be complete, nor can it be attained in a social vacuum. Thus, the kinds of stories I can write will always depend, in some part, on the constraints imposed by the circumstances in which I find myself. [However], social and political arrangements are, we might say, justifiable to the extent that they foster and encourage individual autonomy understood as authorship, and they are suspect to the degree that they obstruct the pursuit of that ideal.

One further warning: just as the ideal of autonomy need not imply total and unconstrained freedom of choice, so it need not imply a single object of choice. The autonomous agent will not be required to make a single, once-for-all decision about how his life should go. As Raz expresses it: 'The ideal of personal autonomy is not to be identified with the ideal of giving one's life a unity. . . . The autonomous life may consist of diverse and heterogeneous pursuits. And a person who frequently changes his tastes can be as autonomous as one who never shakes off his adolescent preferences.' (Raz, 1986, pp. 370–1).

Autonomy, then, understood as authorship, is consistent with limitation on choices, and distinct from any requirement that a life shall have a unity. The story of my life, we might say, will have a setting, and it may well be a story with diverse strands rather than a single 'plot'. It is, nevertheless, an autonomous life to the extent that I am able to mould and fashion it for myself.

In what follows, I want to argue that autonomy, so understood, is less important than is commonly believed. My aim is to show that by giving centrality to the concept of autonomy, moral and political philosophers neglect what is of most significance to many people (particularly to women), that they simultaneously misrepresent the nature of personal relationships, and that, in consequence, they advocate social and political arrangements which are false to the realities of life.

I shall try to substantiate these claims via the examination of a single dramatic case: the case of Nora in Ibsen's play *The Doll's House*. My claim will be that we should not understand Nora as lacking in autonomy. There is an alternative account of her predicament, one which identifies it as problematic not because she is unable to write the story of her own life, but because, and in ways to be explained, she is unable to read the story of her own life.

In Ibsen's play the two central characters are Torvald Helmer and his wife, Nora. Torvald is a successful businessman who, as the play opens, is on the verge of promotion to a high-ranking position in the local bank, which will bring with it wealth and respect from the local community. However, his success and status have been hard-won, and during the early years of his marriage to Nora, he suffered serious ill-health. At that time, and unknown to him, Nora borrowed money to pay for his medical treatment. Because women were not allowed to borrow money without a male guarantor, she forged her father's signature on the official loan documents. As the play progresses it becomes increasingly likely that her misdeed will be exposed, Torvald's career in the bank will be threatened, and his reputation as a pillar of the community will be destroyed. In the final scene, Torvald does, indeed, discover what Nora has done. She hopes that when he discovers this, he will realise how much she has loved him and how much she has been prepared to do for him. To her horror, he receives the news as proof that he has been married to a forger, a liar and a cheat. His wife is not an innocent and guileless 'doll'. Rather, she is a common criminal.

> **ACTIVITY: Think of a situation from your practice experience which parallels Nora's problem. Perhaps you found yourself having to either confront, obey or find a way around a rule that you found unjust. How did you handle the situation? What was the reaction of your colleagues?**

The case of Nora, as the title of the play makes clear, is the case of a woman who is treated as a 'doll', more generally as a child, incapable of making decisions for herself, incapable of understanding, much less handling, financial matters. It is a picture

endorsed as appropriate by the society in which she lives. It is a picture which portrays what is 'suitable' for a married woman in a society such as hers. The final traumatic scene, in which Nora realizes that this is the picture endorsed by her husband and her society, is the focus of most critical discussion.

The autonomy of individuals is, we might say, acknowledged by allowing them a voice in the determination of the rules which are to govern their society. Social institutions are just if they are such that autonomous agents could and would agree to them. However, as a woman, Nora has had no voice in this 'initial conversation' which determines the rules of justice that prevail in her society. In this respect she has been denied autonomy. Where autonomy is understood as authorship, Nora has been denied a voice in writing the rules. Additionally, and yet more worryingly, she has been denied the language in which to express her disagreement with those rules, once they have been decided upon.

What I wish to concentrate on is the quite general assumption that denying individual autonomy is suspect, together with the connected assumption that autonomy is a matter of authorship. It is also part of my aim to provide an alternative model of autonomy, or, more correctly, a model of what makes life valuable which depends much less heavily on autonomy or authorship.

In *After Virtue* Alasdair MacIntyre writes:

Man is in his actions and practice, as well as in his fictions, essentially a story-telling animal. He is not essentially, but becomes through his history, a teller of stories that aspire to truth. But the key question for men is not about their own authorship; I can only answer the question 'What am I to do?' if I can answer the prior question, 'Of what story or stories do I find myself a part?' (MacIntyre, 1981, p. 216).

> **ACTIVITY: Stop here for a moment and think about how this might apply to medical ethics and to clinical practice. What is the importance of the question, 'Of what story or stories do I find myself a part?' One answer might be that it is only by understanding how**

the patient understands the story of his or her life and illness that doctors and nurses can communicate effectively with patients. But the converse is also true: the patient is caught up in the narrative of medicine. In our age this is a story about overcoming illness through the heroic discoveries of modern science and the application of wonder technologies. (In this script Peter Noll refused to play a part.)

Now continue with your reading of Mendus.

In what follows I want to take MacIntyre's central claim (that I can only answer the question 'What am I to do?' if I can answer the prior question 'Of what story or stories do I find myself a part?' and apply it in the case of Nora. I shall argue that Nora's predicament is not essentially that of a woman who is unable to write the story of her life. Rather, it is the predicament of a woman who has systematically misread the story of her life. More generally, and following MacIntyre, I shall argue that successful reading is primary and successful writing only secondary. To that extent, modern emphasis on autonomy is partial and potentially distorting of our understanding of what makes life valuable and what makes political and social institutions legitimate.

Firstly, Nora misreads the relationship between the laws of society and personal attachments. In other words, she misreads the world in which she finds herself. Secondly, and connectedly, she misreads her relationship with Torvald, and thirdly, she misreads herself.

Nora's misreading of her society is seen in her astonishment that the law can forbid an act which is undertaken from love. Although she knows that she has broken the law in forging her father's signature, she nevertheless believes that her act is justifiable because it was done to help her husband. Although, of course, Nora understands that she has acted illegally, she cannot believe that she has acted morally badly. If the law says she has, then the law is wrong. Here, then, we have a sense in which Nora misreads the world. She is mistaken about the status of law relative to personal loyalties, and when she discovers what that status is, she is appalled.

Moreover her misreading of the world brings with it a misunderstanding of her relationship with Torvald, and indeed a misreading of Torvald himself. For her discovery that law takes priority over personal relationships is also a discovery that for Torvald law stands above personal relationships. Thus, when faced with a choice between obedience to the law and loyalty to Nora, he chooses the law, saying: 'Nora, I'd gladly work night and day for you, and endure poverty and sorrow for your sake. But no man would sacrifice his honour for the one he loves.' (To which she replies, 'Thousands of women have.') Here we find another way in which Nora has misread her life: not only has she been mistaken about the relative priority of law and personal attachment, she has also been mistaken about their relative priority in Torvald's eyes, and as a consequence she has been mistaken about Torvald himself. She had imagined that he would sacrifice everything, including honour, for her, as she would sacrifice everything for him. In this she is wrong, and her mistake now leads her to conclude that for eight years she has been married to a stranger.

Thirdly, and most poignantly, in the final scene Nora is brought to a realization that she has misread herself. It follows from her misreading of the relationship between law and personal attachment, and the misreading of the relationship between Torvald and herself (he is exposed as a man who cares more about honour in the eyes of the world than about his own wife) that Nora's own life, her hopes, her plans, her aspirations and her actions have all been a deceit. She concludes, 'I thought I had, but really I have never been happy.' The final remark reveals the extent to which Nora's predicament is more a function of her misreading of the world and her place in it, than it is a function of her inability to write the story of her life. In fact, though in a rather perverse sense, she has written the story of her life. She has attained the things she set out to attain — has helped her husband, brought up her children, earned money and in general 'moulded' her life and theirs. What is tragic in her situation is not that she has lacked autonomy, but rather that she has exercised autonomy in a world she has systematically misunderstood.

The discussion of Nora suggests that the ideal of autonomy does not merely make claims about what makes a life valuable for the person who leads it. It is also an ideal which has implications for the ways in which we relate to one another. Thus the claim that what matters most is that 'I mould and fashion my life' implies a clear distinction between myself and others; my life and my projects are to be distinguished from the projects of other people. Of course, other people may contribute to my projects, but it is my projects to which they are contributing. Conversely, of course, other people can constitute a threat to my pursuit of my projects.

What we have here, I suggest, is an account of what makes an individual life worthwhile which implies something rather worrying about the relationship which will hold between the autonomous person and others. What it implies . . . is that a society premised on the value of autonomy will be, at root, a society of strangers – a society which will have difficulty accommodating 'constitutive' relationships such as those of friendship and love. For it is precisely in such relationships that a clear distinction between my projects and those of another person is least plausible.

Thus, when Nora refers to Torvald as a stranger, there are two ways in which her statement can be interpreted: he is a stranger because he is not what she has always believed him to be, and he is also a stranger because, by giving priority to law over personal loyalty, he indicates that the demands of strangers (lawmakers) are more important than his attachment to his own wife. Faced with a choice between the impersonal laws of society and the needs of his wife, he chooses law, and thus in a quite literal sense 'estranges' Nora. Her demands matter less to him than the demands of strangers. More specifically, by refusing to give up his 'honour' for her, he indicates that his life and his projects are still and always distinct from hers. And, in this sense, too, they are strangers to one another.

There are, I think, some very general conclusions to be drawn from these considerations, and the conclusions have implications for our practical dealings with others. Firstly, if we aspire to encourage and develop autonomy, then we must be aware that autonomy is not simply an individual ideal. It is an ideal which has implications for how we relate to others. Put bluntly, a world of autonomous individuals will be, more or less, a world of strangers.

Secondly, and connectedly, the ideal of autonomy cannot be one which merely enables each person to live whatever life he or she chooses: if autonomy implies something about the ways in which we can relate to others, then some kind of relationships will be deformed by the attempt to render them compatible with autonomy. Nora's understanding of marriage is an example of just this.

Thirdly, and most importantly, the ideal of autonomy presupposes a background of values, and where an individual misunderstands that background, it is not the case that she is damaged by being denied autonomy. She is mocked because her life is based on a deception. Therefore if we are to write the story of our lives, we must first read the context of our lives. We can only answer the question 'What am I to do?' if we can answer the prior question 'Of what story or stories do I find myself a part?' And we must read our own stories accurately.

> **ACTIVITY:** We will end your reading of Mendus at this point. Please go back now to the summary table you were asked to draw up as part of your guided reading, and let's finish filling in the heading under narrative/feminist ethics'. What critiques of autonomy does Mendus suggest? What alternative concepts does she offer? What parts of the autonomy model does narrative ethics retain?

As we saw in the previous section, the dominant principlist school in medical ethics focuses primarily on actions, on particular decisions, on medical dilemmas. In an account like that of Joseph Raz, the autonomous agent's life is not a unity; rather, it is a series of possible diverse decisions. This concentration on life as a string of separate action choices has had several consequences which critics view as undesirable:

- The dilemmas have generally tended to be the 'big issues': abortion, euthanasia, and withdrawal of life-sustaining treatment. This does not adequately convey the tenor of ordinary practice. Day-to-day clinical life is much more about routine cases which may not even be immediately recognizable as ethical dilemmas; at most they may just look like practical questions. So, what sustains clinicians in their everyday work is much more like something that could be called the 'narrative dimension of medicine'.

- In a dilemma-focused approach, the four principles become a sort of 'ready reckoner': apply autonomy, beneficence, non-maleficence and justice to the situation, and hey presto, a decision emerges. This is, of course, a parody, even a travesty to advocates of the principles. But the criticism of narrative ethicists is that the principlist approach lends itself to becoming just such a superficial checklist; indeed, some of its advocates view that as one of its advantages – that it provides a sort of formula for busy clinicians.

- The same principles are to be applied to every situation, in every culture and country. This is insensitive to different institutional structures, to multiculturalism, and to the nuances of relationships – in all of which autonomy is not necessarily the be-all and end-all. People don't make their own lives, particularly not the sick and vulnerable people clinicians encounter in daily practice. It just doesn't feel right in day-to-day practice to accord autonomy the central place; it feels artificial. In Mendus's terms, it means failure to read the situation in which you find yourself: insistence on imposing another script instead.

- It also posits a model in which other people are a threat to 'my' project. Translated to the healthcare context, the autonomy approach is too conflictual. It leads us to expect conflict in the doctor–patient relationship, when doctors stand

in the way of patients' autonomy, and that could turn out to be a self-fulfilling prophecy. Although Mendus does not touch explicitly on the doctor–patient relationship, she does say that 'some kinds of relationships will be deformed by the attempt to render them compatible with autonomy'. Is the doctor–patient relationship one of them? Or does even admitting that it might be land us back with blatant medical paternalism?

- As MacIntyre says, the approach which concentrates on the right action is, in fact, self-defeating unless it asks the sorts of questions about the entire narrative. '*But the key question for men is not about their own authorship; I can only answer the question "What am I to do?" if I can answer the prior question, "Of what story or stories do I find myself a part?"*'

ACTIVITY: What criticisms can be made of the narrative ethics approach?

In a moment we will ask you to begin your second guided reading exercise in this chapter, an article on Virtue Ethics by Justin Oakley, from Monash University in Australia. This paper first appeared in *A Companion to Bioethics*, 1998, Kuhse, H. & Singer, P. As you read, please return to the table and fill in the sections under virtue ethics'.

Before we do that, however, we would like you to read the following case. As you read, ask yourself whether this suicide was an autonomous act and, if so, what sense of autonomy it illustrated.

The Case of Dario Iacoponi

Schoolboy coolly chose suicide: gifted pupil weighed pros and cons in diary, inquest hears (*Guardian*, 3 December 1998)

A brilliant schoolboy and talented musician killed himself after meticulously weighing up the pros and cons in a diary over two months, an inquest heard yesterday. Fifteen-year-old Dario Iacoponi, a pupil at the grant-maintained London Oratory

School, calmly analysed his existence – and recorded just before his death: 'On balance, life is not good.'

The 'deep-thinking' choirboy – who gained six A and A* GCSEs a year early – then took his father's shotgun, wedged a wooden spoon in the trigger, and used his foot to fire a shot through his head, at his family's home in Ealing, West London, last month.

To his family, Dario, who played the violin in a local youth orchestra, showed no signs of depression – but the five volumes of a diary he filled over a year revealed that he was preoccupied with religion, philosophy, life and death.

John Burton, the coroner, told the court: 'On the very last entry in the diary there are two pages of pros and cons, and he came down on the side of suicide. He was very stoical about it. He did not fear death. He described death as neutral. He decided that on balance life is not good, and points out that the mathematics he has used are indisputable and that is his last entry. It was a considered process.'

He continued: 'With some young people, you think they don't appreciate what they are doing, but he had analysed what he was doing. . . . He had been thinking about the way he would die, planning it, organising it, and analysing if there is a purpose in life.'

He realized he needed a 'window of opportunity' when his parents were away to carry out his aim – and killed himself on November 3, as his mother Saleni, a teacher, attended an amateur dramatic society meeting and his father Pietro, a translator, was in Switzerland on business.

He took just one cartridge for the clay-pigeon shooting gun, which he had secretly learned how to use. His body, slumped in the spare room, was found by the family's lodger, a 20-year-old student.

The court heard that his diaries made no mention of bullying and that drugs and alcohol had played no part.

After the inquest, the boy's father, who did not attend, said: 'We had no idea he was planning on taking his life. He never showed any sign of depression. Dario was a most serious boy and very, very clever. He was a very mature young boy – more mature than us. As you can imagine, we are all terribly distraught.'

> **ACTIVITY: What points might the narrative feminist analysis of autonomy raise about this account? Now go on to read the paper by Justin Oakley. As you do so fill in the table, as you did with the article by Mendus.**

A virtue ethics approach

Justin Oakley

The closing decades of the twentieth century have seen a revitalization in ethics of the ancient notion of virtue. The origins of this renewed philosophical interest in the virtues can be traced back to Elizabeth Anscombe's article, `Modern moral philosophy', published in 1958, but the bulk of work on virtue-based approaches to ethics did not begin to appear until the early 1980s, mainly in the writings of Philippa Foot, Bernard Williams, and Alasdair MacIntyre. Nowadays, a virtue-based approach to ethics has been developed to the point where it is widely recognized as offering a coherent and plausible alternative to the mainstream Consequentialist and Kantian approaches. This revival of virtue-based approaches to ethics has led to a corresponding development of a virtue ethics perspective on issues in bioethics.

The rise of virtue ethics

While a virtue-based approach to ethics has its intrinsic merits, the turn towards virtue ethics has, to a significant extent, been motivated by dissatisfaction with certain aspects of mainstream ethical theories. One general complaint which advocates of virtue ethics have made about consequentialist and Kantian theories is that they place too much emphasis on questions about what we ought to do, at the expense of dealing with more basic questions about what sort of person we ought to be and what sort of life we ought to lead. Another general criticism which proponents of virtue ethics make of consequentialist and Kantian theories is that they are deficient even as ethics of action, for they are excessively abstract and thus say too little about what agents ought to do in concrete circumstances. A related charge is that these mainstream theories evaluate all acts in terms of 'right', 'wrong', 'obligatory', or 'permissible', and in doing so leave us with an impoverished moral vocabulary. A virtue ethics approach, by contrast, employs such evaluative terms as 'courageous', 'callous', 'honest', and 'just' – as well as the more familiar 'right' and 'wrong' – and thereby provides a much richer and more finely grained range of evaluative possibilities. More specifically, many have argued that the impartiality characteristic of both consequentialist and Kantian approaches to ethics devalues the ethical importance of personal relationships such as friendship, and that the duty-based approaches of Kantianism and deontology lead to an objectionably minimalist conception of a good life.

The development of a virtue ethics approach to bioethics, in particular, while inspired by these general dissatisfactions with standard ethical theories, has also drawn impetus from some more localised targets. To some extent, virtue-based approaches to bioethics have been developed as a reaction to the dominance of bioethics by utilitarianism, which some have thought over-simplifies certain issues in bioethics (see Hursthouse, 1987). But some writers explain the rise of virtue theory in bioethics as a reaction not so much to utilitarianism in particular but rather as a response to the shortcomings of principle-based approaches to bioethics (or 'principlism'), which usually claim to be founded on common ground between utilitarian and Kantian or deontological approaches to bioethics. Principle-based approaches (and especially that taken by Beauchamp and Childress, 1994) have become a virtual orthodoxy in discussions of many issues in bioethics (and patient care issues in particular), but various writers have recently expressed doubts about whether such approaches adequately capture both the contex-

tual nature of decisions in patient care, and the moral importance of a health professional's character (and these doubts echo some of the general criticisms noted above of consequentialism and Kantianism as ethical theories).

However, it can be misleading to contrast virtue-based and principle-based approaches to bioethics, since this implies that virtue-based approaches reject appeals to principles. But there is no reason why a virtue ethics approach cannot endorse certain principles, both generally – such as 'we ought to repay our debts', and in relation to patient care – such as 'a good general practitioner normally gives priority to his or her own patients, over those of other doctors'. Also, since principle-based approaches are usually put forward more as theories telling us how we are to deliberate about ethical issues, rather than as accounts of what ultimately justifies a certain decision, to contrast principle-based approaches with virtue ethics can create the false impression that virtue ethics is simply a rival theory of deliberation or character, supplementing more fundamental theories of justification.

Further, while there is no essential conflict between a virtue ethics approach to bioethics and the idea (commonly found in principle-based approaches) that patient autonomy is an important value, it is nevertheless possible to see the development of a virtue ethics approach to bioethics as a reaction to the rise of the consumerist movement in healthcare, which places respect for patient autonomy as the paramount value in healthcare decisions. The advance of the consumerist movement has led some writers to assume that the most appropriate role for a health professional is that of the patient's agent, where health professionals have no moral independence from the patients they serve. However, others have expressed concern that such a notion involves a kind of 'de-professionalization' of healthcare workers, and virtue ethics' emphasis on the importance of character (in a morally robust sense) can be seen as an attempt to remedy this tendency.

Some philosophers have regarded the above shortcomings of consequentialist and Kantian approaches as reasons to supplement or modify the accounts of moral motivation and deliberation usually given by those theories, while retaining a basically consequentialist or Kantian criterion of rightness. However, other philosophers have regarded those shortcomings as fatal defects of consequentialism and Kantianism, and have looked to virtue ethics as a thoroughly revisionary theory, capable of providing a criterion of rightness which will replace those given by the standard theories.

Many of virtue ethics' claims have often been put in negative form, and so the approach has become better known for what it is against rather than by what it is for. But focusing only on virtue theorists' critiques of standard ethical theories fails to distinguish the approach from those of others who have made similar criticisms. For example, advocates of feminist approaches to ethics have also attacked mainstream impartialist ethical theories for their inadequate treatment of personal and family relationships, and proponents of particularism have also been critical of the excessive abstraction of conventional principle-based ethical theories. (Particularists argue that the search for general ethical principles leads us to overlook the multiplicity of features which can have moral relevance, and the variations in the moral relevance of those features across different contexts, and so urge us to focus primarily on examining the details of each case as closely as possible.) We therefore need a systematic account of the positive claims made by virtue ethics, in order to show what is essential to and distinctive about the approach. In the next section I will sketch a brief account of those positive claims.

> ACTIVITY: As you read Oakley's account of the positive claims of virtue ethics consider how it might be relevant in the case of Nora described in Mendus' paper.

What is Virtue Ethics?

There are six key claims which are essential to modern forms of virtue ethics. These claims are common to the different varieties of virtue ethics, and also help to distinguish the approach from utilitarianism and Kantianism. The first and perhaps most fundamental claim made by virtue ethics states its criterion of rightness (see Hursthouse, 1991, p. 225; 1996, p. 22):

(a) An action is right if and only if it is what an agent with a virtuous character would do in the circumstances

Thus, according to virtue ethics, reference to character is essential in the justification of right action. A right action is one that is in accordance with what a virtuous person would do in the circumstances, and what makes the action right is that it is what a person with a virtuous character would do here. For example, Philippa Foot (1977, p. 106) argues that it is – other things being equal – right to save another's life, where continued life would still be a good to that person, because this is what a person with the virtue of benevolence would do. Likewise, Rosalind Hursthouse (1996, p. 25) argues that it is ordinarily right to keep a deathbed promise, even though living people would benefit from its being broken, because that is what a person with the virtue of justice would do here.

The primacy given to character in (a) helps to distinguish virtue ethics from standard forms of Kantianism, utilitarianism, and consequentialism, whereby actions are justified according to rules or outcomes. However, more recent advocates of Kantian, utilitarian, and consequentialist theories have suggested that the relevant criterion of rightness can be understood as an internalized normative disposition in the character of the good agent. Such theories can therefore be put in terms of what a virtuous person would do, where such a person is one whose motivation to act is regulated by the correct rules, or is motivated to maximize utility (see Oakley, 1996, pp. 131–2). How does (a) distinguish virtue ethics from those theories?

Unlike those forms of Kantianism, utilitarianism, and consequentialism which tell us to have a certain sort of character, virtue ethics holds that reference to character is essential in a correct account of right action. By contrast, most forms of those other theories which tell us to develop a Kantian, utilitarian, or consequentialist character allow that the rightness of an action can be determined independently of a reference to the character of a good Kantian, utilitarian, or consequentialist agent. For example, act-utilitarianism holds that an act is right if, and only if, it results in the most utility of any act the agent could do. However, some recent versions of Kantianism, utilitarianism, and consequentialism hold that right actions must be guided by a certain sort of character, and so, like virtue ethics, these accounts give character an essential role in the justification of action. Thus, one must look beyond the primacy of character in (a), in order to distinguish virtue ethics from other forms of character-based ethics.

The distinctiveness of virtue ethics compared to other theories is brought out when we turn to the ways in which advocates of the approach ground the normative conceptions in the character of the virtuous agent. Modern virtue ethicists take one of two broad approaches to filling out the notion of a virtuous character. Many virtue ethicists take the Aristotelian view that the virtues are character traits which we need to live humanly flourishing lives. On this view, developed by Foot (1978) and Hursthouse (1987), benevolence and justice are virtues because they are part of an interlocking web of intrinsic goods – which includes friendship, integrity, and knowledge – without which we cannot have eudaimonia, or a flourishing life for a human being. According to Aristotle, the characteristic activity of human beings is the exercise of our rational capacity, and only by living virtuously is our rational capacity to guide our lives expressed in an excellent way. There is a sense, then, in which someone lacking the virtues would not be living a human life. Another approach to grounding the virtues, developed principally by Michael Slote (1992), rejects the Aristotelian idea that the virtues are given by what humans need in order to flourish, and instead derives the virtues from our common-sense views about what character traits we typically find admirable – as exemplified in the

lives of figures such as Albert Einstein and Mother Teresa – whether or not those traits help an individual to flourish.

A second claim made by virtue ethics is:

(b) Goodness is prior to rightness

Contrary to deontological theories and to traditional forms of Kantianism, virtue ethics holds that the notion of goodness is primary. Thus, no account can be given of what makes an action right without having first established what is valuable or good. This sort of priority of the good over the right is also found in utilitarian theories (and in consequentialist theories generally), and so claim (b) brings out a structural similarity between virtue ethics and those theories.

A third claim made by virtue ethics is:

(c) The virtues are irreducibly plural intrinsic goods

The intrinsic goods embodied in the virtues cannot be reduced to a single underlying value, such as utility, but are plural. While this claim distinguishes virtue ethics from older, monistic forms of utilitarianism, it does not distinguish the approach from modern, pluralistic forms of preference utilitarianism. For preference utilitarians can allow that there is a plurality of things which have intrinsic value, at least in so far as people desire to have certain things (such as knowledge, autonomy, and accomplishment) in themselves, and not merely for their good consequences.

Nevertheless, a further claim helps to distinguish virtue ethics from a preference-utilitarian approach:

(d) The virtues are objectively good

Virtue ethics sees the virtues as objectively good in the sense that they are good independent of any connections they may have with desire. The goodness of the virtues is based on their connections with essential human characteristics, or with what we consider admirable, and they remain good, whether or not the agent who has them desires (or would, if suitably informed, desire) to have them. By contrast, a preference utilitarian who accepted the plural value of the different virtues derives their value from the fact that the agent desires (or would, if suitably informed, desire) to have them.

However, some consequentialists allow that there can be plural intrinsic and objective values. On this view, it is valuable for agents, e.g. to be autonomous, even if they do not (and would not, if suitably informed) desire to be autonomous. Two further claims help to distinguish virtue ethics from these forms of consequentialism:

(e) Some intrinsic goods are agent relative

Standard forms of consequentialism claim that all goods are agent neutral. This means that whether a good in question is mine or someone else's, it carries fundamentally the same moral weight. So, for example, pluralistic consequentialists who accord intrinsic value to friendship and integrity tell me to maximize friendship and integrity *per se*, even if doing so is at the expense of my own friendships or integrity. By contrast, virtue ethics holds that certain goods, such as friendship, have agent relative value. That is, the fact that a relationship is my friendship is itself a morally relevant feature, and carries additional moral weight. Thus, if I find myself in circumstances where I must choose between performing a friendly act towards my friend and promoting friendships between others (for example, my friend asks me to help him move house on the day I had been planning to throw a party to welcome new colleagues), I would be justified in acting for my friend.

Finally, unlike standard forms of consequentialism, which hold that we must maximize the good, virtue ethics claims that:

(f) Acting rightly does not require that we maximize the good

Virtue ethics holds that acting rightly does not require agents to bring about the very best possible consequences they can. Rather, many virtue

ethicists argue that we ought to aspire to a level of human excellence. For example, instead of being required to have the very best friendships we can have, virtue ethics tells us that we ought to have excellent friendships.

These six claims do not themselves add up to a substantive ethical theory; they need to be filled out with some account of the virtues themselves before the theory can be applied to practical problems.

> ACTIVITY: In the next part of his paper, Oakley explores the way in which virtue ethics might be said to be relevant to bioethics. As you read it consider what it might have to say about the case of Dario Iacoponi.

Virtue ethics approaches to bioethics

As is becoming clear from the writings of its contemporary exponents, virtue ethics has a great deal to contribute to bioethics. Virtue ethics provides a distinctive new perspective on many familiar issues in bioethics, and it addresses some important questions which standard utilitarian and deontological approaches have shown themselves ill-equipped to deal with, or have neglected altogether. Among the areas of bioethics which have received considerable attention from virtue ethicists are abortion, euthanasia, and the practice of healthcare.

An excellent example of a virtue ethics approach to bioethics is Rosalind Hursthouse's groundbreaking book on the ethics of abortion, *Beginning Lives* (1987). Hursthouse argues that the traditional debate about the competing rights of the mother and the fetus is fundamentally irrelevant to the morality of abortion. Individuals can exercise their rights virtuously or viciously, and Hursthouse argues that the morality of a woman's decision to have an abortion depends importantly on the sort of character which a woman manifests in deciding to have an abortion in her particular circumstances. For example, deciding to terminate a 7-month pregnancy in order to have a holiday abroad would be callous and self-centred, and aborting a fetus because one is fearful of motherhood is cowardly, if one is otherwise well positioned to become a parent; however, an adolescent girl who has an abortion because she does not feel ready for motherhood yet would thereby show a proper humility about her present level of development. Hursthouse argues that these judgements are appropriate because

parenthood in general, and motherhood and childbearing in particular, are intrinsically worthwhile, [and] are among the things that can be correctly thought to be partially constitutive of a flourishing human life (1991, p. 241; see also 1987, pp. 168–9, 307–18).

These virtue-based evaluations of women's abortion decisions also reflect the fact that terminating a pregnancy (unlike, say, having a kidney removed) involves cutting off a new human life, which in most circumstances should be regarded as a morally serious matter (Hursthouse, 1991, p. 237; see also 1987, pp. 16–25, 50–8, 204–17, 331).

Hursthouse's virtue ethics approach to abortion brings out two broad sorts of reasons why a woman may in some circumstances be acting wrongly in deciding to terminate her pregnancy. Firstly, she may be showing a failure to appreciate the intrinsic value of parenthood, and its importance to a flourishing human life. And, secondly, she may be taking the decision to cut off a new human life without due seriousness. Hursthouse discusses briefly how these sorts of failings may also be shown by individuals in making decisions about allowing severely disabled infants to die, and in decisions about experimentation on human embryos.

Another example of a virtue ethics approach in bioethics is Philippa Foot's (1977) influential discussion of euthanasia. Foot analyses the concept of euthanasia, and argues that wanting to die does not necessarily make death a good for that person; rather, death can be a good to a person only when their life lacks a minimum of basic human goods, such as autonomy, friendship, and moral support. Foot argues that the virtues of

justice and charity allow one to fulfil a competent individual's request to be killed, where such basic human goods are absent. Foot also argues that analysing end-of-life decisions in terms of these virtues can bring out an important moral difference between killing and letting die. In normal circumstances, both justice and charity require us not to kill people, and both virtues require that we do not let people die when we could reasonably have helped them. Further, where someone whose life lacks a minimum of basic human goods expresses a sincere request to be killed, both justice and charity would permit such an action to be carried out. However, where such a person demands not to be killed, and wishes to be left to die in agony, the requirements of these virtues diverge – that is, justice would forbid us from carrying out the act of killing which charity would normally permit in such circumstances.

Virtue ethics also offers a promising and insightful approach to many issues in patient care. For example, Edmund Pellegrino and David Thomasma (1993) show how an account of the virtues in medical practice is necessarily based on a philosophy of medicine, in a way that demonstrates what goals are appropriate to and distinctive of medicine as an important human endeavour. Virtue ethics approaches to medical practice typically examine issues in patient care by looking at the doctor–patient relationship, and at the sorts of character traits which are crucial for a doctor in that relationship, such as honesty, compassion, integrity, and justice. Thus, according to this approach, doctors ought to tell the truth, not so much because of the importance of informed consent and respect for patient autonomy, but rather because that is what is involved in their having the virtue of truthfulness (see Drane, 1988, pp. 43–62; Hauerwas, 1995; Pence, 1980; Shelp, 1985). However, some who acknowledge the importance of virtuous character traits in good medical practice do not take a virtue-based approach, but rather see such accounts as providing a necessary practical supplement to a fundamentally deontological or utilitarian morality (see, e.g. Pellegrino and Thomasma, 1993; Beauchamp and Childress, 1994; Hare, 1994).

Criticisms of virtue ethics

A number of criticisms have been made of virtue-based approaches to ethics. I will describe two criticisms which I take to be particularly important, and outline how a virtue theorist might respond to them. Both of these objections centre on virtue ethics' appeal to 'what the virtuous agent would do' as the determinant of right action (as in (a) above).

The first criticism raises doubts about whether the notion of virtue is clear or detailed enough to serve as the basis of a criterion of rightness. Many writers argue that this criterion of rightness is too vague to be an acceptable basis of justification in ethics. What would a virtuous agent do in the great variety of situations in which people find themselves? Also, there is a plurality of virtuous character traits, and not all virtuous people seem to have these traits to the same degree. Moreover, these people might not always respond to situations in the same way. Given a set of circumstances, is the right action here the action which would be done by an honest person, a kind person, or a just person? Further, even if the range of possible virtuous characters is narrower than this suggests, how do we know what a virtuous person would do in a particular situation? As Robert Louden (1984) puts it:

Due to the very nature of the moral virtues, there is . . . a very limited amount of advice on moral quandaries that one can reasonably expect from the virtue-oriented approach. We ought, of course, to do what the virtuous person would do, but it is not always easy to fathom what the hypothetical moral exemplar would do were he in our shoes (p. 229).

Now, to the extent that the criticism here expresses a general worry about appeals to 'what

a certain person would do', it is worth remembering that such appeals are quite commonly and successfully used in justifications in a variety of areas. For example, novice doctors and lawyers being inducted into their professions sometimes justify their having acted in a certain way by pointing out that this is how their professional mentor would have acted here. Also, courts often rely significantly on claims about what a reasonable person would have foreseen, in determining a person's legal liability for negligent conduct. Moreover, any general worry about such appeals would also apply to many modern consequentialist theories, which hold that the rightness of an action is determined partly by appealing to what consequences would have been foreseen by a reasonable person in the agent's position.

However, those who accept reliance on such appeals in other areas might well have misgivings about the particular sort of appeal to such a standard which is made by virtue ethics. For it may be considerably more difficult to determine which of the variety of virtuous character-traits a virtuous person would act on in a given situation, than it is to determine what consequences of a given action a reasonable person would foresee (see Rachels, 1993, p. 178). Now, it is true to say that virtue ethics does not deliver an 'algorithm' of right action (as Aristotle put it), and that a virtue ethics criterion of rightness is perhaps less precisely specifiable and less easily applicable than that given by consequentialist theories (although perhaps not compared to those given by Kantian theories). But it is perhaps an over-reaction to argue that this undermines virtue ethics' claim to provide an acceptable approach to ethical justification. For virtue ethicists often give considerable detail about what virtuous agents have done and would do in certain situations, and these details can help us to identify what it is right to do in a particular situation. (We might not gain any more precision from the directives of contemporary Kantian and consequentialist theories which advise us to do what a good Kantian or consequentialist agent would do.) And further, virtue ethics need not claim that there is only one true account of what a virtuous person would be and do, for it can allow that, sometimes, whichever of two courses of action one chooses, one would be acting rightly. In some situations, that is, whether one does what a kind person would have done, or what an honest person would have done, one would still have acted rightly (see Hursthouse, 1996, p. 34).

The second major criticism of virtue ethics is more fundamental than the first, as it focuses on the plausibility of a purely character-based criterion of rightness, such as that given by virtue ethics in (a) above. That is, many have argued that reference to what an agent with a virtuous character would have done (no matter how precisely specifiable and unitary virtuous character traits are) is not sufficient to justify actions. In support of this criticism, many writers argue that people with very virtuous characters can sometimes be led by a virtuous character trait to act wrongly. For example, a benevolent doctor may be moved to withhold a diagnosis of terminal cancer from a patient, although the doctor reveals the news to the patient's family, and asks them to join in the deception. Or, a compassionate father might decide to donate most of the family's savings to a worthwhile charity, without sufficiently thinking through how his action is likely to result in severe impoverishment for his family in the long term. Likewise, a compassionate nurse caring for a convicted murderer in a prison hospital might be so moved by the story of a patient's deprived upbringing that the nurse may deliberately fail to raise the alarm when the patient makes a dash for freedom. As Robert Veatch (1988) puts the worry:

I am concerned about well-intentioned, bungling do-gooders. They seem to exist with unusual frequency in healthcare, law, and other professions with a strong history of stressing the virtue of benevolence with an elitist slant (p. 445).

If we agree that thoroughly virtuous people can sometimes be led by their virtuous character-traits to act wrongly, then this seems to cast strong doubt on the plausibility of virtue ethics' criterion of rightness in (a) above. Many critics have been led by such examples of moral ineptitude to claim that virtue ethics is incomplete, and must therefore be underwritten by a deontological or a utilitarian criterion of rightness (see Frankena, 1973, pp. 63–71; Pellegrino and Thomasma, 1993; Rachels, 1993; Driver, 1995; Hare, 1994; Beauchamp and Childress, 1994, pp. 62–9).

Now, some virtue theorists would question whether the agent does act wrongly in these sorts of cases (see, e.g. Slote, 1995). However, suppose it is granted that the agent concerned does, indeed, act wrongly in some such cases. There is no reason to think that virtue ethics is committed to condoning such moral ineptitude. For most virtues are not simply a matter of having good motives or good dispositions, but have a practical component which involves seeing to it that one's action succeeds in bringing about what the virtue dictates. Therefore, we might question the extent to which the agent really does have the virtuous character trait which we are assuming he does here. Is it really an act of benevolence to withhold a diagnosis of terminal cancer from a patient, leaving that patient to die in ignorance of his or her true condition? Alternatively, in cases where the action does not seem to call into question the degree to which the agent has the virtuous character trait under scrutiny, it might be that the agent was lacking in some other virtue which was appropriate here. Thus, the father seems to have an inadequate sense of loyalty towards his own family, and the nurse's sense of justice seems defective. However, in some cases, these sorts of responses may not be very plausible, and to that extent, the virtue ethics criterion of rightness in (a) may need to be re-examined.

Conclusion

Because contemporary virtue ethics is a relatively recent arrival in ethical theory and bioethics, it is difficult to assess its future prospects. A virtue ethics approach has already made significant contributions in both areas, but more work remains to be done both to develop the approach itself, and to investigate its applications to ethical issues in healthcare and reproduction. Nevertheless, it is clear that the renaissance of virtue theory has enriched normative ethics considerably, and the emergence of virtue-based approaches to issues in bioethics has created a promising alternative to the rather formulaic methods of the more established approaches.

> ACTIVITY: What are the positive and negative aspects of the virtue ethics approach as outlined by Oakley? What does such an approach have to say about the emphasis on autonomy in many contemporary versions of medical ethics?
>
> Like virtue ethics and narrative ethics, deliberative approaches to ethics are also sensitive to embeddedness in relationships. Like feminist ethics in particular, it does not necessarily seek to jettison the concept of autonomy altogether, but rather to broaden and deepen it: 'Autonomy, the root of ethics . . . has an essential dialogical dimension which must not be forgotten' (Silva, 1997, p. 16). As the third and final reading in this section, we now turn to an article by Michael Parker, 'A deliberative approach to bioethics'. Again, please read this article actively, filling in the remaining boxes on your grid.

A deliberative approach to bioethics

Michael Parker

A 'rivalry of care' case

In their book, *The Patient in the Family*, Hilde and James Lindemann-Nelson describe the case of a man whose daughter is suffering from kidney failure (Lindemann Nelson, H. and J., 1995). She is spending six hours, three times a week on a dialysis machine, and the effects of this are becoming increasingly hard for her and her family to bear. She has already had one kidney transplant, which her body rejected, and her doctors are unsure whether a second would work but are willing to try if they can find a suitable donor. After some tests the paediatrician privately tells the father that he is compatible and therefore a suitable donor.

It may seem inconceivable that a father would refuse to donate his kidney to his daughter under such circumstances. Yet he does refuse and justifies his decision both on the grounds that the success of the transplant is uncertain and also on the basis of his concerns about the implications of the operation itself for him and his family. He is frightened and worried about what would happen to him and his other children if his remaining kidney were to fail. But he is ashamed to feel this way and cannot bear to refuse openly so he asks the paediatrician to tell the family that he is in fact not compatible. However, whilst having some sympathy, she says she cannot lie for him and, after a silence, the father says, 'OK then I'll do it. If they knew that I was compatible but wouldn't donate my kidney, it would wreck the family'.

But, why should this decision wreck the family, ask the Lindemann Nelsons? Does a father have a special obligation to donate his kidney to his daughter? What is it about families and the values that underpin them which leads to the expectation that parents will sacrifice themselves for their children (and, in particular, for the child who is ill)? What is it about modern patient-centred medicine that intensifies such expectations?

The case is used by the Lindemann Nelsons because they believe it suggests that there is a conflict in healthcare between two sets of values: those individualistic values which underlie patient-centred medicine and the communitarian (community-based) values which sustain families and communities. They argue that modern medicine's overriding focus on the benefit of the individual patient has distorted the ways in which family members interact with one another and in particular with those who are sick. They argue that at times of stress families often adopt the individualistic values of the medical world and this leads them unintentionally to trample on the values and concerns that sustain families. It is with this tension, they suggest, that the father wrestles in the case described.

Who am I?

The claim that there are important tensions between the values of patient-centred medicine and those which sustain families and communities reflects an ongoing and important contemporary debate in bioethics (and in ethics more widely) between what have been called 'individualistic' approaches and those which have come to be known as 'communitarian' (Parker, 1999). The conflict is one that is characterized by Michael Sandel and other communitarians as one between two conceptions of what it is to be a moral subject (Sandel, 1982).

The communitarian analysis of the case offered by the Lindemann Nelsons urges the father to seek a resolution of his moral problem in an answer to the question 'who am I?' where his identity is to be seen as informed by his membership of a community (in this case, a family) rather than through an analysis of rights (Lindemann Nelson, H. and J., 1995) or a 'balancing' of principles (Beauchamp and Childress, 1994). For, as Kukathas and Petit suggest,

[For communitarians] the end of moral reasoning is not judgement but understanding and self-discovery. I ask, not 'what should I be, what sort of life should I lead?' but 'Who am I?' [And] to ask this question is to concern oneself first and foremost with the character of the community which constitutes one's identity (Kukathas and Petit, 1990).

Sandel too, argues that,

I [should] ask, as I deliberate, not only what I really want but who I really am, and this last question takes me beyond attention to desires alone to reflect on my identity itself (Sandel, 1982, p. 180).

At the heart of this communitarian approach to the moral which urges us to emphasize the values which sustain families and communities over those of autonomy and patient choice, is the ontological claim that the moral world consists of fundamentally and essentially 'socially-embedded' beings who draw their identities, and their moral values, from their constitutive attachments to a 'community'.

Interestingly, Sandel argues that the individualist too, whose approach it is which is rejected by the Lindemann Nelsons and other communitarians, agrees that the question of who I am is at the core of moral deliberation (Sandel, 1982). In contrast to the communitarian however, the individualist is said to conceive of the moral subject in terms of the autonomy and the free choice of the individual 'free chooser', rather than in terms of a being constituted by his or her embeddedness in a constellation of social and communal values, and this leads to an approach to bioethics which emphasizes the values of autonomy and patient choice over those of community and family.

The individualist argues that the value of such freedom is independently derivable by virtue of the fact that it is a necessary condition of the very possibility of the moral, and hence of the very possibility of a constellation of values at all and it is this which means that autonomy ought to 'trump' other values (Dworkin, R., 1977). As Sandel explains,

For justice to be primary, certain things must be true of us. We must be creatures of a certain kind, related to human circumstance in a certain way. In particular, we must stand to our circumstance always at a certain distance, conditioned to be sure, but part of us always antecedent to any conditions. Only in this way can we view ourselves as subjects as well as objects of experience, as agents and not just instruments of the purposes we pursue (Sandel, 1982, p. 11).

The basis of an emphasis on autonomy is thus not the ends we choose but the capacity of us to choose them and such capacity depends upon the free and independent nature of the subject. As Kant argues, in response to the question of what makes the moral possible,

'It is nothing else than personality, i.e., the freedom and independence from the mechanism of nature regarded as a capacity of a being which is subject to special laws (pure practical laws given by its own reason) (Kant, 1956 [1788]).

Sandel's claim then, is that both the individualist and the communitarian seek an explanation of the moral in an answer to the question of what it means to be a moral subject each rejecting the other on the grounds that it is incapable of providing such an explanation. I shall be going on to argue in the rest of this paper, however, that each of these conceptions must themselves be rejected and that this rejection of both individualism and community has important and far-reaching implications for the practice of bioethics, some of which I shall tease out in the final section.

> ACTIVITY: Parker identifies two different conceptions of the moral subject or of the moral person – the individualistic and the communitarian. Choose the model with which you have most sympathy and then try to identify two arguments for why this ought to be rejected and two for why it ought to be supported.
>
> In the section which follows, Parker goes on to provide reasons for rejecting both of the models in favour of a third, discursive approach.

Three reasons for rejecting the liberal individual moral subject

It seems to me that the communitarian is right to reject the liberal individualist model as conceived in this way and the grounds for such a rejection can, I want to argue, be grouped under three headings.

The first of these grounds might best be collected under the heading, 'The impossibility of moral understanding' and draws together arguments from both philosophy and psychology which suggest that the individualist account of morality must be rejected because it is not possible to provide an explanation of the development of moral understanding from an individualistic epistemological perspective. For, the very possibility of moral understanding and moral language, it is claimed, is dependent upon the social dimension of human experience. Ludwig Wittgenstein's 'private language argument' is one powerful argument to this effect in which Wittgenstein argues that the very possibility of meaning and hence language depends upon the existence of standards of established social practice. (Wittgenstein, 1974, n 150–200). But this is not the only argument to this effect. Alasdair MacIntyre in *After Virtue* argues that,

In so far as persons must be understood as partly individuated by their membership of traditions, the history of their lives will be embedded in the larger narrative of a historically and socially extended argument about the good life for human beings (MacIntyre, 1981).

The second group of arguments are those which claim, against the individualist, that the having of moral problems and moral identity at all depends on the fact that we are all socially embedded. That is, it is claimed, we are all inevitably located in social, intersubjective networks from which we draw our identity and that the liberal conception of the subject as divorced from such networks inevitably comes at a price. For, as Michael Sandel writes,

To imagine a person incapable of constitutive attachments such as these is not to conceive an ideally free and rational agent, but to imagine a person wholly without character, without moral depth (Sandel, 1982, p. 179).

Perhaps the strongest proponent of this type of argument is Charles Taylor who argues that to be a self at all is to be an essentially moral being located within what he calls evaluative frameworks and that such frameworks are inevitably linguistic and hence social.

This is the sense in which one cannot be a self on one's own. I am a self only in relation to certain interlocutor: in one way in relation to those conversation partners who are essential to my achieving self-definition; in another in relation to those who are now crucial to my continuing grasp of languages of self-understanding – and, of course, these classes may overlap. A self exists only within what I call 'webs of interlocution' (Taylor, 1989, p. 36).

The third groups of arguments, are those which attempt to describe the unacceptable social conse-quences of individualism. Communitarians some-times argue that historically the over-emphasis on rights in liberal democracies has had unacceptable consequences both for societies and individuals (i.e. the breakdown of traditional structures such as the family) and for this reason should be rejected (Etzioni, 1993).

Whilst I have my doubts about the strength of the third group of arguments in a world in which perhaps the most striking moral challenge is the oppression of individuals by communities, the combination of these arguments taken together means that communitarians are right, it seems to me, to call for the rejection of what I have called elsewhere 'overly individualistic' approaches to ethics.

Three reasons for rejecting the communitarian 'embedded moral subject'

The communitarian argument for the 'socially embedded subject' must itself be rejected, however, for three sets of reasons which, again for reasons of space, I shall simply state here.

Firstly, the explanation of morality in terms of the 'socially embedded self' and of 'constitutive attach-ments' means that communitarianism is incapable of recognizing the moral status of the individual. Feminists, for example, have argued that, whilst communitarianism is very good at describing the benefits of community, it says very little about the damage caused by families and communities and says nothing for those at the periphery of societies for whom we expect moral theory to have special concern. Taken to its logical conclusion, communi-tarianism seems capable of justifying the oppres-sion of minorities and of the weak by the majority, of the novel by the traditional (Parker, 1996). And,

whilst we might agree with the communitarians that overly individualistic approaches to ethics must be rejected, we would surely not want to reject with it that which is valuable about the indi-vidualistic approaches; namely a recognition of the moral status of the individual. For this would be to throw out the baby with the bathwater.

Secondly, and following from the above, the communitarian approach is, it is argued, incapable of providing an explanation of social change or of the need for the critical moral reflection, creativity and criticism necessary for the change and devel-opment of communities. Another way of saying this is to say that communitarianism is incapable of providing an account of how the individual can come to have an effect upon the society within which they live and upon their constitutive values and relationships (Parker, 1995; Mendus, 1992).

Thirdly, Jürgen Habermas has argued that it is not in fact possible to identify the shared values required by communitarians (Habermas, 1993). The breakdown of shared values and traditions identified by communitarians brings into question the viability of the communitarian project itself. For, when we look around us, there appear few if any candidates for the shared values upon which a communitarian New World might be built. We live in a world characterized by diversity in which can-didates for the role of paradigmatic communities are revealed to be as often the sites of conflict and violence as of mutual support (Campbell, 1995); a world in which it is not possible to identify the kind of shared values or traditions upon which a communitarian morality might be founded.

ACTIVITY: Using the method you used in your anal-ysis of the paper by Juhani Pietarinen at the start of this chapter (writing out the various stages of the argument), assess Parker's argument. Does the argu-ment stand up to scrutiny? If not, why not?

In the next section of his paper, Parker attempts to elaborate a deliberative approach to medical ethics. We would now like you to read this final section and, as you do so, to consider how such an approach might deal with a case such as that of Dario Iacoponi.

A resolution? The deliberative moral subject

Both the individualist and communitarian models of the moral subject (and of the person) in ethics must be rejected. But where does this leave us? If we wish to elaborate a coherent moral theory and, if appeal is no longer possible either to the kind of detached, individual, rational decision making called for by the liberal individualist or to communitarian shared values and traditions as the basis of ethical decision making in healthcare, how are we to approach the making of ethical decisions of the kind confronting the father at the beginning of this paper? What seems clear is that any coherent explanation of the moral will have to be one capable of capturing the insights of both communitarianism and individualism whilst avoiding their weaknesses and pitfalls and what this means is that it must be capable of capturing both the value of the individual voice and the moral status of the individual whilst, at the same time, of recognizing the intersubjective and social context of morality and the value of social relationships and their various manifestations.

It is worth pausing here for a moment to reflect upon the interdependent nature of the relationship between the two sets of arguments I have identified for the rejection of individualism and of communitarianism. For it is an important feature of each of these arguments that such rejection is in each case put in terms of the necessity of the other to any coherent account of the moral. The argument that individualism must be rejected, for example, is based on the claim that recognition of the role of the social is a necessary element of any coherent explanation of morality. The argument for the rejection of overly social accounts on the other hand, is phrased in terms of the necessity of a recognition of the role of the individual.

My point in juxtaposing the arguments in this way is to suggest that both the social and the individual are together necessary and it is their combination that makes a coherent account of the moral possible. I want further to argue that

these features of our moral world are jointly and together only explicable in terms of the actual relations between people in the intersubjective contexts which constitute their everyday lives with others. For it is only here, in the intersubjective relations between people, that the community meets the individual and vice versa. It is here that morality is elaborated and here that the maintenance and the transformation of social practice occur. This is to suggest following Harre and Gillett (1994) and Shotter (1993) and other discursive psychologists that the primary social reality is neither the individual nor the community but people in conversation. To quote Alasdair MacIntyre from *After Virtue*,

Conversation, understood widely enough, is the form of human transactions in general (MacIntyre, 1981).

This must indeed be the case, I suggest, for the reasons above and because it is through such 'conversations' that we are both introduced into the world of human affairs and negotiate our identity and our moral concerns. It is also here that we discover the ethical voice with which we reflect upon, deliberate and change the nature of our relations to our community and other people. From this deliberative perspective, it seems to me, it is possible to begin to recognize the particular value, and indeed the necessity, of the engagement of human beings in deliberation about the moral features of their own lives. And of the nature of their relations with those around them, with those who constitute their communities. For the development of much that is of value in what it is to be human is made possible by such relationships. Hence, within a moral framework of this kind it is possible to capture, as neither individualists nor communitarians are able, both the value of communal life and the moral significance of the individual ethical voice. It is to claim that it is neither the freedom of the abstracted individual nor the emphasis of community values which ought to be given a special place in the constellation of values but the interrelationship between the two. It is also to claim that deliberation is the developmental fundamental of human experience and that it is this that makes the moral possible (Parker, 1995).

Implications for bioethics

What then are the implications of this deliberative approach for bioethics? It seems to me that there are several key features of an approach such as this and I shall attempt to outline these very briefly in conclusion.

(i) The value of deliberation with others

Firstly, to adopt this perspective is to argue, as I have already suggested, that the deliberative search for moral meaning is at the core of what it is to be human in a world with others. This is to locate morality and the search for moral meaning very firmly at the centre of human life. To adopt this perspective therefore is to recognize the particular value of the engagement of human beings in the attempt to 'make moral sense' of their lives and the nature of their relation with those around them. This is necessarily a social process but is also necessarily part of what it is to be and to become autonomous. It is also by these means to recognise as neither individualists nor communitarians are able, both the value of communal life and the moral significance of the individual ethical voice. Whilst placing an emphasis on the social therefore, this approach nevertheless has the advantage of providing, as communitarianism does not, space for a critique of accepted or traditional values on the basis of a respect for the discursive nature of human experience. For, whilst such recognition is capable of capturing our social embeddedness, it is also capable of recognising that individuals need both to be protected from, and to have a voice in, their community.

To assert the value of deliberation is in many respects to follow Alasdair MacIntyre who argues for a conception of the moral life as one which is constituted by engagement in a conversation with history and tradition in an attempt to establish the narrative unity of one's life. It is also to align oneself with Charles Taylor's claim that the identity

of the self is inextricably linked to its sense of the significance and meaning of the situations it encounters in life and this is to see, as does Ronald Dworkin, life as a series of 'challenges' which must be addressed (Dworkin, R., 1986). The good life is at least, to some extent, one in which we are engaged in the attempt to make sense of the challenges with which we are confronted.

(ii) Subsidiarity and participation

Secondly, it follows from the emphasis on the value of 'making sense' that ethical decisions are best made and in fact might only be capable of being made by those most closely involved and this is to suggest that the process of making ethical decisions ought to adhere to a principle of 'subsidiarity'. Nevertheless, such an approach is also, and perhaps primarily, one which emphasizes the participation of all those who have a legitimate interest, and this means that the requirement that decisions be made by those most likely to be affected needs to be balanced against a responsibility to ensure that all who have a legitimate interest are involved. This is to suggest that decision-making in bioethics will need to take a range of different forms, from the establishing of public consensus conferences about ethical issues of widespread public or even global concern, to conversations between doctors, patients and families or within families themselves about the ethical questions raised by a particular case or treatment option and in some cases, perhaps even most, this will mean that decisions will be made by the patient alone, or in collaboration with his or her doctor.

However, whilst taking a variety of forms, such fora would have to share a commitment to recognition of the fundamental value of deliberative involvement and hence would have to place an emphasis on both participation and subsidiarity.

(iii) Openness and truthfulness in ethical decision-making processes

Thirdly, and briefly, the emphases on the values of 'making sense', 'participation' and 'subsidiarity' all imply a requirement both for the openness of the processes of decision making and for truthfulness in the decision making forum. This is clearly crucial to any deliberative approach to ethics and whilst it might be argued that such an emphasis on truthfulness might be captured by the first principle which argues for the engagement in a genuine attempt to 'make sense', it seems to me that having it as a separate principle highlights the formal elements of the deliberative ethical space within which 'making sense' is possible (Habermas, 1993).

(iv) A decentralized bioethics

Finally, and perhaps most importantly, this is an argument for the democratization and decentralization of ethics. For, whilst the philosophical analysis of ethical problems and ethical theory and the elaboration of biomedical principles can be useful in creating a framework for the discussion of ethical problems, the resolution of such problems in an ethical way involves the creation and maintenance of ethical fora of the kind I have described in which those who have a legitimate interest in a case can engage jointly in the process deliberation. This is to argue for a genuinely participatory, democratic and discursive bioethics and such a perspective has, I suggest, profound and radical political implications both for the medical profession and beyond.

ACTIVITY: We began this chapter by discussing the growing importance of the concepts of 'autonomy' and 'patient choice' in modern medicine, and we provided examples of the ways in which these concepts have been integrated into healthcare policy making. Through the rest of the chapter we have explored the limits of these concepts and have looked at some alternative conceptions. As we come to the end of the chapter, and indeed the workbook, we would like you to read through a case and attempt to identify the ways in which this case might be addressed from the perspectives of Mendus, Oakley and Parker.

THE CASE OF OLLE

Olle is 84 years old and suffers from Parkinson's disease. In addition to this, he has poor vision and hearing. Olle has lived in a residential home for several years but he's not happy there. One particular source of discontent is his love of good food and consequent dissatisfaction with the meals provided at the home.

The problem for the staff and for other residents, however, is that Olle has an electric wheelchair which he drives around in, occasionally going too fast to be safe. The other residents have complained about this, saying that they find it frightening and the atmosphere in the home has become tense and irritable as a consequence. Some of the staff and some of the other residents feel that Olle should have his electric wheelchair replaced with an ordinary one because he is a danger to the safety of others.

But this would mean that Olle would become dependent upon the staff for mobility as he is not able to propel himself in a manual wheelchair. The electric chair provides him with freedom.

ACTIVITY: As your final activity of this chapter, we would like you to consider whether these alternative conceptions have added anything significant to the discussion of autonomy as encapsulated in the official statements at the start of the chapter.

In the final analysis, it would seem to be true to say that our best chance of protecting the vulnerable in healthcare and of practising ethical medicine is in fact by an increasing emphasis on and support for 'autonomy and patient choice'. In this chapter we have begun to see, however, that the question of how we are to make this happen effectively in practice demands an increasingly sophisticated understanding of the ethical dimensions of medicine and of medical practice more widely.

Finally make a list of the key points raised in this chapter.

Suggestions for further reading

Kuhse, H. (ed.) (1998). *A Companion to Bioethics*. Oxford: Blackwell.

Lloyd, G. (1993). *The Man of Reason: 'Male and Female' in Western Philosophy* (2nd edition). London: Routledge.

MacIntyre, A. (1991). *A Short History of Ethics*. London: Routledge.

Parker, M. (ed.) (1999). *Ethics and Community in the Healthcare Professions*. London: Routledge.

Sherwin, S. (1993). *No Longer Patient*. Philadelphia: Temple University Press.

Singer, P. (ed.) (1991). *A Companion to Ethics*. Oxford: Blackwell.

Appendix 1: Study guide for teachers

Each of the chapters in this workbook is intended to be a flexible educational resource, and we would encourage both learners and teachers to use the materials in a way which best suits their requirements. In some cases this might mean working through an entire chapter, but more often it might mean using a case study and the related activities as an educational resource to be used in conjunction with other materials. The chapters and the activities within them are intended to be used in a variety of ways at different points in the medical or nursing curriculum or for post-qualifying training; they are equally suitable for use as distance learning materials for self study.

We aim to present a kind of medical ethics and a way of teaching it which we believe doctors and nurses will find highly relevant to their everyday practice. Although we sometimes refer to the 'big' cases and issues, as evidence of legal positions, for example, we concentrate on 'everyday ethics' by beginning each chapter with a very ordinary and typical sort of case. So we answer the question '*why* study medical ethics?' by beginning from examples which will resonate with practitioners, we hope. The headline topics are important, demonstrating that the issues of medical ethics are of widespread interest to the population as a whole – of which healthcare practitioners are, of course, a part. We do not ignore them, but we do not begin from them, as many texts and courses in medical ethics have done. Nor do we start from abstract 'principles' such as 'autonomy', 'beneficence', or whatever, and then work down to cases, in a deductive fashion. Instead, we begin empirically from typical cases and, importantly, from the narratives which practitioners construct around them. They write those stories in different ways according to what professional part they play in them, according to their disciplinary background.

Using a case study

Here is an example of the sorts of cases we use, and of the interactive, experiential way we ask you to look at them. Like almost all the others in this workbook, it is a real-life case which has been heavily anonymized to protect patient confidentiality. After the case you will find an activity with comments; again, this is a typical structure in the chapters, designed to enhance interactive learning. The typical activity in these chapters is not merely a 'quiz' on factual aspects of the case; here, it requires you to do some thinking about the arguments for and against the proposition that, although this is an everyday sort of case, it is not about ethics, but rather simply a matter of good and bad patient management. This sort of activity is common to the workbook as a whole, deriving from our aim of encouraging 'reflective practice'. We would encourage you to enter your reflections on these activities in a learning journal. You might also wish to compare your reactions with those of colleagues; indeed, in a more formal teaching or training setting, the activities are a good focus of groupwork, and a possible means of formative or summative assessment. But they, and the cases on which they centre, can also be read and analysed by individuals working on their own. Later in this guide, we will give some suggestions on different approaches to reading the cases, particularly for those working alone. But first, you should read the case without any such 'coaching'.

THE CASE OF MR P

Mr P, who is 64, has pre-senile dementia of the Alzheimer's type. His condition is deteriorating rapidly, and for the past 4 months he has lived in a nursing home. Now he is confined to a wheelchair and cannot feed himself. His wife Susan comes to visit him every day, bringing a home-cooked evening meal. The nursing home's guidelines for good practice encourage relatives' involvement, and Mr P does seem pleased to see Susan when she first arrives. But, although Mr P has a hot meal at lunchtime in the nursing home, Susan thinks he also needs 'a proper meal' in the evening, rather than the sandwiches and cakes provided at the home. Mr P appears to resist Susan's attempts to feed him, tossing and turning in his wheelchair. She, in turn, has taken to 'playing a little game': holding his nose, so that, when he opens his mouth for air, she can spoon feed him. This seems to make Mr P very agitated, and he is often hard to calm after Susan's visits.

The nursing home staff have asked Susan not to feed Mr P, but this has led to worsening relations. They feel that Mr P is clearly indicating that he does not want to be forcibly fed. Susan, very hurt by this comment, insists that she is handling Mr P in a playful but caring fashion, and that she has to do something about Mr P's weight loss, which she blames on inadequate nutrition in the home. 'If you can't even feed him properly, what else are you doing wrong? He's not getting any better, you know.' The nursing staff themselves are divided, some feeling that Susan is trying to help, and others that she is in denial about her husband's impending death. The doctors at the nursing home, however, are unanimous. They see no reason to allow Susan to continue feeding Mr P, as it is contrary to his medical best interests and indeed risks asphyxiation. The manager of the home agrees with the doctors: this unnecessary trouble is upsetting the smooth running of the home, and should be stopped.

> **ACTIVITY:** Firstly, consider the response that this case has nothing to do with medical ethics, that it is simply a matter of patient management. What are the arguments for and against that view? Secondly, make a list of the ethical issues which you feel this case evokes. In doing so, try to think of what issues would be identified by (a) the nurses on both sides of the question (b) the doctors (c) Susan (d) the home manager and, interestingly, (e) Mr P in his pre-senile condition.

Let's look first at the viewpoint which insists that this case is just an illustration of bad management, and that it does not raise any difficult ethical dilemmas: it is clear what should be done. Arguably, the problem could have been avoided by not allowing Susan to feed Mr P in the first place. There is no medical need, and Mr P's weight loss is due to his condition, which Susan apparently cannot accept. Perhaps her behaviour is due to her denial about his impending death, in that view. Alternatively, the bad practice is seen as lying in poor communication. Better communication might have prevented the breakdown in relations between Susan and the nursing home staff. But the difficulty here is about what should have been communicated, not just how it should have been communicated. If the nursing home staff were obliged to tell Susan that she was not permitted to feed Mr P, it is hard to see how conflict could have been avoided altogether, no matter how tactfully it was done.

These sorts of interpretations are commonly heard, but what is less often realized is that this 'anti-ethics' position itself rests on a value or ethical base. Not allowing Susan to feed Mr P, because it is not in his medical best interests, or because it upsets the routine of the home, is a *paternalistic* stance. It implies that 'doctor (or nurse, or manager) knows best'. The home has, in fact, not taken that stance; the staff have allowed Susan to feed Mr P. Implicitly, they are accepting a different ethical stance, one which gives weight to non-medical factors. It is a more consultative, *egalitarian* position, which accords some rights to the patient's relatives (or alternatively, for competent patients, to patients themselves). This dynamic between *paternalism* and *rights* has been the wellspring of much of modern medical ethics, over the past 30 years. So, this very ordinary case – much more everyday than most of the questions raised in medical ethics during the past three decades, which originally concentrated more heavily on death and dying, abortion, and other 'big' topics – seems to us to prove that no, you can't avoid 'doing ethics' in everyday practice. Ethics, in our view, is also about institutional structures and power relations, not just about individual choices, and when seen in that light, it is difficult for practitioners to avoid.

What about the second question? – that is, the ethical issues which would be identified in different professional 'narratives'. We have already suggested one set of issues, around rights and paternalism. Others might include:

- Consent to treatment, particularly for incapacitated patients
- The prior question of whether feeding is treatment
- Communication of a terminal diagnosis to the patient's relatives
- How actively we should treat patients at the end of life
- The formulation of hospital and nursing home internal guidelines and consultation between different categories of staff
- Resource issues, such as the amount of staff time devoted to calming Mr P after Susan's visits
- Nurse advocacy: what does it mean to be the patient's advocate in this case?
- Best interests of the patient: are they purely medical? Or does Mr P derive some emotional benefit from Susan's visits?

You may also have identified other questions. So, this abbreviated, ordinary case raises a wide range of ethical questions (and 'meta-ethical' ones, about whether something is an ethical matter in the first place).

Once we have identified the sorts of ethical questions which arise in such cases as Mr P's, however, we need to know where to go from there. It is not enough simply to say that an ethical issue

has been raised; we need to know how to get a better purchase on the ethical question. Many people believe that there are no absolute answers to ethical questions, and that each person's point of view is equally valid. This can lead to a crippling form of moral relativism. In clinical practice, teams need to make decisions; clinical and ethics research committees need to decide on guidelines. On what basis can this possibly be done if everyone's opinion is equally good? (Perhaps this, coupled with a view of ethics as abstract and difficult philosophy, is one reason why people are sometimes reluctant to identify a question as a matter of ethical debate; it will be impossible to get agreement once that concession has been made.) And, in terms of ethics education, the dilemma is equally compelling. Doesn't teaching ethics either imply forcing a particular viewpoint on people, or throwing up one's hands in despair and conceding that it's all a matter of opinion? We have tried to avoid either course in these chapters. In the next section, we present a view of ethics as communicative activity which underpins our approach and which we feel forestalls total relativism. Again, we present the substance and the method of the chapters together in the next chapter; you will be asked to read part of an article by the German ethicist Dieter Birnbacher, arguing for the view of ethics not as grand, impenetrable theory but as communicative activity. This illustrates both the ways in which the chapters typically proceed – from case examples to guided reading exercises based on papers – and the 'philosophy' behind the chapters.

Using a reading exercise

Each of the chapters in the workbook starts off with a set of interactive experiential activities structured around real, everyday cases and commentaries upon those cases by practitioners from Europe, the United States and Australia. In addition to this, the chapters also include guided reading exercises based around papers written by participants in the project who may be practitioners, lawyers, philosophers, patients, economists or social policy analysts.

As an example of how we do this, we have included a short extract from a paper below by Dieter Birnbacher in which he discusses the role of medical ethics and how it ought to be taught. We have included this paper in the study guide because this guide is largely concerned with just this question. The papers included in the other chapters such as that on resource allocation are much more case and clinically based. In the other chapters we generally introduce the question of, say resource allocation, by means of an everyday case, such as the one in the previous section. We then lead into a reading exercise in which we would ask the student to read the paper in the light of the issues raised by the case. The activities and the questions we ask are designed to encourage the student to question the thesis which the paper presents. In this case, for example, whilst we largely agree with Birnbacher that ethics ought to be practically based, we would encourage the student to reflect on this question for him or herself.

To see how this would work we would now like you to read the following short extract from the paper which is concerned with a conflict between two quite different approaches to medical ethics. As you do so, we would like you to reflect on the case of Mr P with which we began this study guide. How would you go about analysing the case from each of the two perspectives Birnbacher introduces? Are the two approaches necessarily in conflict or might they be complementary in some respects? What would an ethics as practice look like? To what extent do you think students of medical ethics require a sense of ethics as theory in order to make an ethics of practice possible?

Teaching clinical medical ethics

Dieter Birnbacher

Which aims and functions of medical ethics are achievable by means of an exchange between the views of patients and doctors? Is this kind of exchange a genuine and constitutive part of

medical ethics, or is it an exercise in which concepts, principles and norms of medical ethics are simply applied?

The answer depends on how medical ethics is conceived. A conception of ethics as theory has tended to predominate in the tradition of philosophy. Its task was the theoretical clarification of moral concepts, the study of moral arguments and the development of a maximally coherent and well-founded set of moral principles. Ethics in this sense was academic work done in writing books, giving lectures and holding seminars.

Ever since the times of the Sophists and of Socrates, however, there has also existed a rival conception of ethics according to which ethics is practice rather than theory, more analogous to art than to science. According to this conception ethics (and philosophy generally) is an activity rather than a doctrine, where 'activity' means an essentially communicative activity of problem identification, deliberation and problem-solving. Though making use of methods similar to those of theoretical ethics and requiring similar skills (in fact, some more), this kind of doing ethics is quite different in its performance aspects. Ethics as theory is mainly monologue, ethics as practice mainly dialogue. Ethics as theory deals mainly with intellectual problems and intradisciplinary controversies, whereas ethics as practice deals mainly with real-life problems and extradisciplinary controversies. Ethics as theory deals mainly with potential cases, ethics as practice mainly with real cases. Taken as ideal types, ethics as theory is done in the ivory tower, ethics as practice in the market-place.

ACTIVITY: Stop here for a moment and consider the case of Mr P with which we began this study guide. When you read the case earlier, we asked you to consider the question of the extent to which cases like this are matters of patient management rather than of ethics. We also asked you to list the ethical issues which you felt the case posed. What are the relative advantages and disadvantages of the two approaches, that is, 'ethics as theory' and 'ethics as practice' in the process of case analysis of this kind?

Now continue with your reading of Birnbacher.

The idea of medical ethics as a truly practical discipline derives from the Socratic idea that ethics (and philosophy generally) is an activity, and an activity that is in principle open to everyone prepared to subject himself to the discipline of controlled dialogue. Correspondingly, the role of the professional ethicist radically changes. Far from functioning as a teacher of ethical wisdom, his role is rather that of a catalyst, moderator and mediator. His task is to see to it that the ethical dialogue keeps its aims firmly in view and is not led astray by extraneous motives, without himself prejudging or manipulating its results.

> **ACTIVITY:** Try to make a list of the kinds of aims you think an ethicist should have in view in such a dialogue. What precisely is his or her role *vis-à-vis* the other participants?

Dieter Birnbacher answers this question as follows. As you read through his list, compare it with your own adding any of those that are missing to your list:

(a) A definition of the problem. It must be clear what the problem is. The ethicist can support the group in fixing the object of the debate.

(b) Articulation of views. The ethicist can give help, where needed, in making these views explicit and giving them adequate expression.

(c) Arguing for one's views. 'Arguing' does not mean, of course, rigorous philosophical reasoning. It should be open for all kinds of relevant inner and outer experiences.

(d) An effort to understand the others' views and arguments. This is the task for which the help of the ethicist is probably most needed. He should insist that the reasons others have for their views are not only taken notice of but understood in depth, taking into account their cognitive and emotional background: Which normative principles are presupposed by these views? On which kind of experience do they depend? Which commitments and attitudes do they manifest? How far are they

guided by external (legal, institutional, financial) constraints?

(e) The potential revision of views in the light of Step 4. Confrontation with conflicting views of others may lead to a rethinking of reactions and positions, or to a weakening of claims to absolute truth.

(f) Finding common ground, consensus formation. Ethics is, among others, the endeavour to solve practical problems in a way acceptable to all sides. The ethical standpoint is the 'view from nowhere' (Nagel, 1986) in which the partiality of all particular viewpoints is transcended but in which all particular viewpoints are somehow taken account of. The ethicist may be helpful as a mediator, paving the way to consensus.

Ethics education for practitioners

The structure of each of the chapters varies slightly depending on the topic it addresses. In some, after a reading exercise of this kind, readers might be asked to look at another case, perhaps one which involves the law more directly. In others, they might be asked to read another paper or perhaps a commentary on the case by a practitioner, or they might be asked to relate the issues raised to their own practice.

Nevertheless, despite their differences, the chapters adopt a consistent and coherent overall educational and theoretical approach, and the topics themselves might be said to each relate in a different way to a single theme, which might be expressed as a concern with the nature of relationships as the focus of ethical problems in medical practice. Each of the chapters can be seen to some extent as testing the relationship between practitioners and patients and their families in a variety of ways, illustrating and analysing the various difficulties which arise as a result.

This study guide has told you something about our view of the 'why, how and what' of ethics education; in self-reflexive fashion, it has also illustrated that view by having you do a bit of ethics learning in our preferred experiential, activity-based format. You will have seen that our style uses case material as a base. We think the case-based approach has several advantages.

- It cuts across disciplinary and cultural boundaries. Everyone can 'relate' in some sense to an actual case, even if they come from very distinct religious or cultural traditions which dictate different principles of ethical conduct. Similarly, different healthcare disciplines have increasingly evolved their own forms of healthcare ethics: nursing ethics, for example, sees its concerns and approach as quite distinct from those of medical ethics proper. But in a case approach, the different slants of different disciplines can be explicitly built in.
- It requires little previous knowledge of ethics and reassures students who think of philosophy as abstruse and difficult.
- It encourages students to think of comparable cases of their own, and thus to generalize what they have learned from one case to another, comparing similarities and differences.
- In the broader context, it allows students to learn from practice in other countries.

But, before you begin work on the workbook itself, you may wonder how to approach these cases. Cases, like any other narrative, are constructed by their authors; the facts do not just speak for themselves. Although the Mr P case study comes from a true account, it is a selective account, it also had to be anonymized, and thus 'fictionalized' to some extent. It is always worth asking just how 'realistic' is this case? What has been left out?

From the reader's point of view, it is also true that cases do not necessarily just speak for themselves. So, before ending this study guide, we want to present two possible approaches to reading the case studies. You may choose either or neither! – but it may be helpful to have different frameworks of analysis before you start. Even if you decide to use these frameworks however, it is important not to do so mechanically. It is important to be sensitive to the nuances of the actual case, rather than trying to fit it into a straitjacket of a framework.

In a text written primarily for medical students,

Alan Johnson develops what he calls 'pathways in medical ethics'. These are decision trees which require a choice at several stages among possible responses. For example, the first thing to ask about a clinical situation, in Johnson's framework for ethical analysis, is whether it is a question of ethics at all. The first part of the tree therefore reads: 'Clinical situation: is it:

(a) Technical?
(b) Ethical?
(c) A matter of professional etiquette?
(d) An emotional question?'

Perhaps you can see some problems with this framework already: it assumes 'only one of the above', but a situation could easily manifest all four components. In particular, we have our doubts about the distinction between 'ethical' and 'emotional'. It implies that ethics is divorced from emotion, but this represents an increasingly outdated and out-of-touch view of philosophical reasoning (Blum, 1980; Lloyd, 1993; Lindemann Nelson and Lindemann Nelson, 1995). However, let us continue with Johnson's framework.

If the situation is viewed as 'ethical', Johnson suggests you should subdivide the components of the case next. He limits the components to four again, assuming that any question can be typified as being about one of the following:

(a) Aims of medical care in this situation
(b) Value questions (e.g. about quality of life)
(c) Autonomy (the capacity to determine one's own actions)
(d) Truth, confidentiality and promise-keeping

The next stage is to enunciate the general and specific moral principles which apply, including law and professional codes. If these principles are in conflict, what should be the outcome? Through another series of choices, Johnson eventually suggests applying the standard of best consequences. This implies a particular philosophical slant, generally termed consequentialist or utilitarian (see Glossary at the end of this study guide). It is worth noting, then, that Johnson's framework is not value-free; indeed, no framework is. If cases do not speak for themselves, neither do the analytical frameworks for analysing cases.

An alternative method of case analysis is offered by David Seedhouse and Lisetta Lovett in their *Practical Medical Ethics* (1992). This is the 'ethical grid', which suggests that, in any clinical case, the doctor should take account of each of the following:

(a) The principles behind health work (defined as respecting persons equally, creating autonomy, respecting autonomy and/or serving needs first)

(b) The duties of a doctor (defined as minimizing harm, doing the most positive good, telling the truth and/or keeping promises)

(c) The general nature of the outcome to be achieved (defined as the most beneficial outcome to society, the most beneficial outcome for the patient, the most beneficial outcome for the practitioner, and/or the most beneficial outcome for a particular group)

(d) The pertinent practical features of the situation (such as the law, the wishes of others, resources available, the effectiveness and efficiency of action, the risks, codes of practice, the degree of certainty of the evidence on which action is taken, and disputed facts).

At each level, some aspects will be relevant and others will not; however, all four levels of the grid are always relevant.

As Seedhouse and Lovett write,

In one sense the Grid is merely a reminder that there are at least four separate levels at which to think, and that within these levels there are several different ways of deciding on strategy. As the Grid is used it soon becomes apparent that it is not the Grid that is working – but the doctor. To say 'I am using the Ethical Grid' is simply to say 'I am engaged in moral reasoning.' (p. 19)

Whether or not you choose to use 'pathways' or 'the ethical grid', or some other approach, this point holds. It is not the mechanism for analysing cases and clinical situations that is doing the work: it is you. We hope that this workbook will provide you with the necessary motivation, interest and support to help you to think critically and constructively about medical ethics.

Appendix 2: The UK core curriculum[1]

In 1998 teachers of medical ethics and law throughout the United Kingdom agreed a national core curriculum in medical ethics and law. Our text, *The Cambridge Medical Ethics Workbook*, was at that time in the process of being written. Because keen interest was expressed by the working group of UK teachers in having a single text which would cover all the core curriculum, we have developed this text to integrate with the core curriculum, to as great an extent as possible.

Below, we reproduce the core curriculum, and its correspondence with the sections of the *Cambridge Workbook in Medical Ethics*. In many cases this is a straight one-to-one affair: for example, Chapters 4, 5 and 6 of our text directly parallel key topics in the national core curriculum. In other cases we have covered the core curriculum topics in several chapters, pulled together here in this Appendix. For example, UK Core Curriculum Topic 1, 'Informed consent and refusal of treatment', is covered in Section 4 of our Chapter 4, Section 2 of our Chapter 7, and in all of our Chapter 9. Teachers wishing to use this text to cover a particular module or session on a core curriculum topic should use this 'grid' as a guide.

There are two major differences between our text and the UK core curriculum. Firstly, although the core curriculum includes a topic area on children, we include chapters on both children and long-term care of the elderly. We do so because we wish to equalize the balance between early and late stages of life, and because many of the most common – and also most philosophically interesting problems – arise in relation to long-term care of the elderly. Secondly, we do not deal at great length with UK Core Topic 10, 'Vulnerabilities created by the duties of doctors and medical students', because this text is not written solely for doctors and medical students. However, readers will find some suggested sections under this heading from sections of the *Cambridge Workbook* on conflicting responsibilities.

Core Topic 1: Informed consent and refusal of treatment

Chapter 4: Medical research, Section 4, 'Valid consent'

Chapter 7: Children and young people, Section 2, 'Consent to treatment and the child's best interests'

Chapter 9: Thinking about ethics: autonomy and patient choice

- The significance of autonomy: respect for persons and for bodily integrity
- Competence to consent: conceptual, ethical and legal aspects
- Further conditions for ethically acceptable consent: adequate information and comprehension, non-coercion

[1] Ashcroft, R., Baron, D., Benatar, S., Bewley, S., Boyd, K., Caddick, J., Campbell, A., Cattan, A., Clayden, G., Day, A., Dickenson, D., Dlugolecka, M., Doyal, L., Draper, H., Farsides, B., von Fragstein, M., Fulford, K., Gillon, R., Goodman, D., Harpwood, V., Harris, J., Haughton, P., Healy, P., Higgs, R., Hope, A., Jackson, J., Jessiman, I., Johnson, A., King, J., Lutrell, S., Matthews, E., Meakin, R., Parker, M., Portsmouth, O., Schwartz, L, Shenfield, F., Snashall, D., Somerville, A., Steiner, T., Vernon, B., Ward, C., Zander, L. & DeZulueta, P. (1988). Teaching medical ethics and law within medical education: a model for the UK core curriculum. *Journal of Medical Ethics*, **24**, 188–92.

- Treatment without consent and proxy consent – when and why morally and legally justifiable
- Assault, battery, negligence and legal standards for disclosure of information
- Problems of communicating information about diagnosis, treatment and risks: the importance of empathy

Core Topic 2: The clinical relationship – truthfulness, trust and good communication

Chapter 4: Medical research, Schuklenk, 'Clinical research in developing countries: trials and tribulations'
Chapter 5: Long-term care, Widdershoven, 'Truth and truth-telling,'
Chapter 9: Thinking about ethics: autonomy and patient choice, Parker, 'A deliberative approach to bioethics'

- The ethical limits of paternalism towards patients
- The significance of honesty, courage, prudence and facilitative attitudes in the practice of good medicine
- Legal and ethical boundaries of clinical discretion to withhold information
- Practical difficulties with truth-telling in medicine: inter/intraprofessional conflicts and other barriers to good communication
- The ethical and legal importance of good communication skills and the significance of the patient's narrative (as distinct from other professional narratives) in building relationships of trust. The importance of cultural, gender, intergenerational, religious and racial sensitivity

Core Topic 3: Confidentiality and good clinical practice

Chapter 2: Genetic testing, Chadwick: 'The Icelandic database: do modern times need modern sagas?'
Chapter 4: Medical research, Section 1, 'What counts as medical research' (based on Fulford)
Chapter 5: Long-term care, Section 2, 'Autonomy, competence and confidentiality'

Chapter 7: Children and young people, Section 3, 'Confidentiality and conflicting responsibilities'

- Professional information, privacy and respect for autonomy
- Trust, secrecy and security in the sharing of information: the practical demands of good practice
- The patient and the family: potential moral and legal tensions
- Disclosure of information: public v. private interests
- Compulsory and discretionary disclosure of confidential information: professional and legal requirements

Core Topic 4: Medical research

Chapter : Medical Research
- Historical and contemporary examples of abuses of medical research
- Individual rights and moral tension between the duty of care to the individual and the interests of others. Therapeutic and non-therapeutic research
- Professional and legal regulation of medical research
- The ethical significance of the distinction between research, audit and innovative and standard therapy, as well as between patients and healthy volunteers
- Research and vulnerable groups: ethical and legal boundaries of informed and proxy consent
- Research on animals: ethical debates and legal requirements

Core Topic 5: Human reproduction

Chapter 3: Reproduction
- Ethical debates about, and the legal status of, the embryo/fetus
- The maternal–fetal relationship: ethical tensions
- Abortion: professional guidelines, legal requirements and debates about the use of tissue from aborted fetuses
- Sterilization: ethical and legal issues
- Pre- and post-natal screening and testing: ethical

issues concerning informed consent and the determination of the interests of the future child

Core Topic 6: The 'new genetics'

Chapter 2: Genetic testing
Chapter 4: Medical research, Section 2, 'A case of genetic research'

- Gene therapy: ethical issues concerning the distinction between treating the abnormal and improving the normal
- Somatic versus germline treatment and research: ethical and legal arguments
- Eugenics v. patient-centred care
- Genetic counselling: responsibilities to patients versus responsibilities to families
- Benefits and dangers of genetic testing and screening after birth: the risks of unwelcome information and of genetic stigmatization
- Cloning: genetic v. personal identity – ethical implications

Core Topic 7: Children

Chapter 7: Children and young people
Chapter 2: Dickenson, 'Can children and young people consent to be screened for adult-onset genetic disorders?'

- Respect for the rights of children: evolution of current legal issues
- The relevance of age in the determination of competence to consent to or refuse treatment
- Ethical debates about legal boundaries of consultation with younger and older children as regards consent to treatment
- The doctor/parent relationship: proxy decision-making and protecting children's interests
- Good ethical and legal practice in reporting suspected child abuse

Core Topic 8: Mental disorders and disabilities

Chapter 6: Mental health
Chapter 8: Long-term care

- Definitions of mental disorders and mental incapacity (including mental illness, learning disability and personality disorder)

- Ethical and legal implications of serious mental illness: civil incapacities, vulnerability and reduced responsibility
- Treatment of, legal detention of, and research on the seriously mentally disordered, with or without consent
- Patient, family and community: ethical and legal tensions

Core Topic 9: Life, death, dying and killing

Chapter 1: Decisions at the end of life

- Palliative care, length and quality of life and good clinical practice
- Attempting ethically to reconcile non-provision of life-prolonging treatment with the duty of care: killing and letting die, double effect, ordinary and extraordinary means
- Withholding and withdrawing life-prolonging treatment – and potentially shortening life – in legally acceptable ways
- Euthanasia and assisted suicide: ethical and legal arguments
- Transplantation: ethical and legal issues
- Death certification and the role of the coroner's court

Core Topic 10: Vulnerabilities created by the duties of doctors and medical students

Chapter 4: Medical research, Lotjonen, 'Ethical and legal issues concerning the involvement of vulnerable groups in medical research'
Chapter 7: Children and young people, Section 1, the case of Peter, Section 3, 'Confidentiality and conflicting responsibilities', and Parker, 'The ethical aspects of working with homeless minors in London'

- Public expectations of medicine: difficulties in dealing with uncertainty and conflict. Ethical importance of good inter- and intraprofessional communication and teamwork
- The General Medical Council. Professional regulation, standards and the Medical Register. Implications for students and their relationships with patients

- Responding appropriately to clinical mistakes: personal, legal and ethical responsibilities. Unethical and unsafe practice in medicine: 'whistleblowing'
- The law of negligence, NHS complaints and disciplinary procedures
- The health of doctors and students, and its relationship to professional performance: risks, sources of help and duties to disclose
- Medical ethics and the involvement of doctors in police interrogation, torture and capital punishment

Core Topic 11: Resource allocation

Chapter 8: Resource Allocation
- Inadequate resources and distributive justice within the National Health Service: the law
- Theories and criteria for equitable healthcare: needs, rights, utility, efficiency, desert, autonomy
- Debates about rationing: personal, local, national and international perspectives. Markets and ethical differences between competing healthcare delivery systems
- Boundaries of responsibility of individuals for their own illnesses and ethical implications

Core Topic 12: Rights

Chapter 4: 'Medical research,' sections on Nuremberg and Helsinki codes
Chapter 5: Long-term care, ter Meulen, 'Care for dependent elderly persons and respect for autonomy', and Adshead, 'Autonomy, feminism and psychiatric patients'
Chapter 7: 'Children and young people' sections on United Nations Convention of the Rights of the Child
Chapter 8: Resource allocation, section 5, 'Philosophical models of resource allocation'
Chapter 9: Thinking about ethics: autonomy and patient choice
- Conceptions of rights – what are they?
- Links between rights and duties and responsibilities
- International declarations of human rights
- The importance of the concept of human rights for medical ethics
- Debates about the centrality of rights for good professional practice in medicine
- Rights and justice in healthcare

Glossary

A priori: (Latin, 'what comes before') known to be true without reference to experience.

Advance directive: a document in which a person provides guidance for the making of medical decisions should they become incapacitated. An 'instructional' directive states specific treatment preferences in the case of anticipated decisions. A 'proxy' directive nominates an individual to make decisions on the patient's behalf in such situations.

The legal status of advance directives varies from state to state and between countries, as do the procedural rules governing the validity of such directives. In cases where such directives have no legal status, they may still play a valuable role in the assessment of the patient's best interests and as a reflection of the person's wishes in regard to future healthcare.

Affects: 'a term used in psychology for a feeling or emotion, particularly one leading to action' (*The Oxford Companion to the Mind*, ed. R.L. Gregory, Oxford University Press, 1987, p. 12).

Autonomy: in Greek, literally 'being a law onto oneself', the quality of being self-governing. Autonomy is probably the most frequently used (and misused) concept in medical ethics. One common source of fuzziness lies in the difference between treating autonomy as a description of someone's actual mental state, or viewing it as a prescription that tells us how we should aim to treat people, regardless of whether or not they are fully competent. That is, is autonomy a normative or a descriptive concept? The American philosopher Joel Feinberg (1970) has identified four disparate but frequently confused senses of the term. The concept of autonomy is explored in much greater detail in Chapter 9.

Beneficence: '. . . in ordinary English the term 'beneficence' connotes acts of mercy, kindness and charity. Altruism, love and humanity are also sometimes considered forms of beneficence. We will understand beneficent action even more broadly, so that it includes all forms of action intended to benefit other persons. 'Beneficence' refers to an action done for the benefit of others; 'benevolence' refers to the character trait or virtue of being disposed to act for the benefit of others; and the 'principle of beneficence' refers to a moral obligation to act for the benefit of others. Many acts of beneficence are not obligatory, but a principle of beneficence, in our usage, asserts an obligation to help others further their important and legitimate interests (Beauchamp & Childress, 1994, p. 260).

Coase's theorem: set out by the economist Ronald Coase in an influential article, 'The problem of social cost' (*Journal of Law and Economics*, vol. 3, pp. 1–44 (1960)). Coase held that, regardless of initial entitlements, a pure market would achieve 'Pareto optimality', which means that no one's lot could be improved without worsening someone else's.

Communitarian: communitarians argue that communities and communal values are of value in themselves, over and above the value of the individuals of whom they are constituted. Communitarians such as Etzioni argue that the 'good community' is one in which rights and responsibilities are 'balanced'. Communitarians have criticized 'patient-centred' medicine for what they see as its over-emphasis on the rights of individual patients at the expense of families, communities, social values and so on (see, for example, Callahan, D., 1987).

Consequentialist: pertaining to moral theories that maintain that the morality of actions is to be judged according to their foreseeable outcomes. Utilitarianism is an example of a consequentialist moral theory.

Co-payments: co-payment is a term used to describe the situation in which patients and their families are expected to contribute part of the costs of their treatment or care.

Deontological: pertaining to duty-based systems of ethics, such as Kantianism which maintains that the morality of actions is to be judged in terms of their conformity with moral rules, duties, obligations, rights and so on, rather than in terms of their consequences. More loosely, and as sometimes used in this workbook, the concept of deontology pertains to the medical codes of southern Europe (and Ireland), in which the patient has a positive duty to maximize his or her own health and to follow the doctor's instructions, whilst the physician is constrained more by professional norms than by patient rights.

Efficiency: productive efficiency measures which producer achieves the most favourable ratio of inputs to outputs. Allocative efficiency concerns arranging the societal distribution of resources so as to reward the most productively efficient producers.

Epistemology: the branch of philosophy concerned with the problem of knowledge. Epistemologists investigate questions regarding such matters as, the reliability of claims to knowledge, the scope of knowledge, the nature of knowledge and so on.

External effects: actions of one economic agent which affect the welfare of another but which are not reflected in market prices. For example, an

external cost of burning coal is pollution, for which the firm selling the electricity usually does not pay, and which is therefore not reflected in the price paid for electricity by consumers. However, it affects the welfare of those living near the generating station.

First-order decisions: 'determine the total quantity of resources distributed to various sectors or programmes . . . [whilst] second-order decisions . . . determine the services directed to individual recipients or claimants.' (Thorslund et al., 1997b, citing Calabresi & Bobbitt, 1978).

Hermeneutics: the Webster's dictionary defines hermeneutics as the study of the methodological principles of interpretation (for example, the Bible). In the sense Widdershoven uses it, hermeneutics is intended to mean the study of meaning and interpretation as a philosophical method.

Iatrogenic: literally, created by the doctor (Greek); as in iatrogenic harm, harm to patients caused in the course of treatment rather than by the condition itself.

In arguendo: for the sake of the argument (Latin), e.g. a concession made for the sake of argument.

Incompetence/incapacity: lack of decision-making ability or authority.

Liberalism: in political theory, an enormously influential, wide-ranging and varied doctrine which (a) elevates individual rights over collective interests, on the grounds that liberty is the natural human condition and society an artificial construction, and (b) acknowledges only that political authority which protects individual rights. Government is seen as a contract between the ruler and the ruled, and typically limited by constitutional checks and restraints.

Lumpenproletariat: Marx's term for the residuum of workers with few or no skills, the most impoverished section of the working class.

Marginal cost: The cost of producing each extra unit of goods or services.

Mill, John Stuart (1806–1873): utilitarian philosopher whose *On Liberty* (1859) proposes 'one very simple principle': that society may not coerce individuals against their wills except when other people's welfare is threatened. Paternalism is entirely wrong, on this interpretation, as is legislation for 'one's own good'.

Non-maleficence: 'The principle of non-maleficence asserts an obligation not to inflict harm intentionally. It has been closely associated in medical ethics with the maxim '*primum non nocere*': 'Above all [or first] do no harm'. . . . An obligation of non-maleficence and an obligation of beneficence are both expressed in the Hippocratic oath: 'I will use treatment to help the sick according to my ability and judgement, but I will never use it to injure or wrong them' (Beauchamp & Childress,1994, p. 189).

Opportunity cost: the loss of other opportunities foregone when one alternative is chosen.

Persistent Vegetative State: (PVS) is distinguished from coma in that the patient is awake but not aware of his or her environment. Such patients breathe for themselves, usually have a sleep/wake pattern, and may smile, scream, grunt or move their limbs without obvious reason. The diagnosis of PVS should only be made after 1 year, except under exceptional circumstances according to BMA guidelines. The prognosis is poor: only very occasionally do patients recover enough after a year or more to be able to perceive and respond to stimuli.

Prima facie (Latin for 'at first sight'): pertaining to an assumption, duty or argument which to hold unless proven otherwise.

Principles: in the work of Beauchamp and Childress (1994), the 'four principles' of biomedical ethics are said to be autonomy, beneficence, non-maleficence and justice. These four principles have been widely adopted by ethicists and practitioners as a method of drawing out and expressing the ethical dimensions of problems in healthcare. This approach has come to be known as 'principlism'.

Principlism: an approach to medical ethics derived from the influential work of Tom Beauchamp and James Childress, *Principles of Medical Ethics* (4th edn, 1994) and found also in many subsequent authors, e.g. Raanan Gillon, *Philosophical Medical Ethics* (1986). Principlism attempts to apply and weigh four principles in any decision-making situation: autonomy, beneficence (doing good), non-maleficence (doing no harm) and justice. Critics of principlism argue that it is too rigid; that the principles represent something of a philosophical hodgepodge and form an incoherent whole; that they fail to take the intricacies of relationships into account, being abstract; and/or that what actually motivates practitioners in medical dilemmas is not a mechanical weighing of principles but an attempt to put into practice the virtues of a good doctor or nurse.

Reality Orientation Therapy: this term is used by Widdershoven to refer to a therapeutic approach in psychiatric work with patients suffering from dementia in which the patient is confronted with, or brought to see the truth, as a way of delaying/working with his or her dementia. This is opposed to an approach called validation in which healthcare professionals engage with the patient's world as expressed by him or her, treating his or her expressed desires, wishes, etc. as meaningful in their own right. Several of the writers in this chapter challenge the usual use of the concept of autonomy and argue that autonomous needs to be reconceptualized in a rational sense.

Subsidiarity: a principle, originating in the structure of the Catholic church and later adopted by the European Union, by which decisions are to be made as close and as locally as possible to the place of their effect. This is essentially a decentralizing principle. Expressed in reverse, the principle demands that decisions should be made locally unless they have wider implications and effects in which case they should be referred towards the centre until a point is reached, as far from the centre as possible, at which these effects can be taken into account.

Suttee: self-immolation by a Hindu wife on her husband's funeral pyre. The practice was outlawed by the British Raj but is alleged to have returned in some parts of rural India during the 1980s, for example, in the much reported case of an 18-year-old woman.

Telos: (Greek) goal, aim, end, as in the telos of medicine.

Utilitarian: pertaining to that form of consequentialism which holds that the morally best outcomes (consequences) are those that maximize personal and social 'well-being'. Utilitarianism tends to interpret these 'best outcomes' and hence 'well-being' in either hedonistic terms or in terms of the satisfaction of preferences.

Bibliography

4 All ER 177 (1991).

4 All ER 627 (1992).

Abel, E. (1991). *Who Cares for the Elderly? Public Policies and the Experiences of Adult Daughters*. Philadelphia, PA: Temple University Press.

Abel, E.K. and Browner, C.B. (1998). Selective compliance with biomedical authority and the uses of experiential knowledge. In *Pragmatic Women and Body Politics*, ed. M. Lock and P. Kaufert, pp. 310–26. Cambridge: Cambridge University Press.

Ach, J.S. and Gaidt, A. (1994). Am Rande des Abgrunds? Anmerkungen zu einem Argument gegen die moderne Euthanasie-Debatte. *Ethik in der Medizin*, **6**, 172–88.

Achterhuis, H. (1988). *Het rijk van de schaarste. Van Thomas Hobbes tot Michel Foucault*. Baarn: Ambo.

Adshead, G. & Dickenson, D. (1993). Why do doctors and nurses disagree? In *Death, Dying and Bereavement*, ed. D. Dickenson and M. Johnson, pp. 162–8. London: Open University & Sage.

Agich, G. (1990). Reassessing autonomy in long-term care. *Hastings Center Report*, **20**, (6), 12–17.

Agich, G. (1993). *Autonomy in Long-term Care*. New York: Oxford University Press.

Aiken, W. and LaFollette, H.(eds.) (1980). *Whose Child? Children's Rights, Parental Authority and State Power*. Totowa, NJ: Rowan and Littlefield.

Airedale NHS Trust v. *Bland* [1993] 1 All ER 821.

Airedale NHS Trust v. *Bland* [1993] 1 All ER 882–3.

Alderson, P. (1990). *Choosing for Children*. Oxford: Oxford University Press.

Alderson, P. (1992). In the genes or in the stars? Children's competence to consent. *Journal of Medical Ethics*, **18**, 119–24.

Alderson, P. (1994). *Children's Consent to Surgery*. Buckingham: Open University Press.

Alderson, P. and Montgomery, J. (1996). *Healthcare Choices: Making Decisions with Children*. London: Institute for Public Policy Research.

Allmark, P. (1995). Can there be an ethics of care? *Journal of Medical Ethics*, **21**, 19–24.

Almond, B. (1991). Education and liberty. *Journal of Philosophy of Education*, **25**(2), 193–202.

Almond, B. (1993). Rights. In *Companion to Ethics*, ed. P. Singer, pp. 259–69. Oxford: Blackwell.

American Fertility Society (1990). Surrogate mothers. In *Surrogate Motherhood: Politics and Privacy*, ed. L. Gostin, pp. 307–14. Bloomington: University of Indiana Press.

American Psychiatric Association (1983). Guidelines for legislation on the psychiatric hospitalisation of adults. *American Journal of Psychiatry*, **140**, 622–79.

American Psychiatric Association (1990). Task Force Report: *The Practice of Electroconvulsive Therapy: Recommendations for Treatment, Training and Privileging*. Washington, DC: American Psychiatric Association.

American Psychiatric Association (1994). *Diagnostic and Statistical Manual. Version IV*. Washington, DC: American Psychiatric Press.

Angell, M. (1996). Euthanasia in the Netherlands – good news or bad? *New England Journal of Medicine*, **335**, (22), 1676–8.

Anscombe, E. (1958). Modern moral philosophy. *Philosophy*, **33**, 1–19.

Archard, D. (1993). *Children, Rights and Childhood*. London: Routledge.

Aristotle (1980). *The Nicomachean Ethics* (trans. W.D. Ross). Oxford: Oxford University Press.

Ashcroft, R. (1998). Teaching for patient-centred ethics. Paper presented at the European Society for Philosophy in Medicine Conference, Marburg, Germany, August.

Ashcroft, R.E., Chadwick, D.W., Clark, S.R.L., Edwards, R.H.T., Frith, L.J. and Hutton, J.L. (1997). Implications of sociocultural contexts for ethics of clinical trials. *Health Technology Assessment*, **1**(9), 1.67.

Attanucci, J. (1988). In whose terms: a new perspective on self, role and relationship. In *Mapping the Moral Domain*, ed. C. Gilligan et al., Cambridge, MA: Harvard University Press.

B v. *Croydon HA* [1995] 1 All ER 683.

Baldwin, S. and Oxlad, M. (1996). Multiple case sampling of ECT administration to 217 minors. *Journal of Mental Health*, **5**(5), 451–63.

Baltussen, R., Leidl, R. and Ament, A. (1996). The impact of age on cost-effectiveness ratios and its control in decision-making. *Health Economics*, **5**, 227–39.

Barni, M. (1991). La medicine legale e le ethiche esterna alla legge. *Rivista Italiana di Medicine Legale*, **13**, 375–80.

Barry, R.L. and Bradley, G.V. (1991). *Set No Limits. A Rebuttal to Daniel Callahan's Proposal to Limit Healthcare for the Elderly*, Urbana and Chicago, IL: University of Illinois Press.

Bates, P. (1994). Children in secure psychiatric units: Re K, W and H – 'out of sight, out of mind'? *Journal of Child Law*, **6**, 131–7.

Baylis, F. and Sherwin, S. (2000). Judgements of noncompliance in pregnancy. In *Ethical Issues in Maternal–Fetal Medicine*, ed. D. L. Dickenson. Cambridge: Cambridge University Press.

Beauchamp, T. L. and Childress, J. F. (1989). *Principles of Biomedical Ethics*, 3rd edn. Oxford: Oxford University Press.

Beauchamp, T. L. & Childress, J. F. (1994). *Principles of Biomedical Ethics*, 4th edn. Oxford: Oxford University Press.

Beecher, H. (1966). Ethics and clinical research. *The New England Journal of Medicine*, **274**, (24), p. 1354–60.

Bell, D. (1993). *Communitarianism and its Critics*. Oxford: Clarendon Press.

Benhabib, L. (1997). Ethical issues in child psychiatry in the Algerian community in France. Paper represented at the Seventh EBEPE Workshops, Rome, March.

Bennett, R. and Harris, J. (2000). Are there lives not worth living? When is it morally wrong to reproduce?' In *Ethical Issues in Maternal–Fetal Medicine*, ed. D. L. Dickenson. Cambridge: Cambridge University Press.

Berghmans, R. (1992). *Om bestwil. Paternalisme in de psychiatrie* [For the patient's good. Paternalism in psychiatry]. Amsterdam: Thesis Publishers.

Berghmans, R. (1994). Zelfbinding in de psychiatrie. Ethische aspecten. [Self-binding in psychiatry. Ethical aspects]. *Tijdschrift voor Psychiatrie*, **36**, (9), 625–38.

Berghmans, R. (1996). The Netherlands. In *Informed Consent in Psychiatry. European Perspectives of Ethics, Law and Clinical Practice*, ed. H-G. Koch, S. Reiter-Theil and H. Helmchen, pp. 197–229. Baden-Baden: Nomos Verlagsgesellschaft.

Berghmans, R. (1997a). Physician-assisted death, the moral integrity of medicine and the slippery slope. Paper presented at the seventh European Biomedical Ethics Practitioner Education workshop, Maastricht, 21–22 March.

Berghmans, R. (1997b). Protection of the rights of the mentally ill in the Netherlands. Paper presented at the Tenth EBEPE Conference, Turku, Finland, June.

Berlin, I. (1969). Two concepts of liberty, in Berlin, I. *Four Essays on Liberty*. Oxford: Oxford University Press.

Bertagnoli, M.W. & Borchardt, C.M. (1990). A review of ECT for children and adolescents. *Journal of American Academy of Child and Adolescent Psychiatry*, **29**(2), 302–7.

Binstock, R.H. and Post, S.G. (1991). *Too Old for Healthcare?*

Controversies in Medicine, Law, Economics and Ethics. Baltimore: Johns Hopkins University Press.

Birke, L., Himmelweit, S. and Vines, G. (1990). *Tomorrow's Child: Reproductive Technologies in the 90s*. London: Virago.

Birleson, P. (1996). Legal rights and responsibilities of adolescents and staff in Victorian Child and Adolescent Mental Health Services. *Australian and New Zealand Journal of Psychiatry*, **30**, 805–12.

Black, D. (1991). Psychotropic drugs for problem children. *British Medical Journal*, **302**, 190–1.

Blank, R. and Merrick, J. S. (1995). *Human Reproduction, Emerging Technologies, and Conflicting Rights*. Washington, DC: Congressional Quarterly.

Blasszauer, B. (1993). Ethical issues in institutional care. Paper for the May Conference of the Project Care for the Elderly: Goals and Priorities, Maastricht May 7–8.

Bloch, S. and Chodoff, P. (1993). *Psychiatric Ethics*, 2nd edn. Oxford: Oxford University Press.

Blum, L. (1980). *Friendship, Altruism and Morality*. London: Routledge and Kegan Paul.

Blum, L. (1988). Gilligan and Kohlberg: implications for moral theory. *Ethics*, **98**, 472–91.

Blustein, J. (1982). *Parents and Children: The Ethics of the Family*, Oxford: Oxford University Press.

Bok, S. (1989). *Secrets: On the Ethics of Concealment and Revelation*. Vintage Books.

Bonner v. *Morgan* 126 F2d 121, 122 (DC Cir 1941).

Borst-Eilers, E (1990). Leeftijd als criterium. In *Grenzen aan de Zorg. Zorgen aan de Grens*, ed. J. K. M. Gevers and H. J. Hubben, pp. 66–72. Alphen aan de Rijn: Tjeenk Willink.

Borthwick, C. (1995). The proof of the vegetable: a commentary on medical futility. *Journal of Medical Ethics*, **21**, 205–8.

Bosanquet, N. (1998). The case for investing in quality health services for older people. Paper delivered to British Geriatric Society, October 1998.

Bouman, N. (1997). Ethical issues in child psychiatric consultations and liaison in paediatrics. Paper presented at the eighth European Biomedical Ethics Practitioner Education (EBEPE). workshop, Rome, 7–8 March.

Bowlby, J. (1988). *A Secure Base: Clinical Applications of Attachment Theory*. London: Routledge.

Bracalenti, R. and Mordini, E. (1997). The role of psychiatric and psychological support at the end of life. Paper presented at the Seventh EBEPE Workshop.

Breggin, P. (1991). *Toxic Psychiatry, Drugs and Electroconvulsive Therapy: The Truth and the Better Alternatives*. New York: St. Martin's Press.

Breslau, N., Davis, G.C., Andreski, P., Peterson, E. and Schultz, L. (1997). Sex differences in posttraumatic stress disorder. *Archives of General Psychiatry*, **54**: 1044–8.

British Broadcasting Corporation (1995). Open University course K260 *(Death and Dying)*. radio programme.

British Medical Association (1995). *Medical Ethics Today*. London: BMA.

British Medical Association (1998). *Human Genetics: Choice and Responsibility*. Oxford: Oxford University Press.

British Medical Association (1999). *Withholding and Withdrawing Life-prolonging Medical Treatment*. London: BMJ Publishing Group.

Brock, D. (1993). A proposal for the use of advance directives in the treatment of incompetent mentally ill persons. *Bioethics*, 7, 247–56.

Brody, B. (1988). *Life and Death Decision Making*. Oxford: Oxford University Press.

Brody, H. (1997). Medical futility: a useful concept? In *Medical Futility and the Evaluation of Life-sustaining Interventions*, ed. M.B. Zucker and H.D. Zucker, pp. 1–14. Cambridge: Cambridge University Press.

Brown, D. (1994). Self-development through subjective interaction: a fresh look at ego training in action. In *The Psyche and the Social World*, ed. D. Brown and L. Zinkin, pp. 80–98. London: Routledge.

Brown, G. & Harris,T. (1978). *The Social Origins of Depression*. London: Tavistock.

Brown, L. and Gilligan, G. (1992). *Meeting at the Crossroads: Women's Psychology and Girls' Development*. Cambridge MA. and London: Harvard University Press.

Buchanan, A. and Brock, D. (1989). *Deciding for Others: The Ethics of Surrogate Decision Making*. Cambridge: Cambridge University Press.

Button, E. (1992). *Rural Housing For Youth*. London: Centrepoint.

Calabresi, G. and Bobbitt, P. (1978). *Tragic Choices*. New York: Norton.

Callahan, D. (1987). *Setting Limits. Medical Goals in an Ageing Society*. New York: Simon and Schuster.

Callahan, D. (1990). *What Kind of Life. The Limits of Medical Progress*. New York: Simon and Schuster.

Callahan, D. (1994). Setting limits: a response. *The Gerontologist*, 34, 393–8.

Callahan, D. (1995a). *Setting Limits: Medical Goals in an Ageing Society*, 2nd edn. Washington DC: Georgetown University Press.

Callahan, J. (ed.). (1995b). *Reproduction, Ethics and the Law: Feminist Perspectives*. Indiana University Press.

Calzone, C. (1996). Consent or compliance? From informed consent to the right to informed guidance. Paper presented at the Sixth EBEPE Workshop, Naantali, Finland, 6–7 September.

Calzone, C. and D'Andrea, M.S. (1996). New offspring in a family with a handicapped child. Paper presented at the First EBEPE Workshop, Rome, May.

Campbell, B. (1995). *The London Independent*, March 16th.

Campbell, D.M. and MacGillivray, I. (1985). Pre-eclampsia in a second pregnancy. *British Journal of Obstetrics and Gynaecology*, 92, 131–40.

Capron, A.M. (1995). Baby Ryan and virtual futility. *Hastings Center Report*, 25, (2), 20–1.

Carney T. and Tait, D. (1997). Caught between two systems? Guardianship and young people with a disability. *International Journal of Law and Psychiatry*, 20, 141–66.

Carr, V., Dorrington, C., Schrader, G. and Wale, J. (1983). The use of ECT for mania in childhood bipolar disorder. *British Journal of Psychiatry*, 143, 411–5.

Carse, A. L (1991). The 'voice of care': implications for bioethical education. *Journal of Medicine and Philosophy*, 16, 5–28.

Casey, R.J. and Berman, J.S. (1985). The outcome of psychotherapy with children. *Psychological Bulletin*, 98, 388–400.

Chadwick, R. (1987). *Ethics, Reproduction and Genetic Control*. London: Routledge.

Charmaz, K. (1987). Struggle for a self: identity levels of the chronically ill. In *Research in the Sociology of Health Care*, ed. J. Roth and P. Conrad, vol. 6, pp. 283–321. Greenwich, Connecticut: J.A.I. Press.

Cheon-Lee, E. and Amstey, M.A. (1998). Compliance with centers for disease control and prevention, antenatal culture protocol for preventing Group B streptococcal neonatal sepsis. *American Journal of Obstetrics and Gynaecology*, 179, 77–9.

Chesley, L.C., Annitto, J.E. and Cosgrove, R.A. (2000). The remote prognosis of eclamptic women. *American Journal of Obstetrics and Gynecology*, 182 (1 pt 1), 247.

The Children Act. (1989). London: HMSO.

Choices in Healthcare (1992). Report by the Government Committee on Choices in Healthcare, The Netherlands. Rijswijk: Ministry of Welfare, Health and Cultural Affairs.

Christman, J. (1988). Constructing the inner citadel: recent work on the concept of autonomy. *Ethics*, 99, 109–24.

Cicero (1951). *On Moral Duties, The Basic works of Cicero*, ed. M. Hadas, p. 47. New York: Modern Library.

CIOMS/WHO (1993). *International Ethical Guidelines for Biomedical Research involving Human Subjects*. CIOMS/WHO: Geneva.

Clark, A.E. (1996). Autonomy and death. *Tulane Law Review*, 71, (45), 45–137.

Clark, P.G. (1989). Canadian health-care policy and the elderly: will rationing rhetoric become reality in an ageing society? *Canadian Journal of Community Mental Health*, 8, 123–40.

Clarke, A. (1994). *Genetic Counselling: Practice and Principles*. London: Routledge.

Clinical Genetics Society (1994). The genetic testing of children: report of a working party. *Journal of Medical Genetics*, 31, 785–97.

Cole, T.R. (1988). Ageing, history and health: progress and paradox. In *Health and Ageing*, ed. J.F. Schroots, J.E. Birren and A. Svanborg, p. 45–63. New York & Lisse: Swets.

Cole, T.R. (1992). *The Journey of Life. A Cultural History of Ageing in America*. New York: Cambridge University Press.

Connors, A.F. Jr, Speroff, T., Dawson, N.V. et al. (1996). The effectiveness of right-heart catheterization in the initial care of critically ill patients. *Journal of the American Medical Association*, **276** (11), 889–97.

Consensus statement by teachers of medical ethics and law in UK medical schools (1998). *The Journal of Medical Ethics*, **24**(3), 188–92.

Cook, A. & Scott, A. (1992). ECT for young people. *British Journal of Psychiatry*, **161**, 718–19.

Cooper, D.K. (1997). Juveniles' understanding of trial-related information: are they competent defendants? *Behavioural Sciences and the Law*, **15**, 167–80.

Council of Europe Steering Committee on Bioethics (1999). *The Icelandic Act on a Health Sector Database and Council of Europe Conventions*. Strasbourg: Ministry of Health and Social Security (CDBI-CO-GT2(99)7 1999.)

Council of Europe (1981). *Convention for the protection of individuals with regard to automatic processing of personal data*. Strasbourg: Council of Europe.

Council of Europe (1997a). Convention for the Protection of Human Rights and Dignity of the Human Being with regard to the Application of Biology and Medicine: Convention on Human Rights and Biomedicine (Oviedo 4 April 1997). *European Treaty Series 164*.

Council of Europe (1997b). *Recommendation on the Protection of Medical Data*. Strasbourg: Council of Europe (No R(97)5.)

Council of Europe (1997c). *Recommendation Concerning the Protection of Personal Data Collected and Processed for Statistical Purposes*. Strasbourg: Council of Europe (No R(97)18.)

Crawford, R. (1980). Healthism and medicalization of everyday life. *International Journal of Health Services*, **10**, 365–88.

Crenier, A. (1996). Child abuse and professional secrecy: doctors and the law. Paper presented at the First EBEPE Workshop, Rome, 25 May.

Crisp, R. (ed.). (1996). *How Should One Live? Essays on the Virtues*. Oxford: Clarendon Press.

Crisp, R. (ed) (1997). *Virtue Ethics*. Oxford: Oxford University Press.

Culver, C.M. and Gert, B. (1982). *Philosophy in Medicine*. Oxford: Oxford University Press.

Cushman, G. (1990). Why the self is empty: toward an historically situated psychology. *Journal of Medicine and Philosophy*, **45** (5), pp. 599–611.

Dalla Vorgia, P. (1997). Car driving and insight: commentary on the case of Mr A from a Greek viewpoint. Paper presented at the Tenth Workshop of the European Biomedical Ethics Practitioner Education Project, Maastricht, May.

Daniels, C. (1993). *At Women's Expense: State Power and the Politics of Fetal Rights*. Cambridge, MA: Harvard University Press.

Daniels, K.R., Ericsson, H.L. and Burn, J.P. (1998). The views of semen donors regarding the Swedish Insemination Act 1984. *Medical Law International*, **3**, (2, 3), 117–34.

Daniels, N. (1988). *Am I My Parents' Keeper? An Essay on Justice between the Young and the Old*. New York: Oxford University Press.

Danish Council of Ethics (1998). *Conditions for Psychiatric Patients – a Report*. Copenhagen: Danish Council of Ethics.

Davies, J. (ed) (1993). *The Family: Is it just Another Lifestyle Choice?*, London: Institute of Economic Affairs.

Davison, J.M. (1992). Renal disease. In *Medical Disorders in Obstetric Practice*, ed. M. Swiet. Oxford: Blackwell Scientific Publications.

Davison, J.M. (1994). Pregnancy in renal allograft recipients: problems, prognosis and practicalities. *Baillière's Clinical Obstetrics and Gynaecology*, **8**, 501–25.

Davison, J.M., and Redman, C.W.G. (1997). Pregnancy post-transplant. *British Journal of Obstetrics and Gynaecology*, **104**, 1106–7.

Dawes, R.M. (1986). Representative thinking in clinical judgement. *Clinical Psychology Review*, **6**, 425–41.

de Beauvoir, S. (1972). *The Coming of Age*. Trans. Patrick O'Brien, p. 28. New York: G.P. Putnam's Sons.

Declaration of Helsinki (1964). Adopted by the 18th World Medical Assembly of the World Medical Association in Helsinki (amended in 1975, 1983, 1989 and 1996).

deCODE genetics. www.database.is (Accessed 14 May 1999.)

De Graeve, D., Lescrauwaet, B. and Nonneman, W. (1997). Patient classification and the costs of HIV and AIDS in Belgium. *Health Policy*, **39**, 93–106.

Denney, J.L. and Denson, J.S. (1972). Risk of surgery in patients over 90. *Geriatrics*, **27**, 115–18.

Dennis, N. (1993). *Rising Crime and the Dismembered Family*. London: Institute of Economic Affairs.

Department of Health (1989). *Working for Patients*. White Paper on the National Health Service, CM555. London: HMSO.

Devereux, J., Jones, D.P.H. and Dickenson, D.L. (1993). Can children withhold consent to treatment? *British Medical Journal* **306**, 1459–61.

Devinsky, O. and Duchowny, M.S. (1983). Seizures after convulsive therapy; a retrospective case survey. *Neurology*, **33**(7), 921–5.

Dickenson, D. (1991). *Moral Luck in Medical Ethics and Practical Politics*. Aldershot: Avebury.

Dickenson D. (1994). Children's informed consent to treatment: is the law an ass? *Journal of Medical Ethics*, **20**, 205–6.

Dickenson, D. (1995). Is efficiency ethical? Resource issues in healthcare. In *Introducing Applied Ethics*, ed. B. Almond, pp. 229–46. Oxford: Blackwell.

Dickenson, D. (1997). *Property, Women and Politics: Subjects or Objects?* Cambridge: Polity Press.

Dickenson, D. (1998). Cross-cultural issues in European bioethics. Paper presented at the Fourth International Association of Bioethics Conference, Tokyo, November.

Dickenson, D. (2000). *Ethical Issues in Maternal–Fetal Medicine*. Cambridge: Cambridge University Press.

Dickenson, D. and Jones, D. (1995). True wishes: the philosophy and developmental psychology of children's informed consent. *Philosophy, Psychiatry and Psychology*, **2**, 287–305.

Dickenson, D. and Shah, A. (1999). The *Bournewood* judgement: a way forward? *Journal of Medicine, Science and the Law*, **39**(4), 280–4.

Dingwall, A., Eekelaar, J. and Murray, T. (1983). *The Protection of Children*. Oxford: Blackwell.

Dooley, D. (1997). *Autonomy, feminism and vulnerable patients*. Paper presented at the Tenth EBEPE Conference, Turku, Finland, June.

Drane, J.F. (1988). *Becoming a Good Doctor: The Place of Virtue and Character in Medical Ethics*. Kansas City: Sheed & Ward.

Driver, J. (1995). Monkeying with motives: agent-basing virtue ethics. *Utilitas*, **7**, 281–8.

Drummond, M., Stoddart, G. and Torrance, G. (1987). *Methods for the Economic Evaluation of Healthcare Programmes*. Oxford: Oxford University Press.

Durlak, J.A., Fuhrman, T. and Lampman, C. (1991). Effectiveness of cognitive-behavioural therapy for maladapting children: a meta-analysis. *Psychological Bulletin*, **110**, 204–14.

Dworkin, G. (1988). *Theory and Practice of Autonomy*. Cambridge: Cambridge University Press.

Dworkin, R. (1977). *Taking Rights Seriously*. London: Duckworth.

Dworkin, R. (1986). Autonomy and the demented self. *The Milbank Quarterly*, **64**, suppl.II, 4–16.

Dworkin, R. (1990). The foundations of liberal equality. In *The Tanner Lectures on Human Values*, ed. G. Petersen. Saltlake City: University of Utah Press.

Dworkin, R. (1993). *Life's Dominion: An Argument about Abortion, Euthanasia, and Individual Freedom*. London: Harper Collins Publishers.

Eastman, N. and Peay, J. (1998). Bournewood: an indefensible gap in mental health law. *British Medical Journal*, **317**, 94–5.

Edgar, A. (1999). The Health Service as Civil Association. In *Ethics and Community in the Healthcare Professions*, ed. M. Parker. London: Routledge.

Edwards, R. (1997). *Ethics of Psychiatry*. New York: Prometheus Books.

Eich, H., Reiter, L. and Reiter-Theil, S. (1996). Bioethical problems related to psychiatric and psychotherapeutic treatment of children. Paper presented at the First EBEPE Workshop, Rome, 25 May.

Eisenberg, L. (1971). Principles of drug therapy in child psychiatry with special reference to stimulant drugs. *American Journal of Orthopsychiatry*, **41**, 371–9.

Elias, N. (1971). *Sociologie en geschiedene en andere essays*. Amsterdam: Van Gennep.

Ellertson, C. (1997). Mandatory parental involvement in minors' abortions: effects of the laws in Minnesota, Missouri and Indiana. *American Journal of Public Health*, **87**, 1367–74.

El-Sharif, A. (1992). *Link: Cause for Concern*. London: Granada (video).

Elton, A., Honig, P., Bentovim, A. and Simons, J. (1995). Withholding consent to lifesaving treatment: three cases. *British Medical Journal*, **310**, 373–7.

Emanuel, E.J. & Emanuel, L.L. (1992). Four models of the physician-patient relationship. *Journal of the American Medical Association*, **267**, 2221–6.

Engelhardt, H. T (1986). *The Foundations of Bioethics*. Oxford: Oxford University Press.

Engelhardt, H.T. (1988). Foundations, persons and the battle for the millennium. *Journal of Medicine and Philosophy*, **13**, 387–91.

Enthoven, A.C. (1985). *Reflections on the Management of the National Health Service*. NPHT.

Es, J.C. van. and Hagen, J.H. (1987). Kostenstijging in de gezondheidszorg, externe en interne factoren. In *Verdeling van schaarse middelen in de gezondheidszorg*, ed. A.W. Muschenga and J.N.D. de Neeling, pp. 69–84. Amsterdam: VU Uitgeverij.

Etzioni, A. (1993). *The Spirit of Community*. London: Fontana.

European Parliament (1995). Directive on the protection of individuals with regard to the processing of personal data. Brussels: European Parliament (Directive 95/46/EC.).

Evans, D. and Evans, M. (1996). *A Decent Proposal: Ethical Review of Clinical Research*. Chichester: Wiley.

Evans, M.I., Littman, L., Richter, R. et al. (1997). Selective reduction for multifetal pregnancy: early opinions revisited. *Journal of Reproductive Medicine*, **42**, 771.

Everaerts, N, J. Peeraer and Ponjaert-Kristoffersen, I. (1993). *Zorg om zorg. Misbehandelen van ouderen*. Leuven: Garant.

Evers, A. and Olk, T. (1991). The mix of care provisions for the frail elderly in the Federal Republic of Germany. In *New Welfare Mixes in Care for the Elderly*, ed. A. Evers and I. Svetlik. Volume 3, pp. 59–100. Vienna: European Centre for Social Welfare Policy and Research.

Ex parte Hincks (1980). (*R. v. Secretary of State for Social Services, West Midlands RHA and Birmingham AHA (Teaching), ex parte Hincks*), 1 BMLR 93, 97.

F v. *West Berkshire Health Authority* (1989). 2 All ER 545.

Faden, R. and Beauchamp, T. (1986). *A History and Theory of Informed Consent*. Oxford: Oxford University Press.

Fairbairn, G. and Mead, D. (1990). Ethics and the loss of innocence. *Paediatric Nursing*, **2**(5), 22–3.

Faulder, C. (1985). *Whose Body Is It?* London: Virago.

Feinberg, J. (1970). *Doing and Deserving*. Princeton: Princeton University Press.

Feinberg, J. (1996). *The Moral Limits of the Criminal Law. Volume III: Harm to Self*. Oxford University Press.

Feinstein, A.R. (1990). On white coat effects and the electronic monitoring of compliance. *Archives of Internal Medicine*, **150**, 1377–8.

Fineschi, V., Turillazzi, E. and Cateni, C. (1997). The new Italian code of medical ethics. *Journal of Medical Ethics*, **23**, 239–44.

Finnish Act on the Status and Right of the Patient (1992). (statute no.785, enacted 1993)

Finnish Mental Health Act, 1991

Flanagan, O. and Rorty, A. (eds.) (1990). *Identity, Character, and Morality: Essays in Moral Psychology*. Cambridge, MA: MIT Press.

Fogarty, M. (1998, October). 'Bring down that Berlin wall'. Editorial in *Health and Aging*.

Foot, P. (1977). Euthanasia. *Philosophy and Public Affairs*, **6**, 85–112.

Foot, P. (1978). *Virtues and Vices*. Berkeley, CA: University of California Press.

Ford, C.A., Millstein, S.G. and Halpern-Feischer, B.L. (1997). Influence of physician confidentiality assurances on adolescents' willingness to disclose information and seek future healthcare: a randomized controlled trial. *Journal of the American Medical Association*, **278**: 1029–34.

Frankena, W. (1973). *Ethics*. 2nd edn. Englewood Cliffs: Prentice-Hall.

Frankfurt, H. (1971). Freedom of the will and the concept of a person. *Journal of Philosophy*, **68**, 5–20.

Franklyn, B. (1995). *The Handbook of Children's Rights*. London: Routledge.

French, P., Uehling, T.E. and Wettstein, H.K. (eds.) (1988). *Midwest Studies in Philosophy: Volume 13: Ethical Theory – Character and Virtue*. Notre Dame: University of Notre Dame Press.

Friedman Ross, I. (1999). *Children, Families and Healthcare Decision Making*. Oxford: Oxford University Press.

Fryer, D. (1994). Commentary 'Community psychologists and politics' by David Smail, *Journal of Community and Applied Social Psychology*, **4**, 11–14.

Fulford, K. W. M. and Howse, K. (1993). Ethics of research with psychiatric patients: principles, problems and the primary responsibilities of researchers. *Journal of Medical Ethics*, **19**, 85–91.

Fulford, K. W. M. and Hope, A. (1994). Psychiatric ethics: a bioethical ugly duckling? In *Principles of Healthcare Ethics*, ed. R Gillon. Chichester: Wiley.

Fulford, K.W.M. and Dickenson, D. (2000). *In Two Minds: A Casebook of Psychiatric Ethics*. Oxford: Oxford University Press.

Gadamer, H-G. (1960*). Wahrheit und Methode*. Tübingen: J.C.B. Mohr.

Gadamer, H-G. (1975). *Die Aktualität des Schönen*. Frankfurt am Main: Reklam Verlag.

Garfield, S.L. (1980). *Psychotherapy: An Eclectic Approach*. New York: John Wiley.

Gater, R. and Goldberg, D. (1991). Pathways to psychiatric care in South Manchester. *British Journal of Psychiatry*, **159**, 90–6.

General Medical Council (1993). *Tomorrow's Doctors*. London: General Medical Council.

General Medical Council. *Duties of a Doctor*. London: General Medical Council.

Genetics Interest Group (1994). *GIG Response to the Clinical Genetics Society Report*. London.

Gevers, S. (1995). Physician-assisted suicide: new developments in the Netherlands. *Bioethics*, **9** (3/4), 309–12.

Gillick v. *W. Norfolk and Wisbech AHA* [1985] 3 All ER 402.

Gilligan, C. (1982). *In a Different Voice: Psychological Theory and Women's Development*. Cambridge, Massachusetts: Harvard University Press.

Gillon, R. (1985). *Philosophical Medical Ethics*. New York: John Wiley.

Gillon, R. (1997). Editorial: futility and medical ethics. *Journal of Medical Ethics*, **23**, (6), 339–40.

Gindro, S. (1994). Luci ed ombre sul progetto di uomo. In *L'Adolescenza: gli anni difficili*, ed. R. Bracalenti. Napoli: A. Guida Editore.

Glover, J. (1977). *Causing Death and Saving Lives*. Harmondsworth: Penguin.

Goudriaan, R. (1984). *Collectieve uitgaven en demografische ontwikkeling 1970–2030*. Rijswijk: Sociaal en Cultureel Planbureau.

Graham, P. (1981). Ethics and child psychiatry. In *Psychiatric Ethics*, ed. S. Bloch and P. Chodoff, pp. 235–54. Oxford: Oxford University Press.

Greely, H. and King, M.C. (1999). *Letter to the government of Iceland*. www.mannvernd.is (Accessed 14 May 1999.)

Griffiths, J. (1995). Assisted suicide in the Netherlands: the Chabot case. *The Modern Law Review*, **58**, 232–48.

Griffiths, J., Blood, A. and Weyers, H. (1998). *Euthanasia and Law in the Netherlands*. Amsterdam: Amsterdam University Press.

Grodin, M. and Glantz, L. (eds.). (1994). *Children as Research Subjects: Science, Ethics and Law*. New York: Oxford University Press.

Groenewoud, J.H., Van der Maas, P.J. and Van der Wal, G. (1997).

Physician-assisted death in psychiatric practice in the Netherlands. *New England Journal of Medicine*, **336**(25), 1795–801.

Grubb, A. (1996). Commentary on Re Y, *Medical Law Review*. 204–7.

Grubb, A. (1998). Who decides? Legislating for the incapacitated adult. *European Journal of Health Law*, 5, 231–40.

Gruenberg, E.M. (1977). The failures of success. In *Milbank Memorial Fund Quarterly/Health and Society*, 55(1), 3–24.

Gutmann, A. (1994). *Multiculturalism*. Princeton: Princeton University Press.

Guttmacher, L.B. and Create, P. (1988). Electroconvulsive therapy in one child and three adolescents. *Journal of Clinical Psychiatry*, **49**(1), 20–3.

Haan, M., Rice, D., Satariano, W. and Selby, J. (eds.). (1991). Living longer and doing worse? Present and future trends in the health of the elderly. *Journal of Ageing and Health*, **3**, Special Issue, 133–307.

Habermas, J. (1980). *Theorie des kommunikativen Handelns*. Frankfurt am Main: Suhrkamp.

Habermas, J. (1993). *Justification and Application: Remarks on Discourse Ethics*, Oxford: Polity.

Hagestad, O. (1991). The ageing society as a context of family life. In *Ageing and Ethics*, ed. N. Jecker, pp. 123–46. Clifton NJ: The Humana Press.

Hagger, L. (1997). The role of the human fertilisation and embryology authority. *Medical Law International*, 3 (1), 1–22.

Halliday, R. (1997). Medical futility and the social context. *Journal of Medical Ethics*, **23**, 148–53.

Hamerman, D. and Fox, A. (1992). Responses of the health professions to the demographic revolution: a multidisciplinary perspective. *Perspectives in Biology and Medicine*, **35** (4), 583–93.

Hamm, C. (1996). Diagnosis in dispute. *Guardian Society*, 4 December, 15.

Hannuniemi, A. (1996). The status of minors in healthcare and social care in Finland. Paper presented at Seminar in Medicine and Law, University of Tartu, Estonia, 6–7 December.

Hare, R.M. (1994). Methods of bioethics: some defective proposals. *Monash Bioethics Review*, 1, 34–47.

Harre, R. and Gillett, G. (1994). *The Discursive Mind*. London: Sage.

Harris, J. (1982). The political status of children. In *Contemporary Political Philosophy*, ed. K.Graham. Cambridge: Cambridge University Press.

Harris, J. (1985). *The Value of Life: an Introduction to Medical Ethics*. London: Routledge and Kegan Paul.

Harris, J. (1987). QALYfying the value of life. *Journal of Medical Ethics* **13**, 117–23.

Harris, J. (1993). *Wonderwoman and Superman: The Ethics of Human Biotechnology*. Oxford: Oxford University Press.

Harris, J. (1999a). Embryonic stem cell research. Paper given at the Conference on Ethics and the Transformation of Medicine, University College, Oxford, September 17–18.

Harris, J. (1999b). Stem cells and genetic manipulation. Paper delivered at the Conference on Ethics and the Transformation of Medicine, University College, Oxford, September 17–18.

Harrison, C., Kenny, N.P., Sidarous, M. and Rowell, M. (1997). Bioethics for clinicians: Involving children in medical decisions. *Canadian Medical Association Journal* **156**, 825–8.

Hartogh, G. den (1994). Leeftijdsdiscriminatie bestaat dat? Over leeftijdsgrenzen in de gezondheidszorg. *Tijdschrift voor Gezondheidsrecht*, **3**, 134–49.

Hartouni, V. (1997). *Cultural Conceptions: On Reproductive Technologies and the Remaking of Life*. Minneapolis: University of Minnesota.

Hattab, J.Y. (1996). Ethical issues in child psychiatry and psychotherapy: conflicts between children, families and practitioners. Paper presented at the First EBEPE Workshop, Rome, 25 May.

Hauerwas, S. (1995). Virtue and character. In *Encyclopedia of Bioethics*, 2nd edn, Vol. 5, ed. W. Reich, pp. 2525–32. New York: Macmillan.

Hawks, D. (1994). Commentary 'Community psychology and politics'. *Journal of Community and Applied Social Psychology*, **4**, 27–8.

Haydock, A. (1992). QALYs – a threat. *Journal of Applied Philosophy*, **9**, 183–8.

Hein, K. (1997). Annotation: adolescent HIV testing— who says who signs? *American Journal of Public Health*, **87**, 1277–8.

Helfgott, A.W., Taylor-Burton, J., Garcini, F.J. et al. (1998). Compliance with universal precautions: knowledge and behavior of residents and students in a Department of Obstetrics and Gynecology. *Infectious Diseases in Obstetrics and Gynecology*, **6**, 123–8.

Heller, J-M. (1997). La defense des mineurs en justice, approche ethicojuridique. Paper presented at the Twelfth EBEPE Workshop, Rome, October.

Hendin, H. (1995). Assisted suicide, euthanasia, and suicide prevention: the implications of the Dutch experience. *Suicide and Life-Threatening Behavior*, **25**, 193–204.

Hilberman, M., Kutner, J., Parsons, D. and Murphy, D.J. (1997). Marginally effective medical care: ethical analysis of issues in cardiopulmonary resuscitation. *Journal of Medical Ethics*, **23**, 361–7.

Hofman, A. (1991). Ontwikkelingen in gezondheid en ziekte. In *Ouderen, wetenschap en beleid*, ed. M.A. van Santvoort. Nijmegen: Nederlands Instituut voor Gerontologie.

Hollander, C.F. and Becker, H.A. (eds.) (1987). *Growing Old in the*

Future. Scenarios on Health and Ageing 1984–2000. Dordrecht: Nijhoff.

Holmes, J. and Lindley, R. (1991). *The Values of Psychotherapy*. Oxford: Oxford University Press.

Holt, J. (1974). *Escape from Childhood*. Harmondsworth: Penguin.

Honig, P. and Bentovim, M. (1996). Treating children with eating disorders – ethical and legal issues. *Clinical Child Psychology and Psychiatry*, **1**, 287–94.

Hope, R.A. (1996). Paper delivered at the Fourth Workshop of the European Biomedical Ethics Practitioner Education Project, Maastricht.

Hope, R.A. (1997). Restraints and the elderly: abuse, enforcement and aggression. Paper presented at the Tenth Workshop of the European Biomedical Ethics Practitioner Education Project, Maastricht, May.

Hope, T. (1995). Editorial: Evidence-based medicine and ethics. *Journal of Medical Ethics* **21**, 259–60.

Hope, T. and Oppenheimer, C. (1996). Ethics and the psychiatry of old-age. In *The Oxford Textbook of Old Age Psychiatry*, ed. R. Jacoby and C. Oppenheimer, Oxford: Oxford University Press.

Hope, T., Lockwood, G. and Lockwood, M. (1995). The interests of the potential child. *British Medical Journal*, **310**, 1455–7.

Hosking, M.P., Warner, M.A., Lobdell, C.M., Offors, K.O. and Melton, L.J. (1989). Outcomes of surgery in patients 90 years of age and older. *Journal of the American Medical Association*, **261**, 1909–15.

Human Genome Organization Ethics Committee (1996). Statement on the principled conduct of genetic research. *Genome Digest*, May, 2–3.

Hurka, T. (1992). Virtue as loving the good. In *The Good Life and the Human Good*, ed. E.F. Paul, F.D. Miller and J. Paul. Cambridge: Cambridge University Press.

Hursthouse, R. (1987). *Beginning Lives*. Oxford: Blackwell.

Hursthouse, R. (1991). Virtue theory and abortion. *Philosophy and Public Affairs*, **20**, 223–46.

Hursthouse, R. (1995). Applying virtue ethics. In *Virtues and Reasons: Philippa Foot and Moral Theory – Essays in Honour of Philippa Foot*, ed. R. Hursthouse, G. Lawrence and W. Quinn, pp. 57–75. Oxford: Clarendon Press.

Hursthouse, R. (1996). Normative virtue ethics. In *How Should One Live? Essays on the Virtues*, ed. R. Crisp, pp. 19–36. Oxford: Clarendon Press.

Husak, D.N. (1992). *Drugs and Rights*. Cambridge: Cambridge University Press.

Hutson, S. and Liddiard, M. (1994). *Youth Homelessness: The Construction of a Social Issue*. London: Macmillan.

Ibsen, H. (1992). *A Doll's House*. Dover Publications.

Iglesias, T. (1990). *IFV and Justice: Moral, Social and Legal Issues Related to Human In Vitro Fertilisation*. London: The Linacre Centre.

In re Crum, 580 NE2d 876 (1991).

In re E.G. 133 Ill2d 98, 103 (1989).

International Huntington Association and World Federation of Neurology Group on Huntington's Chorea (1989). Guidelines for the molecular genetics predictive test in Huntington's disease, *Neurology*, **44**, 1533–6.

Jahnigen, D. and Binstock, R.H. (1991). Economic and clinical realities: healthcare for elderly people. In *Too Old for Health Care? Controversies in Medicine, Law, Economics and Ethics*, ed. R.H. Binstock and S.G. Post, pp. 13–43. Baltimore: Johns Hopkins University Press.

Jinnet-Sack, S. (1993). Autonomy in the company of others. In *Choices and Decisions in Healthcare*, ed. A. Grubb, pp. 97–136. Chichester: John Wiley.

Johnson, M. (1993). Generational relations under review. In *Uniting Generations: Studies in Conflict and Cooperation*, ed. D. Hobman. London: Ace Books.

Jones, J. (1994). *Young People in and out of the Housing Market*. Working Papers 1–5, Edinburgh: Centre for Educational Sociology at the University of Edinburgh and Scottish Council for the Single Homeless.

Jones, Y. and Baldwin, S. (1992). ECT: Shock, lies and psychiatry. *Changes*, **10**(2), 126–35.

Jonsen, A.R.,Veatch, R. and Walters, L. (eds.). (1998). *Source Book in Bioethics*, pp. 11–12. Washington: Georgetown University Press.

Josselson, R. (1988). The embedded self – I and thou revisited. In *Self, Ego and Identity: Integrative Approaches*, ed. D.K. Lapsley and F. Clark Power, pp. 91–106. New York: Springer Verlag.

Jouvenel, H. de (1989). *Europe's Ageing Population. Trends and Challenges to 2025*. Guildford: Butterworths.

Jouvenel, H. de (1990). Le grand tournant démographique. In Europe Blanche, *Les Conséquences Médicales et Socio-économiques du Viélissement des Populations*, pp. 23–32. Paris.

Jungers, P., Forget, D., Henry-Amar, M. et al. (1986). Chronic kidney disease and pregnancy. In *Advances in Nephrology Year Book*, ed. J. Grunfeld, M. Maxwell, J. Bach et al. vol. 15, pp. 103–41. Linn, MO: Mosby Inc.

Kaimowitz v *Michigan Department of Mental Health* (1973). 42 USLW 2063.

Kaivosoja, M. (1996). Compelled to help: a study of the impact of the Mental Health Act on coercive treatment of minors, 1991–1993. (in Finnish). *Sosiaali-ja terveysministerion julkai-suja, 2*. Helsinki.

Kane, R. and Caplan, A. (1990). *Everyday Ethics*. New York: Springer.

Kant, I. (1909). Foundations of the metaphysics of morals. In

Kant's Critique of Practical Reason and other Works on the Theory of Ethics, trans. T.K. Abbott, 6th edn. London: Longmans Green.

Kant, I. (1956). *Critique of Pure Reason*. Translated by L.W. Beck. Indianapolis: Bobbs–Merrill.

Kaplan, D. (1994). Prenatal screening and diagnosis: the impact on persons with disabilities. In *Women and Prenatal Testing: Facing the Challenges of Genetic Technology*, ed. K.L. Rothenberg and E.J. Thomson, pp. 49–61. Columbus, Ohio: State University Press.

Kass, L. (1981). The ends of medicine. In *Concepts of Health and Disease: Interdisciplinary Perspectives*, ed. A.L. Caplan and H.T. Engelhardt. Reading, MA: Addison-Wiley.

Kazdin, A.E. (1988). *Child Psychotherapy: Developing and Identifying Effective Treatments*. New York: Pergamon.

Kazdin, A.E. (1994). Psychotherapy for children and adolescents. In *Handbook of Psychotherapy and Behaviour Change*, 4th edn. ed. A.E. Bergin and S.L. Garfield, New York: John Wiley.

Keenan, K. and Shaw, D. (1997). Developmental and social influences on young girls' early problem behaviour. *Psychological Bulletin,***121**, 95–113.

Kennedy, I. and Grubb, A. (1994). *Medical Law: Text with Materials*, 2nd edn. Guildford: Butterworths.

Kennedy, I. and Grubb A. (1998). Research and experimentation. In *Principles of Medical Law*, pp. 714–46, Oxford: Oxford University Press.

Keown, J. (1995a). Physician-assisted suicide and the Dutch Supreme Court. *The Law Quarterly Review*, **111**, 394–6.

Keown, J. (1995b). Euthanasia in the Netherlands: sliding down the slippery slope. In *Euthanasia Examined: Ethical, Clinical and Legal Perspectives*, ed. J. Keown, pp. 261–96. Cambridge: Cambridge University Press.

Keown, J. (1997). *Comments on Berghmans* given at the Seventh EBEPE Workshop.

Keyfitz, N. and Flieger, W. (1990). *World Population Growth and Ageing. Demographic Trends in the Late Twentieth Century*. Chicago and London: University of Chicago Press.

Kiloh, L. G. (1983). Non-pharmacological biological treatments of psychiatric patients. *Australian and New Zealand Journal of Psychiatry*, 17(3), 215–22.

Knapp v. *Georgetown University* 851 F2d 437, 439 (DC Cir 1988).

Koster, R.W. (1990). Cardiologie bij ouderen. In *Ouder worden nu'90.* Almere: Versluys.

Krugman, S., Giles, J.P. and Jacobs, A.M. (1960). Studies on an attenuated measles-virus vaccine. *New England Journal of Medicine* 263, 174–7.

Kruschwitz, R. and Roberts, R.C. (eds.) (1987). *The Virtues: Contemporary Essays on Moral Character*. Belmont: Wadsworth.

Kübler-Ross, E. (1982). *Living with Death and Dying*. London: Souvenir Press.

Kuhse, H. (1991). Euthanasia. In *Companion to Ethics,* ed. P. Singer. Oxford: Blackwell.

Kuhse, H. (1998). *A Companion to Bioethics*. Oxford: Blackwell.

Kukathas, C. and Petit, P. (1990). *Rawls: A Theory of Justice and its Critics*, Cambridge: Polity.

L v. *Bournewood* (See *Regina* v. *Bournewood*)

Lahti, R. (1994). Towards a comprehensive legislation governing the rights of patients: the Finnish experience. In *Patient's Rights – Informed Consent, Access and Equality,* ed. L. Westerhall and C. Phillips. Stockholm: Nerenius and Santerus Publishers.

Lahti, R. (1996). *The Finnish Act on the Status and Rights of Patients.* Paper presented at the Sixth EBEPE Workshop, Naantali, Finland, September.

Lamb, D. (1998). *Down the Slippery Slope: Arguing in Applied Ethics*. London: Croom Helm.

Larcher, V.F., Lask, B. and McCarthy, J.M. (1997). Paediatrics at the cutting edge: do we need clinical ethics committees? *Journal of Medical Ethics*, 23(4), 245–9.

Latham, M. (1998). Regulating the new reproductive technologies: a cross-Channel comparison. *Medical Law International*, **3**, (2, 3), 89–116.

Launis, V. (1996). Moral issues concerning children's legal status in Finland in relation to psychiatric treatment. Paper presented at the First EBEPE Workshop, Rome, 25 May.

Law Commission (1995). *Mental Incapacity.* Report No. 231. London: HMSO.

Lebeer, G. (1998). Paper presented at the Second UNESCO Conference on Medical Ethics and Medical Law, Copenhagen, June.

Leenen, H.J.J. (1988). *Handboek gezondheidsrecht. Rechten van mensen in de gezondheidszorg.* (Handbook healthcare law. Rights of people in health care). Alphen aan den Rijn: Samsom.

Leenen, H.J.J. (1994). Dutch Supreme Court about assistance to suicide in the case of severe mental suffering. *European Journal of Health Law*, **1**, 377–9.

Légaré, J. (1991). Une meilleure santé ou une vie prolongée? Quelle politique de santé pour les personnes agèes? *Futuribles*, **155**, 53–66.

Levacic, R. (1991). Markets: an introduction. In *Markets, Hierarchies and Networks: The Co-ordination of Social Life*, ed. G. Thompson, J. Frances, R. Levacic and J. Mitchell, pp. 21–3. London: Sage.

Lewontin R.C. (1999). A human population for sale. *New York Times*, Jan 23.

Lindemann Nelson, H. and Lindemann Nelson, J. (1995). *The Patient in the Family*. London: Routledge.

Lindheimer, M.D. and Katz, A.I. (1992), Pregnancy in the renal transplant patient. *American Journal of Kidney Disease*, **19**, 173.

Lindley, R. (1986). *Autonomy*, London: Macmillan.

Livingston, G., Hollins, S. and Katona, C. (1998). Treatment of patients who lack capacity: implications of the *L. v. Bournewood Community Trust* ruling. *Psychiatric Bulletin*, **22**, 402–4.

Lloyd, G. (1993). *The Man of Reason: 'Male and Female' in Western Philosophy*, 2nd edn. London: Routledge.

Lockwood, G.M., Ledger, W.L. and Barlow, D.H. (1995). Successful pregnancy outcome in a renal transplant patient following in-vitro fertilization. *Human Reproduction*, **10**, 1528–30.

Lockwood, M. (1988). Quality of life and resource allocation. In *Philosophy in Medical Welfare*, ed. J.M. Bell and S. Mendus, pp. 33–55. Cambridge: Cambridge University Press.

Lombaert, D., de Graeve, D. and Goossens, H. (1997). *Een economische Evaluatie van het Pneumokokkenvaccin voor Belgie.* Antwerpen: UFSIA, Onderzoeksverlag.

Lopez, I. (1998). An ethnography of the medicalization of Puerto Rican women's reproduction. In *Pragmatic Women and Body Politics*, ed. M. Lock and P. Kaufert. Cambridge: Cambridge University Press.

Lord Chancellor's Department (1997). *Who Decides? Making Decisions on Behalf of Mentally Incapacitated Adults*. London: HMSO.

Louden, R. (1984). On some vices of virtue ethics. *American Philosophical Quarterly*, **21**, 227–36.

Lutzen, K. and Nordin, C. (1994). Modifying autonomy: a concept grounded in nurses' experience of moral decision making in psychiatric practice. *Journal of Medical Ethics*, **20**, 101–7

MacIntyre, A. (1981). *After Virtue: A Study in Moral Theory*, pp. 190–203. Notre Dame: University of Notre Dame Press.

MacIntyre, A. (1984). *After Virtue*, 2nd edn. Notre Dame: University of Notre Dame Press.

MacIntyre, A. (1997). *A Short History of Ethics*. London: Routledge.

Macklin, R. (1994). *Surrogates and Other Mothers: The Debates over Assisted Reproduction*. Philadelphia: Temple University Press.

Magno, G. (1996). The rights of minors in international conventions. Paper presented at the First EBEPE Workshop, Rome, 25 May.

Maguire, D.C. (1975). A Catholic view of mercy killing. In *Beneficent Euthanasia*, ed. M. Kohl. Buffalo, New York: Prometheus Books.

Makanjuola, J.D. and Oyerogba, K.O. (1987). Management of depressive illness in a Nigerian neuropsychiatric hospital. *Acta Psychiatrica Scandinavia*, **76**(5), 486–9.

Mannvernd (1999). *Icelanders for Ethics in Science and Medicine.* www.mannvernd.is (Accessed 14 May 1999.)

Marrs, R.P. (ed.) (1993). *Assisted Reproductive Technologies.* Oxford: Blackwell Scientific Publications.

Marshall, A. (1936). *Principles of Economics*. London: Macmillan.

Marteau, T. and Richards, M. (1996). *The Troubled Helix: Social and Psychological Implications of the New Human Genetics.* Cambridge: Cambridge University Press.

Mattiasson, A-C. and Hemberg, M. (1997). Intimacy: meeting needs and respecting privacy. Paper read at the Ttenth Workshop of the European Biomedical Ethics Practitioner Education Project, Maastricht, May.

Mause, de L. (1995). *The History of Childhood*. New York: Jason Aronson Publishers.

Mawby, R.I. and Walklate, S. (1994). *Critical Victimology: International Perspectives*. London: Sage.

McCabe, L. (1996). Efficacy of a targeted genetic screening program for adolescents. *American Journal of Human Genetics*, **59**, 762–3.

McInnis, M.G. (1999). The assent of a nation: genethics and Iceland. *Clinical Genetics*, **55**, 234–9.

McKie, J., Singer, P., Kuhse, H. and Richardson, J. (1998). *The Allocation of Healthcare Resources*. Brookfield, VT: Dartmouth Publishing Co.

McNeil, P. (1992). *The Ethics and Politics of Human Experimentation*. Cambridge: Cambridge University Press.

Meehan, T.M., Hansen, H. and Klein, W.C. (1997). The impact of parental consent on the HIV testing of minors. *American Journal of Public Health* **87**, 1338–41.

Medical Ethics Advisor (1993). 9(12). December.

Mendus, S. (1992). Strangers and brothers: liberalism, socialism and the concept of autonomy. In *Liberalism, Citizenship and Autonomy*, ed. D. Milligan and W. Watts-Miller, Aldershot: Avebury.

Merck's 1899 Manual of the Materia Medica. New York: Merck and Co. Reprinted in *The Merck Manual*. (1999) New Jersey: Merck Research Laboratories, 1999.

Meulen, R.H.J. ter (1995a). Solidarity with the elderly and the allocation of resources. In *A World Growing Old. The Coming Healthcare Challenges*, ed. D. Callahan, R.H.J. ter Meulen and E. Topinkova, pp. 73–84. Washington: Georgetown University Press.

Meulen, R.H.J. ter (1995b). Limiting solidarity in the Netherlands. a two-tier system under way? *Journal of Medicine and Philosophy*, **20**, 607–16.

Meulen, R.H.J. ter (1996). Care for dependent elderly persons and respect for autonomy. Paper presented at the Fifth EBEPE Workshop, Maastricht, Netherlands, June.

Midgley, M. (1991). Rights talk will not sort out child abuse. *Journal of Applied Philosophy*, **8**, (1), 103–14.

Miles, S.H., Singer, P.A. and Siegler, M. (1989). Conflicts between patients' wishes to forgo treatment and the policies of healthcare facilities. *New England Journal of Medicine*, **321**, (1), 48–50.

Mill, J.S. (1993). *Utilitarianism, On Liberty, Considerations on Representative Government*. London: Everyman.

Miller, D.L. (1986). Justice. In *The Blackwell Encyclopaedia of Political Thought*, ed. D. Miller, J. Coleman and A. Ryan, pp. 260–3. Oxford: Basil Blackwell.

Miller, R. (1991). The ethics of involuntary commitment to mental health treatment. In *Psychiatric Ethics*, 2nd edn, ed. S. Bloch and P. Chodoff, pp. 265–89. Oxford: Oxford University Press.

Ministry of Health (Iceland) (1998a).*Bill on a Health Sector Database*. Reykjavik: Ministry of Health.

Ministry of Health (Iceland). (1998b). *Act on a Health Sector Database*. Reykjavik: Ministry of Health (No. 139/1998.)

Mircea, E. (1979). *Histoire de croyances et des idées religieuses*. Paris: Payot.

Mitchell, J.J., Capua, A., Clow, C. and Scriver, C.R. (1996). Twenty-year outcome analysis of genetic screening programs for Tay Sachs and beta-thalassemia disease carriers in high schools. *American Journal of Human Genetics*, **39**, 793–8.

Mohr v. *Williams*, 104 N.W. 12, 15–16 (Minn., 1905).

Momeyer, R. (1995). Does physician-assisted suicide violate the integrity of medicine? *Journal of Medicine and Philosophy*, **20**, 13–24.

Montgomery J. (1993). Consent to healthcare for children. *Journal of Child Law*, **5**, 117–24.

Montgomery, J. (1997). *Health Care Law*. Oxford: Oxford University Press.

Moody, H. (1991a). The meaning of life in old age. In *Ageing and Ethics*, ed. N. Jecker, pp. 51–92. Clifton NJ: Humana Press.

Moody, H. (1991b). Allocation yes; age-based rationing, no. In *Too Old for Health Care? Controversies in Medicine, Law, Economics and Ethics*, ed. R.H. Binstock and S. G. Post, pp. 180–203. Baltimore: Johns Hopkins University Press.

Mordini, E. (1997). Mandatory hospitalisation in mental health. Paper presented at the AGM of the European Association of Centres of Medical Ethics, Coimbra, 25 October.

Motulsky, A.G. (1997). Screening for genetic diseases. *New England Journal of Medicine*, **336**, 1314–16.

Mullen, P. M. (1990). The long-term influence of childhood sexual abuse on mental health of victims. *Journal of Forensic Psychiatry*, **1**, 13–34.

Mullen, P.M. (1991). Which internal market? The NHS White Paper and internal markets. In *Markets, Hierarchies and Networks: The Co-ordination of Social Life*, ed. G. Thompson, J. Frances, R. Levacic and J. Mitchell, pp. 21–30. London: Sage, 21–30.

Muller, M. (1996). Death on request. *Aspects of Euthanasia and Physician-assisted Suicide with Special Regard to Dutch Nursing Homes*. Amsterdam: Thesis Publishers.

Murray, J.E., Reid, D.E., Harrison, J.H., et al. (1963). Successful pregnancies after human renal transplantation. *New England Journal of Medicine*, **269**, 341–3.

Murray, T. (1996). *The Worth of a Child*. Berkeley: University of California Press.

Naaborg, J. (1991). Benodigde en beschikbare middelen, een groeiend porbleem voor de zorgverlening. Rapport in opdracht voor de Commissie Keuzen in de Zorg. Hoek van Holland.

Nagel, T. (1986). *The View from Nowhere*. Oxford: Oxford University Press.

National Children's Home (1992). *Runaways: Exploding the Myths*. London: National Children's Home Central Office.

National Institutes of Health and Centres for Disease Control and Prevention (1997). *The Conduct of Clinical Trials of Maternal–Infant Transmission of HIV Supported by the United States Department of Health and Human Services in Developing Countries*, July. Available at http://www.nih.gov/news/mathiv/mathiv.htm

Nelson, RM. (1997). Ethics in the intensive care unit: creating an ethical environment. *Critical Care Clinics*, **3**, 691–701.

Neuberger, J. (1992). *Ethics and Healthcare: The Role of Research Ethics Committees in the UK*. King's Fund.

Niakas, D. (1997). Commentary on the case of Mr K. Paper submitted to the Ninth European Biomedical Ethics Practitioner Education (EBEPE) Workshop, Maastricht, April.

Nicholl, C. (1998). *Somebody Else: Arthur Rimbaud in Africa, 1880–91*. London: Vintage Books.

Noddings, N. (1984). *Caring: a Feminine Approach to Ethics and Moral Education*. Berkeley: University of California Press.

Noll, P. (1989). *In the Face of Death*. London: Viking Penguin.

Nuremberg Code (1947). Is included in the judgement of *United States of America* v. *Karl Brandt* et al. Also found in e.g., Annas G. J. and Grodin M. A. (eds.) (1992) *The Nazi Doctors and the Nuremberg Code*, New York: Oxford University Press.

Oakley, J. (1992). *Morality and the Emotions*. London: Routledge.

Oakley, J. (1996). Varieties of virtue ethics. *Ratio*, **9**, 128–52.

O'Neil, O. and Ruddick,W. (eds). (1979). *Having Children: Philosophical and Legal Reflections on Parenthood*. Oxford: Oxford University Press.

Overall, C. (2000). New reproductive technologies and practices: benefits or liabilities for children? In *Ethical Issues in Maternal–Fetal Medicine*, ed D.L. Dickenson. Cambridge: Cambridge University Press.

Parfit, D. (1984). *Reasons and Persons*. Oxford: Clarendon Press.

Paris, J. and Reardon, P. (1992). Physician refusal of requests for futile or ineffective intervention. *Cambridge Quarterly of Healthcare Ethics* 2, 127–34.

Parker, G., Roy, K., Hadzi-Pavlovic, D. and Pedic, F. (1992). Psychotic (delusional). depression: a meta-analysis of physical treatments. *Journal of Affective Disorders*, **24**(1), 17–24.

Parker, M. (1995). *The Growth of Understanding*, Aldershot: Avebury.

Parker, M. (1996). *Communitarianism and Its Problems*. Cogito, November.

Parker, M. (1999). *Ethics and Community in the Healthcare Professions*. London: Routledge.

Parker, M.G. (1997). *Commentary on the case of Mr K*. Paper submitted to the Ninth European Biomedical Ethics Practitioner Education (EBEPE) Workshop, Maastricht, April.

Paul, M. (1997). Children from the age of 5 should be presumed competent. *British Medical Journal*, **314** (7092), 1480.

Pearce, J. (1994). Consent to treatment during childhood: the assessment of competence and avoidance of conflict. *British Journal of Psychiatry*, **165**, 713–16.

Pearce, J. (1996). Ethical issues in child psychiatry and child psychotherapy: conflicts between the child, parents and practitioners. Paper presented at the First EBEPE Workshop, Rome, 25 May.

Pellegrino, E.D. (1992). Doctors must not kill. *Journal of Clinical Ethics*, **3**, 95.

Pellegrino, E. D. (1994). The four principles and the doctor–patient relationship: the need for a better linkage. In *Principles of Health Care Ethics*, ed. R. Gillon, pp. 353–65. Chichester: John Wiley.

Pellegrino, E.D. and Thomasma, D.C. (1993). *The Virtues in Medical Practice*. New York: Oxford University Press.

Pence, G. (1980). *Ethical Options in Medicine*. Oradell: Medical Economics Company.

Pence, G. (1984). Recent work on the virtues. *American Philosophical Quarterly*, **21**, 281–97.

Pence, G. (1991). Virtue theory. In *A Companion to Ethics*, ed. P. Singer. Oxford: Blackwell.

Peonidis, F. (1996). A moral assessment of patients' rights in Greece. Paper presented at the Sixth EBEPE Workshop, Naantali, Finland, September.

Perrett, R.W. (1996). Killing, letting die and the bare difference argument. *Bioethics*, **10**, (2), 131–9.

Persaud, R. D. and Meus, C. (1994). The psychopathology of authority and its loss: the effect on a ward of losing a consultant psychiatrist. *British Journal of Medical Psychology*, **67**, 1–11.

Pincoffs, E. (1986). *Quandaries and Virtues*. Lawrence: University Press of Kansas.

Psychiatric Bulletin (1990). *Guidelines for Research Ethics Committees on Psychiatric Research Involving Human Subjects*. London: Royal College of Psychiatrists.

Purdy, L.M. (1994). Why children shouldn't have equal rights. *The International Journal of Children's Rights*, **2**, 223–41.

R. v. *Cambridge Health Authority, ex parte B* (1995). 2 All ER 129 (CA).

R. v. *Secretary of State for Social Services, ex parte Walker* (1987). 3 BMLR 32.

R. v. *Secretary of State for Social Services, W. Midlands RHA and Birmingham AHA (Teaching), ex p. Hincks* (1980) 1 BMLR 93.

Rachels, J. (1980). Active and passive euthanasia. In *Killing and Letting Die*, ed. B. Steinbock. Englewood Cliffs: Prentice-Hall.

Rachels, J. (1986). *The End of Life: Euthanasia and Morality*. Oxford: Oxford University Press.

Rachels, J. (1993). *The Elements of Moral Philosophy*, 2nd edn. Englewood Cliffs: Prentice-Hall.

Rapp, R. (1998). Refusing prenatal diagnosis: the uneven meanings of bioscience in a multicultural world. In *Pragmatic Women and Body Politics*, ed. M. Lock and P. Kaufert, pp. 143–67. Cambridge: Cambridge University Press.

Rawls, J. (1971). *A Theory of Justice*. Oxford: Oxford University Press.

Raz, J. (1986). *The Morality of Freedom*. Oxford: Clarendon Press.

Re C [1994] 1 All ER 819 (FD).

Re E (1993). 1 FLR 386

Re K, W and *H* [1993] 1 FLR 854.

Re MB [1997] 2 FCR 541.

Re R (1991). 4 All ER 177.

Re R [1996] 2 FLR 99.

Re T [1992] 4 All ER 649.

Re W [1992] 4 All ER 627.

Re Y [1997] 2 WLR 556 (Connell J*).*

Re v. *Bournewood Community and Mental Health NHS Trust, Ex parte L, 2* WLR 764, opinions in the House of Lords delivered 25 June 1998.

Reich, W. (1998). Psychiatric diagnosis as an ethical problem. In *Psychiatric Ethics*, 3rd edn, ed. S. Bloch and P. Chodoff. Oxford: Oxford University Press.

Reiser, S.J., Dyck, A.J. and Curran, W.J. (eds.) (1977). Pope Pious XII. The prolongation of Life. In *Ethics in Medicine – Historical Perspectives and Contemporary Concerns*, pp. 501–4. Cambridge, MA: MIT Press.

Renard, J. (1997). Cloning in animal biology and research. Paper presented at the Societal, Medical and Ethical Implications of Animal Cloning Conference, London, 24–25 November.

Ridley, M. (1996). *The Origins of Virtue*. London: Viking.

Robertson, D.W. (1996). Ethical theory, ethnography and differences between doctors and nurses in approaches to patient care. *Journal of Medical Ethics*, **22**, 292–9.

Robertson, J.A. (1994). *Children of Choice: Freedom and the New Reproductive Technologies*. Princeton: Princeton University Press.

Robine, J-M. and Colvez, A. (1991). Quelle espérance pour la vie? *Futuribles*, **155**, 72–6.

Rodota, S. (1996). *Tecnolgie e Diritti*, Bologna, 11 Mulino.

Roth, L.H., Meisel, A. and Lidz, C.W. (1977). Tests of competence to consent to treatment, *American Journal of Psychiatry*, **134**, (4), pp. 279–84.

Rowland, R. (1992). *Living Laboratories: Women and Reproductive Technologies*. Bloomington: University of Indiana Press.

Royal College of Paediatrics and Child Health (1997). *A Framework for Practice in Relation to the Withholding and Withdrawing of Life-saving Treatment in Children*. Report of the Ethics Advisory Committee. London: Royal College of Paediatrics and Child Health.

Royal College of Physicians (1990). *Research Involving Patients*. London: Royal College of Physicians of London.

Royal College of Physicians (1991). *Ethical Issues in Clinical Genetics: A Report of a Working Group of the Royal College of Physicians Committees on Ethical Issues in Medicine and Clinical Genetics*. London: Royal College of Physicians.

Rylance, G. (1996). Making decisions with children: a child's rights to share in health decisions can no longer be ignored. *British Medical Journal*, **312**, 794.

S v. *S*, *W* v. *Official Solicitor (or W)*. [1972] AC 24, [1970] 3 All ER 107.

Sandel, M. (1982). *Liberalism and the Limits of Justice*. Cambridge: Cambridge University Press.

Savulescu, J. and Dickenson, D. (1998). The time frames of preferences, dispositions, and the validity of advance directives for the mentally ill. *Philosophy, Psychiatry and Psychology*, **5**, 225–46.

Scarre,G.(ed.)(1989). *Children, Parents and Politics*. Cambridge: Cambridge University Press.

Schaefer, C.E., Briesmeister, J.M. and Fitton, M.E. (eds). (1984). *Family Therapy Techniques for Problem Behaviours of Children and Teenagers*. San Francisco: Jossey-Bass.

Schwartz, S. (1991). Clinical decision-making. In *Handbook of Behaviour Therapy and Psychological Science: An Integrative Approach*, ed. P.R. Martin. New York: Pergamon.

Scitovsky A.A. (1984). The high cost of dying: what do the data show? *The Milbank Quarterly*, **62**, 591–608.

Scitovsky, A.A., (1988). Medical care in the last twelve months of life: the relation between age, functional status and medical expenditures. *The Milbank Quarterly*, **66**, 640–60.

Scitovsky, A.A. and Capron, A.M. (1986). Medical care at the end of life: the interaction of economics and ethics, *Annual Review of Public Health*, **7**, 59–78.

Scotland, N.L. (1997). Refusal of medical treatment: psychiatric emergency? *American Journal of Psychiatry*, **154**, 106–8.

Scourfield, J., Soldan, J., Gray J., Houlihan, G. and Harper, P.S. (1997). Huntington's disease: psychiatric practice in molecular genetic prediction and diagnosis. *British Journal of Psychiatry*, **170**, 146–9.

Scutt, J.A. (1990). Epilogue. In *The Baby Machine: Reproductive Technology and the Commercialisation of Motherhood*, ed. J.A. Scutt, pp. 274–320. London: Merlin.

Seedhouse, D. (1994). *Fortress NHS: A Philosophical Review of the National Health Service*. Chichester: John Wiley.

Shah, A. and Dickenson, D. (1998). The Bournewood case and its implications for health and social services. *Journal of the Royal Society of Medicine*, **91**, 98–134, 1–3.

Shelp, E. (ed.) (1985). *Virtue and Medicine*. Dordrecht: Reidel.

Shelter (1992). *Homelessness: The Facts*. London: Shelter.

Sherwin, S. (1993). *No Longer Patient: Feminist Ethics and Healthcare*. Philadephia: Temple University Press.

Shotter, J. (1993). *Conversational Realities*, London: Sage.

Showalter, E. (1987). *The Female Malady: Women, Madness and English Culture 1830–1980*. London: Virago.

Sidaway v. *Board of Governors of Bethlem Royal Hospital* [1985] 1 All ER 643.

Sikan, A., Schubiner, H. and Simpson, P.M. (1997). Parent and adolescent perceived need for parental consent involving research with minors. *Archives of Pediatric and Adolescent Medicine*, **151**, 603–7.

Silva, M. L. P. (1997). Conceptual questions raised by the principles of current medical ethics: on the principle of autonomy. Paper presented at the Tenth EBEPE Conference, Turku, Finland, June.

Singer, P.A. and Siegler, M. (1990). Euthanasia – a critique. *New England Journal of Medicine*, **322**, 1881.

Singer, P. (ed.) (1991). *A Companion to Ethics*, Oxford: Blackwell.

Skoe, E.E and Marcia, J.E. (1991). A measure of care based morality and its relation to ego identity. *Merrill Palmer Quarterly*, **37**, 289–304.

Slote, M. (1992). *From Morality to Virtue*. New York: Oxford University Press.

Slote, M. (1995). Agent-basing virtue ethics. In *Midwest Studies in Philosophy: Volume 20: Moral Concepts*, ed P. French, T.E. Uehling and H.K. Wettstein. Notre Dame: University of Notre Dame Press.

Smail, D. (1994). Community psychology and politics. *Journal of Community and Applied Social Psychology*, **4**, 3–10.

Smith, M.L. and Glass, G.V. (1977). Meta-analyses of psychotherapy outcome studies. *American Psychologist*, **32**, 752–60.

Smith, M.L., Glass, G.V. and Miller, T.I. (1980). *The Benefits of Psychotherapy*. Baltimore: The Johns Hopkins University Press.

Smith, T. (1999). *Ethics in Medical Research: A Handbook of Good Practice*. Cambridge: Cambridge University Press.

Snowden, R. and Mitchell, G.D. (1983). *The Artificial Family: A Consideration of Artificial Insemination by Donor*. London: Unwin Paperbacks.

Södergård, C.-G. (1996). Patients' rights in Finland. Paper presented at the Sixth EBEPE Workshop, Naantali, Finland, September.

Spallone, P.(1989) *Beyond Conception: The New Politics of Reproduction.* Granby, MA: Bergin and Garvey Publishers.

Specter, M. (1999). Decoding Iceland. *New Yorker* Jan 18, 40–51.

Spiegler G.E. (1997). Genetic screening of adolescents. *New England Journal of Medicine*, **337**, 639–40.

Spiker, D.G., Weiss, J.C., Griffin, S.J., Hanin, I, Neil, J.F., Perel, J.M., Rossi, A.J. and Soloff, P.H. (1985). The pharmacological treatment of delusional depression. *American Journal of Psychiatry*, **142**, 243–6.

Stanko, E. (1990). *Everyday Violence.* London: Pandora.

Statman, D. (ed.) (1997). *Virtue Ethics.* Edinburgh: Edinburgh University Press.

Steinberg, D.L. (1997). *Bodies in Glass: Genetics, Eugenics, Embryo Ethics.* Manchester: University of Manchester Press.

Stichting Patiëntenvertrouwenspersoon Geestelijke Gezondheidszorg (1994). *Verslag 1993* ('Report 1993'). Utrecht: SPGG.

Strathdee, R. (1992). *No Way Back.* London: Centrepoint.

Strathdee, R. (1993). *Children Who Run.* London: Centrepoint.

Sturgiss, S.N. and Davison, J.M. (1992). Effect of pregnancy on long-term function of renal allografts. *American Journal of Kidney Disease*, **19**, 167–72.

Sutton, A. (1997). Authority, autonomy, responsibility and authorisation: with specific reference to adolescent mental health practice. *Journal of Medical Ethics*, **23**, 26–31.

SW Hertfordshire v. *KB* [1994] 2 FCR 1051 (FD).

Szasz,T. (1974). *The Myth of Mental Illness.* New York: Harper & Row.

Taket, A.R. (1992). Resource allocation problems and health services for the elderly. *World Health Statistics Quarterly*, **45**, 89–94.

Tauer, C. (1990). Essential considerations for public policy on assisted reproduction. In *Beyond Baby M: Ethical Considerations in New Reproductive Techniques*, ed. D.M. Bartels, R. Priester, D.E.Vawter and A.L Caplan, pp. 65–86. Clifton, NJ: Humana.

Taylor, C. (1989). *Sources of the Self.* Cambridge: Cambridge University Press.

Taylor, C. (1991). *The Ethics of Authenticity.* Cambridge: Cambridge University Press.

Taylor, M. (1996). A rebellious boy. Paper presented at the First EBEPE Workshop, Rome, 25 May.

Thomasma, D.C. (1996). When physicians choose to participate in the death of their patients: ethics and physician-assisted suicide. *Journal of Law, Medicine and Ethics*, **24**, 183–97.

Thompson, A. and Chadwick, R. (1999). *Genetic Information: Acquisition, Access and Control.* New York: Kluwer.

Thomson, J. J. (1971). A defence of abortion. *Philosophy and Public Affairs*, **1**, 47–68.

Thorslund, M., Bergmark, Å. and Parker, M.G. (1997a). Allocation decisions concerning care and services for elderly people: the need for open discussion. Paper submitted to the Ninth European Biomedical Ethics Practitioner Education (EBEPE). Workshop, Maastricht, April.

Thorslund, M., Bergmark, Å. and Parker, M.G. (1997b). Difficult decisions on care and services for elderly people: the dilemmas of setting priorities in the welfare state. *Scandinavian Journal of Social Welfare*, **6**, 197–206.

Tormans, G., Carrin, G., Lauwers, P. and Martens, L. (1990). Coronary heart disease and the cost-effectiveness of simvastatin and cholestyramine therapy – the case of Belgium, UFSIA, Studiecentrum voor economisch en sociaal anderzoek, 128p.

Traugott, I. (1997). In their own hands: adolescents' refusals of medical treatment. *Archives of Pediatric and Adolescent Medicine* **151**, 923–6.

Treece, S.J. and Savas, D. (1997). More questions than answers? R v. Human Fertilisation and Embryology Authority *ex parte* Blood. *Medical Law International*, 3, (1), 75–82.

Trew, A. (1998). Regulating life and death: the modification and commodification of nature. *University of Toledo Law Review*, **29**, (3), 271–326.

Tronto, J.C. (1993). *Moral Boundaries. A Political Argument for an Ethic of Care.* New York/London: Routledge

Turner, T. (1992). The indomitable Mr Pink. *Nursing Times*, **88**(24), 26–9.

UK Government White Paper (1999). *Making Decisions.* The Government's proposals for making decisions on behalf of mentally incapacitated adults. (Cm 4465). October.

UKCC (1988). *Ethical Guidelines for Nursing.* London: UKCC.

Unesco (1997). *Universal Declaration on the Human Genome and Human Rights.* Geneva: Unesco.

United Nations (1989). *Convention on the Rights of the Child.*

Välimäki, M. and Helenius, H. (1996). The psychiatric patient's right to self-determination: a preliminary investigation from the professional nurse's point of view. *Journal of Psychiatric and Mental Health Nursing*, **3**. 361–72.

Välimäki, M., Leino-Kilpi, H. and Helenius, H. (1996). Self determination in clinical practice: the psychiatric patient's point of view. *Journal of Nursing Ethics*, **3** (4), 329–44.

Van den Eynden, B. and Van Bortel, P. (1997). Palliative care and ethics. Presented at the Seventh EBEPE Workshop. Maastricht.

Van der Maas, P.J. (1988). Ageing and public health. In *Health and Ageing*, ed. J.F. Schroots, J.E. Birren and A. Svanborg. New York and Lisse: Swets, pp. 95–115.

Van der Maas, P.J. Delden, J.J.M. van, Pijnenborg, L. and Looman, C.W.N. (1991). Euthanasia and other medical decisions concerning the end of life. *Lancet*, **338**, 669–74.

Van der Maas, P.J., Van Der Wal, G., Bosma, J.M. et al. (1996). Euthanasia, physician-assisted suicide, and other medical practices involving the end of life in the Netherlands. *New England Journal of Medicine*, **335**, (22), pp. 1699–705.

Vanderpool H.Y. (ed.), (1996). *The Ethics of Research Involving Human Subjects: Facing the 21st Century.* Frederick, MD: University Publishing Group

Van Tongeren, P. (1990). Longevity and meaning of life: philosophical–ethical considerations of the theme 'extension of life'. *Tijdschrift Gerontologie Geriatrie* **21**(5), 223–8.

Van der Wal, G. and Van der Maas, P.J. (1996a). *Euthanasie en andere medische beslissingen rond het levenseinde. De praktijk en de meldingsprocedure.* Den Haag: Sdu uitgevers

Van der Wal, G. and Van der Maas, P.J. (1996b). Evaluation of the notification procedure for physician-assisted death in the Netherlands. *New England Journal of Medicine*, **335**, (22), 1706–11.

Van der Wal, G.A. (1991). Geestelijk lijden. In *De dood in beheer. Morele dilemma's rondom het sterven*, ed. R.L.P. Berghmans, G.M.W.R. de Wert and C. van der Meer, pp. 112–37. Baarn: Ambo BV.

Varmus, H. and Satcher, D. (1997). Ethical complexities of conducting research in developing countries. *New England Journal of Medicine*, **337**(14), 1003–5.

Veatch, R. (1988). The danger of virtue. *Journal of Medicine and Philosophy*, **13**.

Veatch, R. (1989). *Death, Dying and the Biological Revolution.* Revised edn. New Haven, CT: Yale University Press.

Verkerk, M. (1990). *De Mythe van de leeftijd. Ethische kwesties rondom het ouderenbeleid.*'s Gravenhage: Meinema.

Verkerk, M. (1998). Paper presented at the Fourth International Association of Bioethics Conference, Tokyo, November.

Vogel. G. (1997). Scientists probe feelings behind decision making. *Science*, **275**, 1269.

Vygotsky, L.S. (1978). *Mind in Society*, Harvard: Harvard University Press.

W. v. Egdell [1990], 1 All ER 835.

W. Midlands RHA and Birmingham AHA (Teaching), *ex parte* Hincks (1980). 1 BMLR 93.

Walker, A. (1996). *The New Generational Conflict.* London: UCL Press.

Walker, A. (1997). Let the people have their say. *Guardian Society*, 19 November, pp. 6–7.

Walrond-Skinner, S. (1986). *Dictionary of Psychotherapy.* London: Routledge & Kegan Paul.

Warren, M. (1991). Abortion. In *Companion to Ethics*, ed. P. Singer. Oxford: Blackwell.

Washington DC: US Government Printing Office, (1949). *Trials of War Criminals Before the Nuremberg Military Tribunals Under Control Council Law No. 10*, Volume 2, Nuremberg, October 1946 – April 1949 pp. 181–2.

Watchtower Bible and Tract Society of New York (1992). *Family Care and Medical Management for Jehovah's Witnesses.* Brooklyn NY: International Bible Students Association.

Webster, C. (1994). Conservatives and consensus: the politics of the National Health Service. In *The Politics of the Welfare State*, ed. A. Oakley and A.S. Williams. London: UCL.

Weir, R.F. & Peters, C.(1997). Affirming the decisions adolescents make about life and death, *The Hastings Center Report*, **27**, (6) 29–45.

Welie, S. (1996). Contribution to EBEPE Workshop, Turku.

Wertz, D.C. Fanos, J.H. and Reilly, P.R. (1994). Genetic testing for children and adolescents: who decides? *Journal of the American Medical Association*, **272**, 875–81.

Widdershoven, G. (1996). Contribution to the Fourth Workshop of the European Biomedical Ethics Practitioner Education Project, Maastricht, September.

Wikler, D. (1987). Personal responsibility for illness. In *Health Care Ethics*, ed. D. Vanderveer and T. Regan, pp. 326-58. Philadelphia: Temple University Press.

Wilde, G. de and Bijl, R. (1993). *Afwenden van gevaar. Mogelijkheden om buiten het psychiatrisch ziekenhuis gevaar af te wenden.* (Aversion of dangerousness. Possibilities to avert dangerousness outside the mental hospital.) Utrecht: Nederlands centrum Geestelijke volksgezondheid.

Wilkie, T. (1993). *Perilous Knowledge.* London: Faber and Faber.

Williams, B. (1973). A critique of utilitarianism. In *Utilitarianism: For and Against*, ed. J.J.C. Smart and B. Williams. Cambridge, Cambridge University Press.

Williams, B. (1985). *Ethics and the Limits of Philosophy.* London: Fontana.

Wilson, G. (1993). *The Moral Sense.* New York: Free Press/Macmillan.

Winkler, E. (1995). Reflections on the state of the current debate over physician-assisted suicide and euthanasia. *Bioethics*, **9**, (3/4), 313–26.

Wittgenstein, L. (1974). *Philosophical Investigations*, 2nd edn. Oxford: Blackwell.

Wolf, R. (1996). Contribution to the Fourth Workshop of the European Biomedical Ethics Practitioner Education Project, Maastricht, September.

World Health Organization (1989). *Cancer Pain Relief and Palliative Care.* Report of WHO Expert Committee. Geneva: World Health Organization.

Young, I.M. (1989). *Polity and Group Difference: a critique of the ideal of universal citizenship*, Ethics 99.

Zola, I.K. (1975). *De medische Macht.* Meppel: Boom.

Index